# Habit Forming

# Habit Forming

## Drug Addiction in America, 1776–1914

ELIZABETH KELLY GRAY

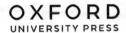

# OXFORD
## UNIVERSITY PRESS

Oxford University Press is a department of the University of Oxford. It furthers
the University's objective of excellence in research, scholarship, and education
by publishing worldwide. Oxford is a registered trade mark of Oxford University
Press in the UK and certain other countries.

Published in the United States of America by Oxford University Press
198 Madison Avenue, New York, NY 10016, United States of America.

© Oxford University Press 2023

CIP data is on file at the Library of Congress

ISBN 978–0–19–764669–4 (pbk.)
ISBN 978–0–19–007312–1 (hbk.)

DOI: 10.1093/oso/9780190073121.001.0001

1 3 5 7 9 8 6 4 2

Paperback printed by Sheridan Books, Inc., United States of America
Hardback printed by Bridgeport National Bindery, Inc., United States of America

*To my father, Bill, my sister, Courtney, and*
*my late mother, Peggy, for their love and support*

# CONTENTS

# ACKNOWLEDGMENTS

This book is the culmination of many years' work, over which time I have benefited extensively from the advice and encouragement of others. To all those with whom I have discussed the book or who have shown interest in my work, thank you.

I am grateful for the grants that I received to conduct archival research for this project and for the wonderful support from the staff at these institutions. My research has benefited from a William M. Helfand Fellowship at the Library Company of Philadelphia and the Historical Society of Pennsylvania, an Andrew W. Mellon Fellowship at the Massachusetts Historical Society, a Charles Donald O'Malley Short-Term Research Fellowship at UCLA's Louise M. Darling Biomedical Library, and a Ferenc Gyorgyey Research Travel Grant at Yale University's Cushing-Hay Library. Thank you to those who attended the colloquia about my project at the Library Company of Philadelphia, the Massachusetts Historical Society, and UCLA. I am grateful for your interest in my work and for your helpful suggestions. For their advice and assistance during my visits, thank you to Linda August, Flo Gillich, Melissa Grafe, James Green, Elaine Grublin, Russell Johnson, Teresa Johnson, Connie King, Marcia Meldrum, Wendy Woloson, and Conrad Wright.

Thank you also to the anonymous readers of the book manuscript for their close attention to it, their encouragement, and their thoughtful suggestions. Thank you to others who have helped to strengthen this project with their advice and assistance, including Diana Ahmad, the late Gert Brieger, David Courtwright, Michael A. Flannery, Dean Grodzins, and the late Bill Rorabaugh. Thank you also to staff at the Albert and Shirley Small Special Collections at the University of Virginia, the Houghton Library at Harvard University, the Maryland Center for History and Culture, the New-York Historical Society, and the New York Public Library. I received valuable feedback on my work in presentations at the meetings of the Alcohol and Drugs History Society, the Baltimore History

Writing Group, the Society for Historians of the Early American Republic, and the Organization of American Historians.

Thank you also to colleagues at Towson University for helpful comments on earlier drafts, including Ben Alexander, Omar Ali, Patricia Anderson, Rita Costa Gomes, Kimberly Katz, Christian Koot, Mike Masatsugu, Steve Phillips, Akim Reinhardt, Nicole Dombrowski Risser, the late Pat Romero, and Bob Rook. I am also grateful for the assistance from librarians at Albert S. Cook Library, including Sara Nixon, Megan Browndorf, and Elizabeth De Coster.

Special thanks to both of my advisers, with whom I discussed this project: the late Arthur P. Dudden, of Bryn Mawr College, and the late Edward P. Crapol, of the College of William and Mary. I am grateful for their encouragement of me and my work.

I extend deep thanks to Susan Ferber and Alexandra Dauler at Oxford University Press for their careful attention to my manuscript, their encouragement, their answers to my many questions, their advice, and all that they did on my behalf. My manuscript has benefited enormously from their work, and I am so grateful.

Thank you to Jean Baker for her encouragement of this project and to Amy Ruth Allen and Bill Walker for their helpful advice.

For helping to ensure that I balance work with relaxation, thank you to Meri Andriesse, Christina Boretos, the late Deborah Davis, David Dubeau, Courtney Gray, Virginia Green, Paul Hollis, the late Louise Hutchinson, Elizabeth Kearney, John Kearney, Jack Kernick, Elizabeth Niemeyer, Debbie Nolan, Lori Offergeld, Catharyn Turner, and the members of the Moist Towelettes trivia team.

And, of course, my deepest thanks for their love, support, and encouragement to my father, Bill, my late mother, Peggy, and my sister, Courtney.

# NOTE ON TERMINOLOGY

Some explanation is in order regarding terminology. As the book's title suggests, American understanding of drug addiction and of people who were addicted transformed over the almost one hundred fifty years that *Habit Forming* covers. Changing perceptions inspired new vocabulary, though some early terms endured. "Habitual" use suggested that the practice was a bad habit—that the response had become automatic as a result of repetition. It did not, however, indicate that the activity was beyond the user's control. The related term "habitué" tended to signify a genteel user. "Addiction" connotes the condition whereby a person continues to use a drug despite negative consequences—that the use is beyond the person's control. The word "addiction" appeared occasionally in eighteenth- and early nineteenth-century sources to refer to the compulsive use of a substance, but its use did not come into frequent parlance until the late nineteenth century.[1] I have sought to adhere to the period terms because those word choices convey the understandings of dependency at the time.

# Habit Forming

# Introduction

"All nations have their stimulants," a writer for *Frank Leslie's Popular Monthly* stated in 1882. "China has its opium, Germany its beer, France its wine, America its tobacco, and Syria and India their hasheesh." At the time, "stimulant" connoted anything that quickened a vital process, such as the user's pulse.[1] Other nineteenth-century Americans also listed various populations' substances of choice. In 1862 Dr. David Cheever, a professor at Harvard Medical School, stated that "the South American ascends the weary slopes of the Andes with lighter step and freer breath under the influence of Coca," an alkaloid of which is cocaine.[2] In 1858, New Yorker Fitz Hugh Ludlow stated that "Hemp, or Hasheesh" was "the narcotic of all Africa." He mentioned additional associations to emphasize that the use of psychoactive substances was indeed universal: "Siberia has its narcotic fungus; the Polynesian Islands their ava, [and] New Granada and the Himalayas their thornapple." The fly-agaric mushroom can produce feelings of well-being. Ava, also known as kava, is an intoxicating drink that was also popular in the Sandwich Islands, or Hawaii, while thornapple is a plant that can cause hallucinations.[3]

These commentators underscored a shared quality among the world's peoples: despite their differences, all of humanity seemed to need something to help them to relax or to cope with life's challenges. Former president James Madison had alluded to this idea in 1819 in a letter to a temperance advocate who had sought his support. Attaining a "*compleat* suppression of every species of stimulating indulgence," he wrote, would be "a work of peculiar difficulty" if, indeed, it were possible at all. He believed that every population used something and that temperance therefore challenged "human nature." "In every age & nation," he stated, "some exhilarating or exciting substance seems to have been sought for, as a relief from the languor of idleness, or the fatigues of labor."[4]

While partaking of psychoactive substances seemed universal, many American writers on the topic—members of the white middle class, primarily—asserted that white and "civilized" people used them more responsibly than did others and

*Habit Forming*. Elizabeth Kelly Gray, Oxford University Press. © Oxford University Press 2023.
DOI: 10.1093/oso/9780190073121.003.0001

that use by some people of color could be dangerous. Madison, for example, saw gentility as having a sobering effect. He suggested that a "passion for ardent spirits" was practically "universal" in "the rudest state of Society." "In the progress of refinement," however, he believed that it became more common to find "beverages [that were] less intoxicating."[5] Others focused on race. Cheever had reflected on reports of opium's effects on its users. He concluded, "Race has a powerful influence in determining the nature of the delirium, which is fierce in the Malay, sensual in the Turk, abject in the East Indian, or intellectual in the Caucasian."[6]

Others opined about the broader implications of widespread use, as they saw a correlation between a society's drug of choice and its apparent degree of advancement. In 1858, a writer for *Scientific American* suggested that people in the Ottoman Empire and in China had an "indolent character" and that their "use of powerful narcotic drugs" helped to render them inactive.[7] Illinois physician Leslie Keeley regarded "opium dreaming" as incompatible with America in the 1880s. "The sluggish nations of the Orient may be content to let to-day be as yesterday and to-morrow as to-day," he supposed. Arab men, he believed, lived much as their ancestors had thousands of years earlier. He insisted that if an American became addicted to opium, he was exchanging a life of forward-looking change for one devoid of achievement. "He passes from the living, progressive world," he warned, "into a desert . . . whose dry and dreary pathways have no end."[8] The impact of Chinese opium use, which appeared to have halted the progress of an ancient and accomplished nation in the nineteenth century, added to the perception of Eastern lassitude. As historian Alan Baumler has observed, China became "the classic example of the decadent, stagnant East against which the modern, active West was contrasted."[9]

For most of the century, there was little public recognition of habitual drug use as an American problem. Although it was less visible than drug use in other countries, such consumption grew extensively throughout much of the nineteenth century. In 1840, for example, the value of opium imported into the United States was just under $41,000. By 1865, it had reached more than $932,000—far out of proportion to population growth. Despite medical demand having increased significantly during the Civil War, a writer for New York's *Journal of Commerce* insisted that most of the increase was unrelated to the conflict—that there had been "a very heavy consumption of opium previous to the war." Those consumers, he added, "use the drug habitually, in some form."[10] In 1868, Ohio physician Lewis Barnes explained that the public was largely unaware of problems associated with opium dependency, because opium users hid their habit. In America, he wrote, the "victim of opium" was "ashamed of his habit, and indulges in solitude. . . . He recoils and hides, and eats and suffers and dies in secret."[11] This book, in part, seeks to reveal that hidden but extensive usage.

* * *

*Habit Forming* examines the addictive psychoactive substances, other than alcohol, that Americans used between 1776 and 1914 when there was almost no federal regulation of drugs. The study begins with the creation of the nation and ends with federal passage of the Harrison Narcotic Act, which restricted the public's access to cocaine and opiates. Except for a 1909 law that banned the importation of the form of opium that is smoked, the Harrison Act was the first federal measure restricting access to drugs. This work places the topic in a global context because many Americans learned about drug habituation and pleasure-seeking drug use by reading accounts from abroad. In addition, international considerations inspired the earliest US laws on narcotics.

*Habit Forming* makes several important contributions to the understanding of this topic. Its emphasis is earlier than that of previous histories, with two-thirds of the chapters focused on the era before domestic drug addiction was widely discussed. It pays extensive attention to Americans' knowledge of compulsive drug use gained from reading about habitual use abroad. The global context is crucial in exploring early Americans' understanding, and misunderstanding, of the subject, due to the general silence regarding domestic use. *Habit Forming* includes all the prominent psychoactive substances—except for alcohol, which other historians have addressed extensively—that Americans used habitually in the era under review that would later be regulated.[12] Assessing the topic with this broad scope brings into clearer relief the patterns of use and the opinions of such use. This work also makes the case that, alongside medical and pleasure-seeking drug use, it is important to consider a third category: the "restorative" use of a drug—use that facilitates relaxation after a difficult day or that helps the user to endure adversity. Because restorative use is neither pleasure-seeking nor clearly therapeutic in nature, there was wide latitude for people to decide whether to condone such use. Overwhelmingly, the tendency was to accept restorative use by members of the white middle class while criticizing such use by marginalized members of society. This aligns with the assertion of other historians that attitudes toward race and class have molded views of drug use and, thus, of drug policy and its enforcement.

\* \* \*

*Habit Forming* builds on the work of scholars who have noted that perceptions of nonmedical drug use, and the drug policies that resulted, have only partially derived from their dangers to users and to those around them. In *Drugs in America, 1800–1980,* historian H. Wayne Morgan concluded that opposition to pleasure-seeking drug use stemmed from the perception that such use threatened society's "values and aspirations." Many Americans believed that efficiency, productivity, and emotional stability were necessary for their nation to thrive, he asserted, and many feared that inessential drug use would endanger that vision. Morgan also noted that Americans looked abroad—to opium use in China and to cannabis use in the Near East, for example—and concluded that widespread drug use could arrest the progress of a society.[13] In *Dark Paradise: A History of Opiate Addiction in America,* historian David Courtwright noted that attitudes toward addiction—including whether an addicted person would receive sympathy or would be treated like a criminal—have depended on widely held perceptions of the "typical" habitué. As he observed, "What we think about addiction very much depends on who is addicted."[14]

Other scholars have focused on the extent to which users' gender and race have shaped drug dependency and perceptions of it. For much of American history, drug habituation was primarily an issue for women. Dr. Stephen Kandall observed that American society has long been unable to address women's addiction "in effective and comprehensive ways." Looking at the second half of the nineteenth century, he points to doctors' "inappropriate and often excessive" medicating of women and the extensive degree to which these patients endured "guilt and shame, both self-imposed and societal," for their dependency.[15] Historian Diana Ahmad has studied native-born Americans' hostility toward opium smoking, a practice common among Chinese immigrants. She noted that doctors, who themselves identified as middle and upper class, regarded opium smoking as "a threat to American values and the economic structure of the nation."[16]

The tendency to accept middle-class addiction and to criticize habitual use by marginalized members of society remained evident into the twentieth century, when national regulation began. Historian Timothy Hickman saw this tendency around 1900. Members of the middle class were spared "the moral responsibility for their condition," he observes, on the theory that they were more susceptible to drug use than others were. Meanwhile, "nonwhite and demimonde others" lacked such an excuse for their use, due to the notion that they were "free of the commercial and cultural strains of modern life." As he notes, the Harrison Narcotic Act divided habitués into "*patients*" and "*criminals*."[17] In his study of drug regulation, historian David Musto also found that while some of the momentum for these laws came from problems resulting from their use, it derived primarily from "profound tensions among socio-economic groups, ethnic minorities, and generations." The greatest enthusiasm for banning a drug, he observed, appeared when advocates believed that its use by members of a nonwhite group made it more difficult to keep them "under control." Examples included the form of opium that was smoked, which was associated with Chinese immigrants, and cocaine, which in the early twentieth century was identified with African American users.[18]

Yet most of this scholarship focuses on the late nineteenth century and subsequent decades, when the issue garnered public attention. In the period before 1867, which *Habit Forming* considers at length, popular publications only occasionally presented drug habituation as an American problem. In 1824, for example, newspapers had reported the case of a female habitué in Philadelphia who stole opium from drugstores.[19] In the 1850s, New Yorker Fitz Hugh Ludlow described his cannabis use in his memoir *The Hasheesh Eater*, and that same year, a writer for *Harper's Weekly* insisted that habitual opium use had become widespread in New York City.[20] Such accounts were, however, few and far between, and most of them, by focusing on an individual's circumstances, did not suggest that dependency was extensive. Also, none of these items launched a succession of similar works. When Dr. David Cheever wrote a lengthy article about habitual drug use for the *North American Review* in 1862, he included Ludlow's book and two British publications, one of which—Thomas De Quincey's *Confessions of an English Opium-Eater*—was more than forty years old. But in 1867, with domestic drug use escalating, Ludlow published an essay in *Harper's New Monthly Magazine* about opium habitués and their agonizing efforts to end their use, titled "What Shall They Do to Be Saved?" Horace B. Day's *The Opium Habit, with Suggestions as to the Remedy* was released the following year, and many additional works on the topic appeared soon thereafter. The conclusion of the Civil War likely provided an opportunity for extended attention to this topic. Although sources for these later decades are more readily available, plumbing the newspapers, periodicals, and personal sources such as letters and diaries before 1867 makes it possible to explore this earlier era in depth.

Rather than emphasizing government policies, *Habit Forming* focuses on how everyday Americans—habitués, their family members, doctors, druggists, and others—experienced drug dependency in the era before national regulation. There were patterns of use among habitual users, but some suppositions were untrue. Many Americans in the late nineteenth century, for example, regarded habitual opiate use as an urban problem, but it was also common in the countryside. In 1871, Dr. Alonzo Calkins insisted that "opium-mania, far from being restricted within the purlieus of our cities and rural centres, is fast pervading the country-populations."[21] Editor George Parsons Lathrop agreed. Criminal trials in western Massachusetts, he pointed out in 1880, had revealed that "great quantities of opium in the form of morphine are consumed by the inhabitants of the lonely hills of that region."[22] Many families in rural areas, with limited access to doctors, kept opiates on hand for their painkilling or soporific qualities but also used them to quell worry or boredom or to provide exhilaration. Some Americans were more likely than others to become habituated. Doctors were disproportionately inclined to become compulsive users, in part because easy access to drugs correlates with the likelihood of usage.[23] For most of the nineteenth century, however, American users were typically middle-aged, middle-class white women. Their use often began with a doctor's recommendation for treating a gynecological problem or a nervous condition. Women were more likely than men to seek medical treatment, due to the notion that men should endure their afflictions instead. Middle-class women, unlike those who were less well off, could afford medical care. And while a woman who drank alcohol risked reproach, she could take opiates without raising eyebrows.[24] The lack of regulation, meanwhile, made it easy for habitués to access their drugs of choice—in ever-increasing quantities, if need be.

This work is not an exhaustive look at global drug use, nor does it include every drug or, for that matter, every addiction. There will be no references to the thornapple. This study focuses on what is now termed "substance abuse" but does not address other behavioral addictions such as gambling addiction, although there is evidence that some nineteenth-century Americans contended with these problems, and some means of social control resembled responses to drug addiction.[25] Tobacco is omitted since it does not produce a psychoactive effect, and other historians have documented its history well.[26] This study includes peyote, a cactus that some Native Americans consumed and that is the source of mescaline. Although there are ongoing questions as to whether its use can become addictive, some asserted in the late nineteenth century that it had this potential.[27]

*  *  *

Addiction is a "chronic, relapsing illness," as psychologist Alan Leshner has pointed out. As public understanding of addiction has changed over time, so has the public response. Some people during the period under review recognized addiction as a disease, but they did not understand that ongoing drug use changes a user's brain. Many drugs mimic neurotransmitters, chemical substances that the human body naturally produces. Morphine, for example, emulates endorphins, which help the body to endure pain. ("Endorphins" is a portmanteau term, combining "endogenous"—or self-produced—with "morphine.") The drugs, however, are much more powerful than their endogenous alternatives. If a person uses morphine regularly, the person's brain will respond by producing fewer endorphins and more receptors—neurons that receive the neurotransmitters. Unoccupied receptors can cause anguish for the person, who then has to take increasing amounts of the drug to avoid experiencing withdrawal.[28] This is how drug users develop a tolerance for a drug and why they consume it in larger and larger amounts. It is also why addiction can be classified as a brain disease.

Drug users typically begin their use voluntarily but once the use has changed their brains, ongoing use does not represent a mere refusal to exercise self-control.

Instead, they suffer from a disease that results in "compulsive drug seeking and use, even in the face of negative health and social consequences," as Leshner has explained. Behavioral treatments can sometimes address the changes to the brain, and medications are sometimes effective. In other cases, the condition is managed, rather than cured, and the drug use continues at a diminished level.[29] In the nineteenth century, however, neither doctors nor scientists—let alone the public at large—understood these aspects of habitual use or were aware of these treatments.

* * *

*Habit Forming* contends that racism and classism have long shaped dominant American attitudes toward drug use and habituation and that those attitudes, in turn, have shaped drug laws and their enforcement. Popular sentiments regarding drug use have typically depended on why habitués first used their drug of choice. Were they taking them to restore well-being, so they could meet their obligations, or did they feel fine and take them seeking enjoyment, knowing that their use would render them idle? People in the first category, such as those who sought pain relief, tended to receive sympathy, even if they became addicted, as they had focused on their health and, therefore, on their ability to meet their social obligations. Those in the latter category, meanwhile, were often criticized, as they had placed their own gratification above other considerations. (There was minimal support, at best, for pleasure-seeking use. Instead, there was the tacit notion that people who were able-bodied should sustain their potential to be productive. Even drug users who advocated nonmedical use emphasized the productive potential of such use, such as users' enhanced ability to explore their minds.) Although the reasons for first use—restoring well-being and seeking euphoria—would appear to be clear-cut, popular racist and classist claims would make it almost impossible for marginalized members of society who had become habituated to garner sympathy, regardless of how their use originated.

Between medical and pleasure-seeking drug use, there was restorative use: a person's use of a drug to cope with sorrow, aggravation, or fatigue. In these cases, people who were weary but not physically ill used drugs with the goal of restoring well-being. Classist and racist notions could shape perceptions of restorative use and, therefore, shape responses to it. Some conditions were medicalized. "Neurasthenia," for example, was a diagnosis of exhaustion in the late nineteenth century. According to Dr. George Miller Beard, neurasthenics sought relief from their enervation, a condition that he maintained was "more distressing than pain." Consequently, they would take "anything that gives ease, . . . such as chloral, chloroform, opium or alcohol," and many became drug dependent. Beard regarded these cases of dependency as unfortunate but understandable. Neurasthenia, however, was regarded as an ailment that afflicted only white people who were members of the middle and upper classes.[30] For more marginalized members of society, no comparable malady existed. Instead, there was the belief that those who worked with their hands—members of the working class and people of color—led healthy and carefree lives. Some suggested that so-called brain workers, such as businessmen, became exhausted, as they endured the hectic pace of work in industrial America while others were spared such headaches. Adherents of this theory, of course, did not consider that physical work can also be exhausting and that people's weariness and unease could derive from sources outside of their work. Their reductionist take misrepresented reality while allowing members of the middle class, and them alone, to use drugs in a manner that garnered approval.[31]

Perceptions of ill health were also malleable with regard to physical ailments. Many white Americans believed that members of the white middle class were susceptible to physical complaints but questioned the purported infirmities of people of color. As a result, there was widespread belief that white Americans deserved extensive and unique license to use narcotics, due to their therapeutic potential. Some middle-class women were frail, in part because social pressures regarding their clothing, diet, and physical activity were not conducive to well-being. There was general acceptance that they needed drugs to cope with their condition, and many came to regard ill health as a sign of gentility.[32] Meanwhile white people, North and South, tended to be skeptical when black people claimed to be ill. Many slaveowners believed that any enslaved people who asserted that they were ill or injured were feigning their condition to avoid work. While visiting the South, landscape architect Frederick Law Olmsted found that when an enslaved field hand maintained that he was unwell, "the proprietor or overseer has, I think, never failed to express his suspicion that the invalid was really as well able to work as anyone else on the plantation."[33] Later in the century, racism affected the treatment of Union Army veterans. When veterans claimed to suffer from ailments that a doctor could not easily verify, the Pension Bureau was more than twice as likely to believe a white veteran as his black counterpart. According to political scientist Sven E. Wilson, when black veterans applied for a pension, "they were not extended the leniency and benefit of the doubt that Whites often received."[34]

Alongside these notions were recurring falsehoods that the use of various drugs caused members of marginalized groups—and, it was implied, them alone—to become violent. Drug use can affect users' behavior negatively. Cocaine use, for example, can lead to increased aggression and therefore to violent behavior.[35] Many white commentators inaccurately implied that drug users' race determined whether they would become destructive, and they asserted that use by people of color was especially worrisome. Sometimes, they provided no examples; at other times, they magnified scant documentation. In the 1880s, for example, white Americans near Indian Territory expressed concern that Comanche Indians' peyote use, which elicited hallucinations, would prompt destructive behavior. Although they offered meager evidence for their concerns, US officials sought to end the use.[36] Around 1900, government reports included allegations that black men's cocaine use caused them to commit rapes. These claims were widely reprinted, but they had no basis.[37] And in the 1910s, newspapers ran stories that stated that marijuana use by Mexicans and Mexican immigrants led to violence. Frequently, however, such statements, despite the stridency of the claims, were revealed to be only suspicions rather than assertions of fact.[38] Nonetheless, these reports accentuated an apparent distinction between those whose drug use would and would not be condoned.

As a result of these beliefs, there was a propensity to accept or forgive almost all drug use by members of the middle class—oftentimes with a reference to the user's great potential—while use by others was deemed indulgent at best and, at worst, as a threat that should be addressed. These views became engrained. When the federal government passed drug regulations in the early twentieth century, the concept of two classes of drug users—one that deserved medical treatment and another whose use should be criminalized—bolstered the passage of legislation and shaped how it was interpreted and enforced.

For almost the entire time covered in this study, all drugs in America were legal at the national level, and state and municipal restrictions rarely interfered with sales and use. While there were multiple reasons for this permissiveness, it derived in part from naïveté regarding the drugs' dangers, the fact that most of these psychoactive substances had medical value, and the lack of better alternatives for those who were ill. Laudanum and morphine, for example, were effective in allaying pain and promoting sleep, and they could be purchased over the counter. Employers sometimes gave cocaine to workers to enhance their productivity, as it would enable them to work long hours. Cocaine was also included in some soda fountain drinks, and preparations of it were sold to treat severe colds with congestion.[39]

Some writers criticized drug use by the upper class. They typically attributed such use to their indolent lives but did not present it as a topic of social concern. The wealthy reportedly took drugs to treat ailments that resulted from their irresponsible habits, such as the late hours they kept—which caused them to need sleeping aids—and their consumption of rich, spicy food, which could cause indigestion.[40] Similarly, their recreational use of hashish in the 1860s led to some eye-rolling by observers, but it was not regarded as a serious problem for the community at large.[41]

Members of the white middle class who were deep in addiction were treated leniently—and regarded as "unfortunate victims"—even if their use did not have a medical origin and even if it led to lawbreaking. In 1920, for example, a judge overturned the conviction of a young British immigrant who was addicted to morphine because he believed that she "came from a refined, high-class family," according to a reporter who covered the case. This bolstered the judge's hope that she could end her drug use.[42]

Patterns of criticism and sympathy, condemnation and forgiveness that were associated with habitual drug use before the era of federal regulation helped to make possible the passage of carefully tailored drug laws. Perceptions of "typical" users forestalled and then enhanced support for federal measures. While many drug users in the 1880s were middle-class morphine habitués, by the 1910s the image had changed to that of young, marginalized men whose use was initially pleasure-seeking in nature. As habitual drug use increasingly became identified with the working class and the demimonde, support for outlawing it increased.[43] This was bolstered by deceptive warnings that drug use by people of color led to violence and false claims that passage of the law would not cause habitués to suffer, because they allegedly could end their use easily or find an illicit drug supply.[44]

These perceptions also shaped enforcement of the Harrison Act. The 1914 law permitted a doctor to prescribe opiates or cocaine only in "the course of his professional practice," a phrase that did not address whether providing doses to a habitué to prevent withdrawal or to stave off craving for the drug was permitted.[45] For a few years, physicians had leeway with such decisions. The Supreme Court then permitted maintenance doses only if the goal was to cure patients—that is, ultimately to end their use. In multiple ways, the legislation challenged long-held tenets. The justices deemed the Harrison Act constitutional, despite the fact that the measure encroached on police powers, which resided with the states. Physicians became increasingly unwilling to regard addiction as a disease or to treat it as such. Some asserted that addiction resulted from a personality disorder, which implied that the problem lacked a physical basis and that those who were addicted posed a threat to society.[46] For these reasons, there was willingness to support national legislation to regulate use by some habitués, but not all.

Legislators and judges divided people who were addicted into two groups, and classist and racist notions continued to affect perceptions of habitués while reinforcing the laws.[47] Some commentators expressed compassion for professionals who were addicted even when they lacked an underlying medical condition. In the words of the Washington, DC, health officer in 1923, such men should not be classed with "underworld persons" whose goal was to "gratify certain sensual pleasure."[48] As policymakers in subsequent decades added new drug laws and amended old ones, they and other authorities continued to design and enforce the legislation in ways that shielded white, middle-class lawbreakers while ensnaring people of color and other marginalized members of society in a manner far out of proportion to their involvement in drug-related crimes.[49]

\* \* \*

Apart from alcohol, opiates were the psychoactive substances that nineteenth-century Americans were using the most, and they consequently receive more attention than other drugs in *Habit Forming*. Opiates are medicines that derive from the opium poppy. (The term "opioids," meanwhile, refers to synthetic narcotics whose effects are akin to that of morphine, an alkaloid of opium.)[50] Opiates were valuable painkillers and sleep agents, and they inspired euphoria in users. They include

- laudanum, the most popular medicinal form in nineteenth-century America, a combination of opium, alcohol, and spices;
- paregoric, a tincture of opium with camphor that was given to restive infants;
- morphine, which was administered as a powder and, later, with a syringe. Because it contained only the active element of opium, it operated more efficiently than opium or laudanum did;
- smoking opium, a preparation of opium that differed significantly from raw opium. Although rarely used in a medical context, it was said to help in the treatment of asthma and migraine headaches;[51] and
- heroin, a semi-synthetic opiate that was initially promoted as a medicine to treat respiratory ailments.

The list does not include raw opium, because few Americans consumed the drug in that form. Some referred to the oral consumption of an opiate as "opium eating," even when it was a liquid preparation.[52] Thomas De Quincey, for example, called his memoir *Confessions of an English Opium-Eater*, but he primarily drank laudanum. Journalist Laura Miller has suggested that he chose the phrase for dramatic effect. Describing himself as a laudanum drinker, she opined, would have been humdrum, since many Britons used laudanum. But the phrase "opium-eater" was "exotically transgressive."[53]

Americans also availed themselves of other drugs that had medical value, sometimes for nonmedical purposes. Hashish, for example, was promoted as an anti-convulsive remedy and as beneficial in treating rabies infections and tetanus. Fitz Hugh Ludlow first found it in a druggist's shop.[54] Chloroform and ether were used as anesthetics. Chloral hydrate promoted sleep. Later in the century, many Americans regarded cocaine as effective in clearing sinuses, and it was used to treat morphine addiction.[55] Many Native Americans found peyote effective in treating ailments including tuberculosis and bronchitis.[56]

A focus on opiates alone could demonstrate the degree to which people's perceptions of drug users shaped attitudes toward restorative drug use. One night in 1805, for example, Dolley Madison could not sleep because she was worried about her husband, who was traveling in poor weather. In a letter, she told him that a friend had given her "several drops of laudanum," which helped to ease her mind.[57] At the time, few would have objected to her use of laudanum in such a situation, even though she was not treating an illness. A few decades later, Chinese immigrants smoked opium to help them endure homesickness and threats of violence, as they competed for jobs with native-born Americans.[58] There was, however, extensive criticism of opium smoking, including from some morphine habitués. For some, it was because smoking opium did not have a medical use. For those who opposed Chinese immigration, the practice underscored the extent of their cultural differences.[59]

Adding other drugs can bring the patterns into clearer focus, since almost all the preparations had medical applications, were unregulated at the federal level, and had a diverse group of users. Writers in the 1860s tended to present hashish experimentation as an enjoyable pastime of the well-to-do, for example, but later, when it was associated in the American West with Sikhs and Mexicans, there was support for outlawing it, based on a concern for the safety of white neighbors.[60] Similarly, many accepted when a white clientele drank the early Coca-Cola or Vin Mariani, drinks that initially contained cocaine. When black Americans had access to cocaine, however, some people exaggerated and fabricated claims that the drug made those users violent. This contributed to a successful push to regulate cocaine strictly.[61]

\* \* \*

Because drugs during the period under review were unregulated at the national level and local regulations were only moderately—sometimes selectively—enforced, many Americans tried a variety of compounds to treat their maladies, though others recognized the riskiness of such experimentation. Americans endured many ailments that medical science has since alleviated, and many lacked access to a physician—some due to the early nation's rural character, others for financial reasons, and others because few doctors would treat non-white patients. Before passage of the 1906 Pure Food and Drug Act, companies could market products as remedies without having to reveal their components or prove their safety or efficacy. Experimentation sometimes led to compulsive use. When an opium habitué described his plight in an 1876 memoir, he explained that he was sharing his story because he feared that opiates would replace alcohol as Americans' drug of choice. The 1870s were "an inquisitive, an experimenting, and a daring age," he observed, in which "restless" people were "prying into everything." He regarded this as a recent development, which he attributed to the hectic pace of industrial America. He contrasted Americans' behavior at that time with the "timorous inactivity" of previous eras.[62]

States and municipalities began passing laws in the 1870s to restrict the use of psychoactive substances in response to growing awareness of addiction as a domestic issue. In the early twentieth century, the US government began passing national legislation restricting the availability of drugs. Beginning in 1915, cocaine and opiates were strictly regulated, and the federal government considered regulating marijuana and chloral hydrate at that point.[63]

Medical advances, rather than restrictive laws, account for the noticeable decrease in drug addiction in the country around the turn of the century.[64] Imports of opium—which was never produced domestically to a significant extent—peaked in 1897 and then began to decline significantly.[65] The decline resulted from the acceptance of germ theory, which helped to keep people healthier; the advent of alternative painkillers, such as aspirin; the demise of people who had been addicted to morphine; and doctors' increasing reticence to use morphine, which slowed the initiation of new habitués.[66]

\*\*\*

Part I of *Habit Forming* describes drug use in early America. Chapter 1 covers opiate use and drug habituation from 1776 to 1842, when it received little attention in the popular press. Most habitués in this era began their use when their doctors recommended opiates. Because habituation was not discussed, few understood the nature of dependency or how to treat it. Chapter 2 focuses on opium use in the United States between 1842 and 1867, an era in which—as import statistics indicate—domestic opiate use was escalating greatly. In large part, it resulted from doctors' excessive prescribing of it, self-medication that sometimes culminated in habitual use, and some drinkers' decision to switch to opiates in response to the temperance movement. The increase likely also derived from the dearth of public attention that domestic habitual use was receiving, as there were few warnings regarding such use. Chapter 3 explores the popularity of hashish in 1860s America. There was a tendency to associate its use and the resulting intoxication with Eastern nations and to associate Western nations with the sober and practical use of the non-narcotic hemp fiber. Some Americans—especially well-to-do white people—used it in a nonmedical context, and Ludlow published his memoir on the topic in the late 1850s. Again, however, little on the topic was published overall at that time.

The middle three chapters, which constitute Part II, focus on the global context that informed American understanding of nonmedical drug use and addiction during the decades when reports of domestic use were, at best, sporadic.

Chapter 4 describes habitual and pleasure-seeking drug use in parts of Asia, Africa, and the Middle East from the sixteenth through the nineteenth centuries by focusing on travelers' accounts that were quoted in American publications, including medical journals. While some observers likened nonmedical opium or cannabis use to the Western use of alcohol, others suggested that such widespread use had prevented or halted the advancement of those societies. Chapter 5 explores Americans' reactions to the writings of English habitués Thomas De Quincey and Samuel Taylor Coleridge, both of whom detailed their stories of compulsive use. Their experiences showed that white, educated Westerners were susceptible to addiction, a fact that some Americans found surprising. Chapter 6 focuses on how the First Opium War, fought between Great Britain and China from 1839 to 1842, introduced to Americans the idea that widespread drug use could devastate a country. From this conflict, Americans also learned about the international commerce in opium and the fact that those who sold the drug would find ways to justify their involvement, since they could profit greatly.

Part III focuses on the era from 1867 to 1914, when American drug habituation received extensive public discussion. Chapter 7 focuses on opium smoking in America and shows that, although Chinese immigrants were not the most numerous drug users in America, they were the most visible, since those who partook did so in dens that, though secluded, were public. Some native-born Americans also patronized the dens. Chapter 8 focuses on other forms of domestic drug use that were prevalent in the 1870s and 1880s, including morphine use. Doctors and recovering habitués penned accounts to help those who were addicted and to implore the curious not to dabble in drugs. Chapter 9 explores the move to regulate drugs at the federal level. In 1914, the national regulation of opiates and cocaine was voted into law. The impetus for this derived primarily not from domestic concerns but from foreign policy considerations, as the United States pursued global agreements regarding the opium trade. By this point, the perception of the typical American habitué had changed from that of a middle-class, middle-aged female morphine user to that of a lower-class young man addicted to heroin, an image that garnered little sympathy and that therefore facilitated the passage of restrictive drug laws. The Conclusion addresses the consequences of that legislation—primarily, how a tax act became the basis of a national prohibitory measure. It also explores the extent to which attitudes toward drug use from the founding era to the Progressive era endured for the subsequent century.

* * *

And those attitudes, including the fiction that users' race determined how drug use would affect them, would endure. In 1914, a physician falsely told readers of the *Medical Record* that any black man who became a cocaine habitué would remain "a constant menace to his community until he is eliminated."[67] At the same time, many regarded excessive drug use by well-to-do white people as amusing. In the spring of 1922, a *Vanity Fair* writer penned a satire about drugs at Hollywood parties—in particular, at "the more exclusive functions," where guests would have been white. The humorist described a " 'Snow'-ball" that featured a "miniature 'Drug-store,' " where guests received "little packages of cocaine, morphine, and heroin."[68] The author presented such use as excessive and indulgent but not as threatening.

In the latter half of the twentieth century, white, middle-class youth who sold and used illegal drugs were far more able than their nonwhite counterparts to evade legal consequences. The white community tended to regard white youth as "victims who must be shielded from both the illegal drug markets and the criminal drug laws," as historian Matthew Lassiter observes. Newspapers focused on nonwhite sellers. According to Lassiter, papers in Los Angeles contributed to a "panic" as they "chronicled Mexican American 'peddlers' who smuggled narcotics (heroin and marijuana) across the border" and " 'preyed' " on white teenagers by selling marijuana to them. When a high school student with marijuana was arrested in southern California in 1953, a local paper headlined the article "Tijuana Dope Bust." By the late 1960s, white middle-class youth were increasingly the defendants in marijuana-related cases. Arrests of white youth, however, "prompted angry protests from parents," and juries were reluctant to convict them. California's legislature removed some of the mandatory sentences pertaining to marijuana in 1968, because the laws threatened the freedom of these youth, and there was widespread support for shielding them.[69]

The racial divide endures in the twenty-first century. Journalists, for example, typically humanize white people who sell or use drugs but exclude that softening context when writing about black or Latino users. Stories about the latter groups tend to be arrest reports, as sociologist Julie Netherland and psychiatrist Helena Hansen have observed. In 2001, for example, a Missouri paper reported that "fourteen men from St. Louis and St. Louis County were arrested early Wednesday as part of a large-scale effort by federal and local authorities cracking a heroin trafficking operation." The journalist named the people arrested, along with their ages and addresses, but provided no further information about them. Those who were arrested included a nineteen-year-old and a twenty-year-old. Meanwhile, articles about white dealers typically explain how their drug involvement began, information that can inspire forgiveness. A story from Minnesota in 2011, for example, focused on Ashton—his last name was omitted—a white twenty-year-old in the Minneapolis suburbs who had grown up with "a loving, supportive family." The journalist explained that he was "a stellar student and athlete until he found a new crowd in middle school" who smoked marijuana.

"Seeking acceptance, he became a user, then a dealer" with access to cocaine and methamphetamine. The context provides a partial defense, while the starker presentation typically given for black dealers has "a dehumanizing effect," as Netherland and Hansen observe. And as they note, the contrasting depictions correlate with the consequences that their subjects face. In 2016, although African Americans used illegal drugs at the same rate as white people, they were "6–10 times more likely to be incarcerated for drug offenses."[70]

The impact of racism and classism on attitudes toward drug use is not new, and it was not new in the 1950s or in the 1910s. Those attitudes have long been entwined with the public's understanding of drug dependency and opinions of pleasure-seeking drug use. These views have always informed what policies are created and how they are enforced. To attain a more complete understanding, it is enlightening to focus on an earlier time, when opiates were widely used medicines, prescriptions were not required, domestic dependency was rarely addressed, and public knowledge drew largely from accounts of overseas use. This is the time in which *Habit Forming* begins.

# PART I

# HIDDEN DRUG USE IN AMERICA

# American Use of Opiates, 1776–1842

In his essay, "Narcotics," Dr. David Cheever emphasized opium's value as a sleep aid and painkiller. "No other narcotic is so trustworthy, and so sure . . . to produce sleep, soothe pain, [and] relax painful spasm," he insisted. He added that opium provided "comfortable intervals and . . . calm nights" to many people in their final days.[1] Opiates would remain the nation's most valuable painkiller until the early twentieth century, when aspirin became widely available.[2]

Cheever also informed his readers that people used some drugs publicly while consuming others in secret. He stated, for example, that perhaps three-fourths of humanity used tobacco and that Europeans and Americans used it openly. With others, the use was furtive, especially if it was an indulgence rather than something that was medically necessary. "Opium and hemp, if indulged in," he pointed out, "are concealed by the Western nations."[3] Cheever's statement had long been true. For decades, Americans had been secretive about their indulgence in opium use.

* * *

Richard Dorsey, a forty-six-year-old Baltimore merchant and financier, spent the evening of Saturday, January 27, 1827, at the Water Street home of his brother-in-law, Robert Gilmor Jr. Gilmor was a respected merchant and one of the nation's earliest art collectors; his three-story, five-bedroom house lacked sufficient wall space for him to display the hundreds of paintings he had amassed.[4] On that winter evening, Dorsey socialized with his host and other guests, including Gilmor's brother, agents of a British merchant house, and John Marshall, the son of the nation's chief justice. The men discussed prominent politicians' "scholarship"—that is, how thoroughly they knew the classics. They concluded that Virginia senator John Randolph of Roanoke was "a man of genius," Gilmor wrote in his diary, but "not one of perfect classic attainments." The late Maryland senator Robert Goodloe Harper, on the other hand, had been "a scholar, particularly

*Habit Forming.* Elizabeth Kelly Gray, Oxford University Press. © Oxford University Press 2023.
DOI: 10.1093/oso/9780190073121.003.0002

a latin one." The men also discussed Rufus King, who had served as a New York senator and as the US minister to Great Britain.[5]

Richard Dorsey was a product of his region, his time, his race, and his class. According to Gilmor, Dorsey's father was a "respectable country gentleman," and Dorsey had worked as a clerk for Gilmor's father before marrying into the family.[6] He had also been employed as a tobacco inspector.[7] Around 1810, he and Gilmor had lost a large and valuable shipment of cotton, tobacco, sugar, and pimento when the French, in the midst of the Napoleonic Wars, seized ships carrying Gilmore and Dorsey's merchandise.[8] Dorsey was also a slave owner. In 1839, two of the men he enslaved, Lloyd and Nicholas Howard, would escape by covering the twenty-odd miles to Pennsylvania by traveling up York Road in a hired hack. The *Baltimore Sun* would chronicle Dorsey's successful lawsuits against two men who had helped the Howards to escape.[9] The following year, he attended a slaveholders' convention in Annapolis.[10]

For most of his adult life, while Dorsey inspected tobacco, ran his business, endured the hazards of international trade in wartime, and took measures to defend and reinforce the institution of slavery, he was preoccupied by a family matter. At the time he sat in his brother-in-law's home discussing politicians, he had already spent twenty years caring for his sister Rebecca, who suffered "Insanity from the use of Opium," as a member of the Pennsylvania Hospital staff attested.[11] She had begun taking the drug, a popular painkiller and sleep agent, early in the century to treat intense and chronic indigestion—a "dyspeptic complaint"—that could cause "excruciating" pain.[12] Then, she kept using it. In 1808, Richard had put Rebecca in a year-long in-patient rehabilitation program in Philadelphia's Pennsylvania Hospital, under the care of Dr. Benjamin Rush, the nation's most respected physician, to try to end her dependency. Around the time that French pirates were seizing Richard's merchandise, he was corresponding with doctors at the hospital, inquiring about her progress. Rebecca had become "more communicative, and rational," William Hammond informed him in December 1809, but Rush believed that "nothing has yet been effected towards a cure."[13] When the program was unsuccessful, Richard arranged for her long-term care back in Maryland.

Rebecca Dorsey, like thousands of other Americans at the time, had become dependent on opium. Typically, habitués first took it as a painkiller or soporific, and then found that they could not forgo it. Historian David Courtwright has estimated that in the 1830s, there were fewer than eleven thousand American habitués, based on the amount of opium that was imported into the country and the quantity necessary to sustain a habit; almost no opium was produced domestically.[14] To find others who were habituated, however, only requires learning about the men who Gilmor and his guests discussed at their gathering. Virginia senator John Randolph of Roanoke had been using opium at least since 1805, when he was twenty-one, and he continued for the rest of his life. Although he was candid with friends regarding his dependency, his condition would not be generally known until after his death, in 1833.[15] Senator Robert Goodloe Harper had married the daughter of Marylanders Charles and Molly Carroll. By the time Harper had married into the family, Molly was long dead. She had become dependent on laudanum, a combination of opium, alcohol, and spices, in the mid-1770s, when she took it to help her sleep, and she never stopped using it. And Rufus King's sister, Paulina King Porter of Maine, had also been a habitual opium user, as King discussed in correspondence with his brother-in-law, Dr. Robert Southgate. Their letters reveal that her dependency had impaired her ability to care for her children. They also stress the difficulty of ending the habit. "Mrs. Porter of Biddeford is to my surprise Restord [*sic*] to a state that Enables her to pay some Attention to her Family," Southgate informed King in 1800. "But she lives still on Opium; & cannot pass a Day with out it."[16]

These four—Rebecca Dorsey, John Randolph, Molly Carroll, and Paulina King Porter—were representative of the drug habitués in early nineteenth-century America. All four began their drug use in a medical context and then found themselves unable to stop. They were white and well-to-do, and most were women, as were most users. White women predominated because of access, which always helps to determine who will become habituated. In the nineteenth century, most dependency began with visits to doctors, as they often prescribed opiates to allay pain or to help a patient sleep. Mainly the prosperous consulted physicians when they were ailing, and almost all Americans who were well-off were white. Women were more likely than men to seek help, due to notions that women were less able than men to endure pain and that it was "unmanly" to consult a doctor.[17] Some habitués ended their usage. While the four women mentioned earlier tried to do so, however, it appears that none of them succeeded.

In late eighteenth- and early nineteenth-century America, opiate habitués and their families were dealing with a problem that they did not understand. Domestic drug dependency was rarely discussed publicly, and while this helped users to hide their condition, it also meant that they had to address the problem with little guidance. Knowledge about the ways that drug use changes the brain's reward system, thus intensifying dependency, would not be acquired for more than a century.[18] In the seventeenth and eighteenth centuries, however, people throughout the world, and members of all classes, were using psychoactive substances to have a "euphoric, delirious, or simply *altered* subjective experience," as historian Benjamin Breen has observed.[19] Some then became dependent on their drug of choice. Americans writing about problems with opiates sometimes described habitual use in distant lands, but they almost never addressed causes or treatments. With regard to domestic drug issues, writers focused on overdoses and debates about administering drugs to babies and young children. Since opiates were widely used medicines that rarely caused noticeably erratic behavior, most habitual users could avoid ignominy. At the same time, they did not grasp why they could not end their use with willpower. Their continued use could complicate relationships by giving the impression that they did not want to quit.

Those who wrote about domestic habitual use early in the century tended to sympathize with habitués whose use had begun with a doctor's advice and to regard other users as selfish. The response was typically based on users' intentions. Did they take the drugs to restore health and productivity and thus fulfill their obligations, or did they take them for pleasure's sake, placing their enjoyment ahead of their responsibilities? There was sympathy for those whose use began in a medical context. Ailing, they had consulted physicians and taken drugs on the advice of these doctors so they could feel better and thus return to their previous activities. Conversely, those who simply wanted to take drugs so they could feel better than normal were criticized for apparently focusing more on their enjoyment than on their commitments.

Some also criticized the idle rich, whose drug use appeared to result from unhealthy habits. They used opium to allay pain and to aid sleep. Their stomachaches, however, resulted from fondness for spicy meals, while their unproductive days and late-night soirees led to insomnia. Many commentators advocated working hard, eating plain food, remaining sober, and enduring minor aches and pains. These behaviors, they suggested, obviated the need for opiates. People who wrote in this vein often associated the countryside with virtue and cities with decadence, even though habitual opiate use was increasing in both places.

* * *

With the important exception of alcohol, Americans who used a drug compulsively before 1914 were most likely dependent on an opiate. Doctors prescribed these drugs, and many people self-administered them. They were available over the counter, and there were no national regulations on medical opium before 1914. The most popular type was laudanum. To get babies to fall asleep, mothers and nannies administered paregoric, a "camphorated tincture" of opium.[20] Other opiates would gain popularity later on: a smokable form of opium in the 1850s; morphine, an alkaloid of opium, in the 1860s; and heroin, a semi-synthetic opiate, in the late 1890s. Before then, the drugs of choice were opium, laudanum, and some proprietary medicines that contained opiates, such as Godfrey's Cordial, Bateman's Pectoral Drops, and Squire's Elixir.[21]

Access to doctors was limited in the early nineteenth century, and most medical care took place within the home, typically administered by women.

They could share medical advice with each other and find it in newspapers, journals, and home remedy guides. In his guide Dr. John Theobald, for example, recommended using "as much as a large pin's head" of both opium and camphor, in a "hollow tooth," to treat a toothache.[22] Newspapers such as the *Pennsylvania Gazette* provided practical medical information, since many readers "are at a considerable Distance from proper Advice."[23] Others lacked the funds to visit a physician. When John Tennent published *Every Man His Own Doctor* in 1734, he explained that he was writing for "the Poor . . . those whom Fortune has placed below the Regard of our *Doctors*."[24] And while some could not summon professional help, others—especially in rural areas—lacked easy access to shops that sold them. It was not uncommon for such families to keep opiates on hand. In August 1800, Philadelphia merchant John Harrison recorded selling four and a half ounces of laudanum for 90 cents, "for A Family Medicine Chest."[25]

Americans' opium was primarily Turkish in origin, though opium poppies were also cultivated in India, Persia, Egypt, and elsewhere. Workers would plant poppy seeds in the fall and collect the raw, gummy opium a few months later. To do this, they would make incisions in the poppy heads, which were "about the size of hens' eggs," as New York clergyman Edward Dorr Griffin Prime explained in the memoir of his international travels.[26] The poppy juice—a "milky latex," in the words of chemist Daniel Perrine—would then exude from the capsules, and laborers would gather it the following morning. This process would be repeated until all the raw opium had been collected. It was then dried, and workers formed it into balls "as large as a cocoanut," according to the Reverend Isaac Pierson. They would pack the raw opium in dry leaves so the balls would not stick together.[27] Opium produced in different locations could vary by color, smell, taste, and morphine content. Most Indian and Persian opium was shipped to China. The "Turkey opium" imported by the United States arrived mainly from the port city of Smyrna, now Izmir. Pharmacists and others regarded Turkish opium as superior to other varieties due to its high morphine content.[28]

Several American doctors promoted the domestic cultivation of poppies for opium since demand was high, test samples of American poppies were of good quality, and domestic production would end dependence on foreign suppliers. In the early nineteenth century, farmers and doctors from New England to Georgia to Ohio experimented with opium production and encouraged others to do likewise. In 1800, for example, the Medical Society of North Carolina offered $25 to the person who could produce the most opium in the state.[29] Catharine Henry Laurens Ramsay cultivated it in South Carolina, and in 1809 her father pointed out that the drug, ounce for ounce, cost more than silver.[30] A warm southern clime was not required. In 1812 Moses Dennison, a farmer in Shirley, Massachusetts, produced a quantity that was "equal to the best Turkey opium" in quality, according to the *New England Journal of Medicine and*

*Surgery*.[31] Others highlighted domestic production as a matter of national independence. In 1810, Georgia physician Milton Anthony insisted that when it
came to supplying necessities, it was "better to be dependant [*sic*] on ourselves
than on our enemies, or doubtful friends."[32]

Although some saw domestic cultivation as a smart move economically,
Americans never produced it on a large scale, due to labor costs. Early on, some
suggested that opium poppies could replace crops for which demand had diminished. In 1811, Dr. James Mease of Williamsburg, Virginia, recommended that
planters "apply a portion of the labour of their slaves to . . . the cultivation of the
poppy." He insisted that it would be profitable and pointed out that "cotton and
rice, and tobacco, are scarcely saleable."[33] At that time, an impasse with Great
Britain over trading rights—which would culminate in the War of 1812—had
deprived the United States of an important market.[34] In 1831, Georgia physician Alexander Jones suggested that opium could become an American export
and thus "make amends for the very depressed prices of our staple commodity,
cotton."[35] He asserted that "women and children" could perform much of the
labor and that opium, unlike cotton, was almost market-ready as soon as it was
collected.[36] Such visions, however, were never realized. Some worried that domestic opium cultivation would lead to increased use.[37] The main issue, however, was the cost of labor. In 1898, naturalist Charles Frederick Holder would
state that cultivation efforts in Virginia, Tennessee, and California had failed due
to frost and "the lack of cheap labor."[38] In 1908, apothecary M. I. Wilbert agreed
that opium never became a permanent domestic commodity "entirely due to the
relatively high cost of labor."[39] The failure of these plans would shape perceptions
of drug dependency. The fact that opium continued to be imported would bolster a tendency, when discussing domestic habitual drug use, to blame people in
other countries for the damage to Americans' lives.[40]

American laws between 1776 and 1842 did not regulate access to narcotics,
though the marketplace and middle-class notions about sickness and health restricted their availability and determined the contours of those restrictions. There
were no age requirements for buying these drugs, for example, and no prescription was required. Sometimes, however, narcotics were priced beyond the reach
of the poor. Free African Americans had to contend with financial concerns and
with racial prejudice, which made it difficult for them to find doctors who would
treat them. Also, people who were enslaved had little access to physicians. There
are occasional references to enslaved people receiving opiates as painkillers.
A writer for a commerce journal in New Orleans, for example, recommended
that plantation owners keep "one ounce of powdered opium" on hand if they
enslaved between fifty and a hundred people.[41] Slave owners, however, could decide whether the people they enslaved would receive opiates when they were ill,
and many dismissed complaints of ill health as attempts to avoid work.[42]

Medicine was not dispensed solely to human patients. Throughout the century, writers for farmers' journals, veterinarian columns, and farriers' guides shared treatments for animals' ailments. Farmers used opium to treat domestic and farm animals that had diarrhea and to treat hogs that refused to eat; laudanum was frequently recommended for horses that suffered from colic or from bots, an internal parasite.[43]

There were numerous opiate overdoses, many of them fatal, but accounts of tragic accidents were not accompanied by calls for regulation. In large part, this was because opiates were the only effective painkillers available. Requiring a prescription would have put them beyond the legal reach of most people, who would have lacked the money to pay a doctor or the proximity to visit one. There were tragedies, but requiring prescriptions would not just have been impractical—it would have been, in its own way, cruel. No state would require a prescription for the purchase of any drug until Nevada placed such a restriction on opium sales, in 1877. Three other states followed in the 1880s, with Montana also adding cocaine and morphine to the list. Otherwise, drugs in the United States retained over-the-counter status at the state and federal levels until the late 1890s.[44]

Opiates were crucial for the ailing. Thomas Lee Shippen, for example, was a late eighteenth-century gentleman who suffered from pulmonary consumption, also known as tuberculosis. The illness had rendered him an invalid. On one occasion, when he felt as if his family had forgotten him, Shippen wrote in his journal, "My old friend the laudanum bottle stands by me, and gives me all my strength and all my spirits."[45] In 1811, John Burns recommended the use of "a suitable dose of laudanum" to treat the pain that resulted from "SCALDS or burns."[46] Around 1820, playwright Royall Tyler was taking heavy doses of laudanum to ease the pain of a facial cancer.[47] In 1845, a medical journal reported that opiates treated ailments including intermittent and typhus fevers; inflammations; rheumatism; gout; "*Catarrhal* complaints"—that is, excessive mucus in the nose and throat; some "*Morbid fluxes*," such as cholera, dysentery, and diarrhea; "*Morbid retentions*," such as colic and the retention of urine; some "*spasms and pains*"; "*Neuroses*," a category that included hydrophobia and delirium tremens; gangrene; syphilis; and some cases of poisoning.[48] They were also used as an anesthetic in surgeries. Opium was the only anodyne used when Abigail "Nabby" Adams Smith, the daughter of John and Abigail Adams, underwent a mastectomy in 1811.[49]

Doctors recommended opiates to treat anxiety, and many people self-administered to secure peace of mind. Such usage was not new. In *Mysteries of Opium Reveal'd* (1701), English physician John Jones noted that opium had, in ancient times, been used to "*take off Sadness, Melancholy, and Anxiety*."[50] Opiates remained useful in this respect. John Quincy Adams, for example, was "prone to bouts of morose self-criticism," as neurologist George Paulson has observed.

In 1787, the twenty-one-year-old wrote in his diary that he felt "a depression of spirits to which I have hitherto been entirely a stranger." A doctor gave him an opiate to treat his anxiety and insomnia, and it allowed him "to quiet his nerves and to enable him to sleep," according to Robert East. It does not appear that he resorted to opiates frequently.[51] In *The Married Lady's Companion* (1804), Dr. Samuel Jennings noted that a young lady might experience "misfortune," such as "the loss of a friend, or a disappointment in love." Although he recommended exercise and the company of "chearful, but sober companions" as part of the treatment, he also recommended "tincture of opium"—that is, laudanum—to help her sleep.[52] And when Mary Hatch's husband left her alone on their Alabama plantation for a time in 1833, she admitted in a letter to her grandmother that she had taken "a great deal of Laudanum."[53]

According to Dr. Benjamin Rush, opium was also appropriate for the bereaved. "The first remedy that is indicated in recent grief, is opium," he wrote in 1812. "It should be given in liberal doses in its first paroxysm"—that is, the onset or first attack—"and it should be repeated afterwards, in order to obviate wakefulness."[54] Many women used opiates to try to find solace following the loss of a child.[55] In 1785, Elizabeth Powel—whose father and husband both served as mayor of Philadelphia—referred to laudanum when she insisted that "this Globe would not be habitable to Thousands was it not for that heavenly Medicine."[56]

Opiates also provided comfort for patients toward the ends of their lives. Benjamin Franklin's doctor wrote that when the statesman endured "extremely painful paroxysms" associated with bladder stones in his later years, "large doses of laudanum" helped to "mitigate his tortures."[57] In a letter to his sister a month before he died, Franklin mentioned how glad he was that, despite his "severe" ailment, he had "every convenience to palliate it, and to make me comfortable under it."[58] "Liberal doses of laudanum" would also assuage Alexander Hamilton's pain in his last twenty-four hours, following his duel with Aaron Burr.[59] And when Nabby Adams Smith's cancer reappeared in 1813, according to writer David McCullough, "opium provided her only relief" before she died.[60] Its palliative benefits extended beyond the relief of physical pain. "Opium has a wonderful effect in lessening the fear of death," Rush observed in 1812. He had seen patients who were "cheerful in their last moments" because they had taken the drug.[61]

Those who oversaw the care of people who were mentally ill used opiates to mollify unruly patients. In some cases, the drugs took the place of mechanical restraints and helped ensure that patients neither harmed anyone nor experienced "fatal exhaustion," as historian Gerald Grob has observed.[62] In 1806, William H. Simmons, a medical student at the University of Pennsylvania, wrote of a case in which doctors had used "a large quantity of opium" to get a "Lunatick" to sleep, after the man had thrown himself out a window and struck his head. They also put him in a straitjacket and withdrew blood. The man fell asleep and "awoke perfectly tranquil, and perfectly rational."[63] In the early 1840s, a thirty-year-old merchant was widowed and lost a great deal of his property. The devastation left him "deranged"—noisy, violent, and threatening others' lives. In 1843, he entered the New York State Lunatic Asylum. After trying other treatments, the staff gave him laudanum "morning, noon and night" for eight months. By then, he was "much improved," according to an asylum report. They reduced the doses and then ended them altogether.[64]

In all these ways—as a painkiller, a sleeping aid, an anesthetic, an anti-anxiety drug, and a sedative—Americans would have regarded opiates as crucial medicines. They helped to restore health to the ailing and brought peace of mind to those who were grieving and those who were beyond health. They were valuable, despite their side effects and dangers.

\* \* \*

There were side effects, though, and these led some doctors to provide alternative treatments. Dr. Benjamin Smith Barton observed that with some patients, opium or laudanum "produces sickness at stomach, head-ache, and other disagreeable effects." In such cases, he instead used "the tincture of the hop"—that is, the plant used to brew beer—and found that it worked well as a substitute.[65] The 1768 edition of *Poor Richard's Almanac* recommended pills of Asafoetida, the gum that exudes from the Ferula plant, as a way "*To procure* REST, *where* OPIUM *is improper.*" Benjamin Franklin added that it had all the benefits of opium, including "appeasing Anxieties and Oppressions; and procur[ing] Rest."[66]

In some severe cases, opiates were ineffective. Early in 1768, a seventeen-year-old servant in Hampton, New Hampshire, had to have a leg amputated as well as the foot of the other leg as a result of overexposure during a New England winter. Over eighteen days, the *New Hampshire Gazette* reported, the patient was given medicine including "one Ounce two Drams of solid Opium," but the drug did not have its intended soporific effect: he "did not sleep one Hour in twenty-four during the whole time."[67] In 1812, Dr. Jacob Bigelow recalled treating a man who had been "violently burnt over the whole of the back and both arms." Although Bigelow gave him a large dose of laudanum, he reported that "the patient complained of severe pain in the left arm during a great part of the subsequent night."[68] Yet the writer of an almanac summed up a widely held view of the drug, stating in 1779, "In all acute and vehement pain, opium is the sovereign relief."[69]

Opium also had a "darker side in the public imagination," as historian H. Wayne Morgan has noted, because there were many overdoses, some of them intentional.[70] In *Primitive Physick*, a medical guide for laypersons published in England and America, English theologian John Wesley explained that he did not include opium in his study because it was "*extremely dangerous.*" Even when administered by capable doctors, he asserted, it often had "*fatal Effects.*"[71] In 1828, scientist and druggist George W. Carpenter praised opium's "extensive usefulness," but he noted that it was often given inappropriately and that druggists' preparations of opiates varied, leading to "many injuries and distressing consequences."[72] In 1839, a fellow druggist agreed with Carpenter. He warned readers of the *American Journal of Pharmacy* against prescribing Godfrey's Cordial, a popular elixir for children, because the amount of opium in it "varies in a very dangerous degree."[73]

Overdoses, however, garnered the most attention; because they were often fatal, they were difficult to hide. In 1803, University of Pennsylvania medical student Franklin Scott acknowledged that "excessive doses" of opium could kill the user and even small quantities could "produce death in those unaccustomed to its use."[74] In 1809, Dr. James Cocke noted that the "fatal effects of [taking] a large quantity" of laudanum were "well known."[75] And in 1832, a writer for the *Boston Medical and Surgical Journal* insisted there was "little doubt" that many "pay with their lives" for taking excessive doses of opium.[76] Overdoses frequently resulted from carelessness. In 1829, "Mrs. G." was suffering from "violent" colic. One of her daughters gave her an opium pill and a dose of laudanum. A few minutes later, another daughter—unaware of what her sister had done—gave their mother another dose. When Mrs. G. began to demonstrate symptoms of having been poisoned, the family sent for a doctor, who was able to save her.[77] In 1838, an eighty-year-old veteran of the Revolutionary War accidentally drank a "wine glassful of laudanum," when a servant brought him the wrong medicine. A doctor revived him with the aid of a stomach pump, coffee, and tea.[78] Sometimes, a doctor administered the improper dose of a drug. Historian Franklin B. Hough tersely noted that Thomas Kilham died in Lewis County, New York, in 1825 "from an opiate given in over dose by a drunken physician."[79]

On many occasions, mothers or nurses—women who were hired to take care of babies or young children—unwittingly gave excessive opiate doses to their charges. Many mothers used paregoric to get them to sleep, or to allay pain, but even a small dose could be lethal. In 1732, the *South Carolina Gazette* reported the deaths of "two Brothers, of about 5 and 7 Years old." The surgeons who conducted the autopsy named the cause as the "excessive Does [*sic*] of some Opiate."[80] In the 1760s, a writer for the *Pennsylvania Gazette* noted that Godfrey's Cordial was "so much used in the Country, and . . . by being injudiciously given, very frequently does Harm."[81] Even a carefully measured dose could be dangerous, because sediment would collect at the bottom of a laudanum bottle over time, or the drug could partly evaporate, rendering the last doses highly concentrated, and therefore intensely potent.[82]

There were few if any calls to regulate opiates to prevent future tragedies, but many people offered instructions as to how to treat overdoses. In 1800, Pennsylvanian Sarah Waln kept on hand a treatment for when "a Person has taken an over Dose of Laudanum or any Narcotick Medicine which makes the Stomach Sick." Lime juice or lemon juice, she suggested, would "destroy the Force of the Anodyne & remove the Sickness."[83] Other treatments included the use of stomach pumps, emetics, flagellation, and "cold affusions"—that is, pouring cold water over the patient's head, as Dr. James Conquest Cross explained in 1824. Cross would sometimes then use "forced exercise" to keep the person awake.[84]

Many overdoses were accidental, but others were intentional.[85] In 1741, Thomas Hall, a twenty-five-year-old resident of Marlborough, Massachusetts, "premeditately [*sic*] and designedly poisoned himself," according to the *New England Weekly Journal.* One evening, he filled a wine glass two-thirds full with laudanum and drank it. He told a neighbor "that he had drank his *Death's Dose*" and had done so because he was a "*Reprobate, a damned Creature.*" A doctor's efforts to save him were in vain.[86] Dr. Barent Staats had greater success when, in the summer of 1824, he was asked to treat "a mulatto fellow" in Albany who had taken opium with suicidal intent and was found unconscious in the woods. Staats "drew away twenty ounces of blood" from the man's neck and doused him with cold water. The man survived.[87] Opium came to be closely associated with suicide. In 1830, Dr. David B. Slack of Providence, Rhode Island, believed people had a "superstitious fear about opium, from its being so often used as an instrument of self-destruction." Concerns with the drug, he added, were obscuring its "salutary effects."[88]

Opiate use was sometimes linked to cases of shoplifting and disorderly conduct in these early years. In 1824, a woman was convicted of stealing opium from several establishments in Philadelphia after entering the stores "under the pretence of purchasing the article." In her confession, she stated that she was "in the habit of eating from *thirty* to *forty* grains of opium per day" when two grains, which would be fifty drops, or about a teaspoon, was a typical medical dose.[89] Although laudanum typically had a sedating effect, it could also make the user disruptive. In 1830, the *Saturday Evening Post* reported the arrest of "A foreigner who called himself Shon King (John King)" for disorderly behavior. The household servant "had a bottle of laudanum in the street on Sunday night," the writer explained, "with which . . . he was cutting many flourishes until arrested by the watchman." King was discharged.[90]

Some people did use opiates as weapons. A jury in Schoharie County, New York, found Abraham Kesler guilty of murdering his wife with laudanum and arsenic, and he was executed in 1818 for the crime.[91] Some women were convicted of using opiates to kill their young children, though juries could be reluctant to accept that the acts were intentional.[92] In 1852, an enslaved woman in Virginia was arrested for poisoning her master's son with morphine.[93] And in 1849, a young lady in New Hampshire was arrested on suspicion of having poisoned four family members with morphine, two of them fatally.[94]

* * *

The concept of drug dependence would have been unfamiliar in early America, but the diagnosis of what later generations would call alcoholism was beginning to emerge. Changing patterns of alcohol consumption had heightened public concern with its use. The cost of rum, for example, had dropped in the 1720s and 1730s. As a result, "a common laborer could afford to get drunk every day," as historian W. J. Rorabaugh has noted. Later in the century, many Americans drank more and more as they endured the consequences of social changes. In the late eighteenth and early nineteenth centuries, for example, rapid population growth led to extensive migration west, but transportation was poor. Many western settlers drank to cope with their isolation. Others on the East Coast reached for the bottle as they withstood the effects of early industrialization. The advent of factories diminished the status of skilled craftsmen, and the new jobs often paid little and demanded long hours. Moreover, these workers came to realize there was little chance that they would eventually own their own businesses. And some artisans and laborers drank to cope with health concerns, friction at home, and seasonal unemployment.[95] Between 1800 and the 1830s, Americans were annually drinking "more distilled liquor than at any other time" in American history, according to Rorabaugh.[96]

Many colonial Americans had regarded excessive drinking as a moral failing, but after the Revolution, some began to see it as the sign of a malady.[97] In his widely read pamphlet *An Inquiry Into the Effects of Ardent Spirits upon the Human Body and Mind*, which first appeared in 1784, Dr. Benjamin Rush asserted that the "habitual use of ardent spirits" should be characterized as an "odious disease."[98] He stated that some people became intoxicated increasingly frequently and reached a phase at which they seemed always to be inebriated. In that state, they could neither work nor interact with others. Such a person became "an object of pity and disgust to his family and friends." Habitual drinking could lead to physical ailments, such as diabetes and liver problems, and psychological issues, such as memory loss and problems with comprehension. Rush also asserted that "drunkenness" had a hereditary component. He knew of one family in which the predilection went "from a father to four out of five of his children," and he knew of other, similar examples. Researchers have since established that alcoholism does have a genetic element.[99] Scottish physician Thomas Trotter, in 1804, agreed that "drunkenness" was "strictly speaking . . . a disease."[100] Sociologist Harry Gene Levine has noted that Rush's observations were valuable because he presented the problem as a "loss of control over drinking behavior—as compulsive activity"; he identified liquor as the problem, and he asserted that it was a disease for which abstinence was the only remedy.[101]

As would happen with other cases of addiction to drugs, perceptions of excessive alcohol use often fell along lines of class. People who were intemperate came "from all walks of life," as historian Matthew Warner Osborn has noted. However, while poor people were "stigmatized as intemperate and degenerate," those who were considered to be "socially respectable" were diagnosed with a disease—delirium tremens—and thereby avoided the odium that was often associated with habitual drunkenness. The distinction was unmerited. Temperance advocates tended to suggest that problem drinking induced the downfall of those who drank, but the circumstances often included challenges beyond the users' control. Most inebriates who died at the Philadelphia almshouse between 1825 and 1850, for example, were admitted due to illness, injury, or the loss of a husband—not because they drank.[102]

Reformed drinkers who shared their stories of intoxication and sobriety were sometimes better able to persuade tipplers to support total abstinence than were ministers who characterized drunkenness as sinful. In 1840, Baltimore artisans who formed the Washington Temperance Society signed total abstinence pledges, and members of their group who attained sobriety recalled for audiences their earlier, excessive drinking, to make the case for teetotalism. One former baker, for example, spoke of his many stints in jail, and he characterized his inability to stop drinking as a "chain of servitude." The approach had appeal because the speakers demonstrated that "intemperance did not destroy their moral nature," as historian Katherine A. Chavigny has observed. The sessions' broad appeal suggested that supporting the intemperate was more effective than condemning their behavior as sinful. The group was in decline by 1845, in part because some who had attained sobriety did not remain sober, but subsequent temperance groups learned from the Washingtonians the value of supporting and sympathizing with those whom they hoped to help.[103]

\* \* \*

Although overdoses had long garnered most of the attention as a risk of opiate use, dependence had been documented by around 1800. Most Americans in this situation were women, including those who self-administered large doses to treat chronic pain, a practice that appeared to be becoming more common. Opium was "formerly given in disguise, or with a trembling hand," Rush recalled. By 1805, however, doctors were prescribing it, and it was "often purchased, and taken without their advice, by many of the citizens of Philadelphia. They even occupy a shelf in the closets of many families."[104] In 1839, a doctor wrote to the

*Boston Medical and Surgical Journal* about "Mrs. R.," who had been in severe pain for several years due to tumors in her uterus. Her doctor noted that "she has accustomed herself to large doses of opium to allay the severity of bearing down pains."[105] At the time, twenty-six-year-old Eliza Turner was consuming large amounts of opium daily to lull the pain of an abdominal tumor. It appears that doctors only learned of her habit when she entered Philadelphia Hospital to be treated for dysentery.[106]

Most habitual users were women not only because they were more likely than men to visit a doctor when ill, but also because they used opiates—and many doctors recommended them—during pregnancies and to address gynecological problems. In his *Treatise on the Management of Female Complaints* (1792), Dr. Alexander Hamilton suggested that a woman be given "30 drops of Laudanum, or a grain opium pill" "immediately" after delivering a child, to help her rest and to alleviate pain.[107] Propriety at the time forbade physicians from doing the research necessary to find a cure for so-called "female complaints"— venereal diseases, uterine cancer, and injuries resulting from childbirth.[108] Consequently, oftentimes the best that male doctors would do was to make their patients more comfortable. Many women, as a result, self-administered laudanum as a painkiller. In the early 1790s, Theodosia Prevost Burr suffered from an "incurable disorder of the uterus" that, as historian Nancy Isenberg has noted, might have developed into cancer. She took laudanum to treat her pains while her husband, Aaron, was representing New York in the US Senate.[109] Because women were more likely than men to use opiates, due to social mores and doctors' inclinations, women were also more likely than men to become habituated and, consequently, frail. Although this condition resulted from inaccurate assumptions of women's inherent delicacy, it appeared to confirm those beliefs.[110]

The ongoing use of an opiate to treat chronic pain often built up the user's tolerance: over time, a given dose would have a diminished effect, thus impelling the user to take larger and larger doses. Some doctors recognized this phenomenon. As Thomas W. Ruble explained in his *American Medical Guide for the Use of Families* (1810), "Like spirits, tobacco, and other substances called narcotics, by frequent use the system becomes accustomed to its stimulus, and refuses to obey without an increase of the quantity."[111] In his *Tracts on Medical Jurisprudence* (1819), Thomas Cooper included the observation of British physician George Edward Male, who said that while some people could consume only small amounts of opium safely, "others, from habit, are enabled to bear considerable quantities, without sustaining inconvenience from it."[112]

Some people interpreted drug tolerance as a sign that a drug was safe— not that a dependency had formed. In 1794, for example, an acquaintance of Philadelphian Elizabeth Drinker asked her for some laudanum to give to his wife, Mary. Drinker's comments suggest that Mary drank laudanum frequently and had perhaps become dependent on it, given that the doses had little effect. Drinker, however, believed the requested laudanum dose

> would do no harm, if it did no good, as she had been us'd to take it, I went in some time after to see her and gave her, by her own urgent desire 50 drops more in about an hour after the 25—I then left her, in hopes it would still those useless pains that she suffer'd—it appear'd to have little or no effect.[113]

Thirty years later, Dr. James Carmichael of Virginia received a letter from a man who asked for an alternate medicine to treat his wife's diarrhea, since laudanum was not working. "My wife has taken laudanum until I believe her system is completely saturated with it," he explained. "It seems to have no effect upon her." He hoped another drug "would perhaps have a better effect."[114] And in 1832, a doctor mused that the "regular and systematic use" of opium by some people rendered such usage "apparently innoxious." Due to tolerance, the opium lost its efficacy, so the greatest concern, the risk of overdose, appeared to be remote.[115]

Doctors and users also encountered cases of withdrawal, when habitués took less of an opiate than their systems craved. In *The Mysteries of Opium Reveal'd*, Dr. John Jones had warned that for a longtime opium user, the "*sudden Leaving off*" of the drug could cause "*Great, and even intolerable Distresses, Anxieties, and Depressions of Spirits*" and that such abstinence could be fatal.[116] In 1820, Philadelphia physician J. C. Rousseau agreed, asserting that when habitués stopped using their drug—or did not increase the size of their dose—they would experience an "alarming state of debility."[117] Poet John Lofland attested to this, describing his suffering when he was deprived of laudanum in a Baltimore hospital in 1838. He could not fall asleep for "thirteen days and nights," he recalled, because he could not remain still. "My limbs jerked violently," he wrote, "cramps seized me in every limb; my nerves crawled like worms." He escaped from the hospital and found a druggist who sold him laudanum. An hour after doing so, he wrote, he was "as happy a man as ever existed."[118]

Other longtime users were also keenly aware of their dependence, and some longed to end it, even if use of the drug did not impede their productivity. Throughout his life, Congressman John Randolph of Roanoke suffered from an array of serious ailments, for which he took opiates. According to physician Alonzo Calkins, Randolph was an invalid from an early age, suffering from a "severe spinal malady," and Calkins attributed Randolph's temper and demeanor, in part, to his "all-controlling habit."[119] In his biography of the congressman, David Johnson noted that Randolph "endured waves of nausea, blinding headaches, and chronic diarrhea," "ailments in his lungs, kidneys, liver, stomach, and intestines," and "lumbago, angina, sciatica, rheumatism, and 'pains almost end-less.'" A few months before he died, he told John Taliaferro, a longtime friend and fellow Virginia politician, that he was "never . . . free from pain except by an excessive use of brandy and opium." Although his behavior was sometimes erratic, he had a lengthy and demanding career. From 1799 to 1833, he served twelve terms as a Virginia congressman, two years as a senator, and a brief stint as the US minister to Russia.[120]

Some others who were drug dependent were less productive, and those around them often did not know why. Because few Americans understood how intractable drug dependency could be, people tended to blame habitués for their continued use, and the habitués, to some extent, blamed themselves. Ignorance of the nature of dependency could devastate marriages, because it appeared that users, rather than struggling with an illness, had prioritized their pleasure over their responsibilities to their families. When New Yorker Daniel Hale married Catalina Dyckman soon after the American Revolution, for ex-ample, he had expected that she would make his life easier—that he could "ex-pect and demand" her to "soothe [his] peace of mind" whenever he suffered "disappointments in business and any other cause," he wrote. Her dependence on laudanum, however, strained their marriage. A doctor recommended that she take it as a painkiller, and her use became habitual. For years, according to James Thomas Flexner, she "kept much to her room as an invalid," and Hale paid someone else to take care of their home. When he learned of her depend-ency, he insisted that Catalina stay with her brother while she tried to end her use. Nobody in the family, however, appreciated how acute her problem was, nor knew how to treat her effectively. Her brother believed she just needed to exert self-control, so while she lived with him, he allowed her to come and go as she pleased. As a result, despite her wish to quit, she continued to buy and consume laudanum. With the aid of three doctors, she reduced her laudanum usage but did not end it. Daniel and Catalina never divorced, but they never again lived together.[121]

Other habituated women also had difficulty taking care of their household responsibilities. In 1800, even the incremental improvement in the condition of Paulina King Porter was cause for mention in her family. The intractability of her situation was indicated not only by her daily need for the drug but also by the fact that her brother-in-law, Robert Southgate, considered her ability to pay "some Attention" to her family to be good enough news to share. Porter and her husband had twelve children.[122] Their niece saw her aunt's improvement. In 1801, she wrote to Rufus King that "my Aunt Porter is not wholly restored to her former health, but is much better than she has been for many years past."[123] Her dependency, though unwitting, had come at the expense of her family obligations.

Others also misunderstood how acute dependency could be. Molly Carroll, for example, began taking laudanum in 1776 to treat insomnia, and three years later she was still taking it. When her father-in-law, Charles Carroll of Annapolis, learned of her continued usage, his reaction suggests that he knew of similar cases and appreciated the seriousness of the situation. He pleaded with his son: "Tel [*sic*] Her I beg Her never to touch Laudanum wh[ich] I hear she stil [*sic*] takes, it is as bad as Dram drinking"—that is, as bad as consuming small amounts of hard liquor. He added that she should avoid anything "wh[ich] may give only present ease."[124] Discussions of Molly's dependency were confined to her family. Almost certainly, her father-in-law learned of her usage from her mother, who lived with him as his housekeeper.[125] His comment indicates the naïveté of the times. He knew that her usage was problematic but believed, like Catalina Hale's brother, that willpower would suffice, as he believed she would end it if she were implored "never to touch Laudanum." Her habitual use continued.[126]

While drug dependency rendered users unproductive, their habituation could strain or even destroy relationships between other family members, if they did not work together in addressing the situation. For almost thirty years, Richard Dorsey assisted his sister, first by paying Pennsylvania Hospital for a year of inpatient rehabilitation—which was unsuccessful—and then by paying women to serve as live-in nurses. After Rebecca's death, Richard's relationship with their brother became strained. Richard had covered the costs of Rebecca's treatment and care—"upwards of $2000," he calculated—and their brother had promised to help. When both men stood to inherit her estate, however, Richard's brother refused to surrender any of his share to repay him. Richard admitted he was "much surprised" to hear that he would not "receive Payment for my Acc't or any part thereof against our unfortunate sister Rebecca." Her estate, he added, was valuable: "I allude to her Slaves." One way or another, he asserted, he would be reimbursed.[127]

\* \* \*

Although most early-American opiate dependency derived from ongoing medical need, some people who used opiates discovered that these drugs could inspire feelings of euphoria. Dr. John Jones had shared this information in 1701, explaining that a grain of opium could have the same impact on a person as "several *Glasses* of *Wine*" and would inspire "a *Pleasure* so sweet, and *delicious*" that he was tempted to compare it with "a continual *Venereal Pleasure*." He believed, however, that it was impossible to capture in words the feeling of "*charming Complacency*" that it inspired.[128] In 1765, Dr. Samuel Bard—who would later serve as President George Washington's doctor—reported that opium could "induce hilarity" in its users.[129] Maryland senator John Henry referred to laudanum as "the Divinity itself," as Vice President John Adams recalled in 1795.[130] It was for this reason that at the time, physicians disagreed as to whether opium was a stimulant or a sedative.[131]

Some men who experienced euphoria were, literally, experimenting with drugs. Around 1780, for example, Dr. James Ramsay felt tired one night and took laudanum at 11 P.M. For two hours, the dose put the Virginian in a "cheerful situation." As he felt inclined to sleep he took another dose, and he marveled at the initial, positive effects. "I soon found myself so exhilarated, as to grow careless of my occupation, and rather inclined to indulge in an excess of gaiety; which was gratified for some time by ridiculous excesses of dancing, singing, &c.," he recalled. Despite ingesting the drug, he attested that the "powers of my mind still remained so perfect" that he could continue to monitor his pulse.[132] At the dawn of the nineteenth century, Franklin Scott found much the same thing. He gave one of his subjects forty drops of laudanum. Forty-five minutes later, the man felt "an exhilaration of the spirits."[133]

Opium dependency became a more noticeable problem in the early nineteenth century, as public sentiment toward alcohol soured. In *Medical Inquiries and Observations* (1805), Dr. Benjamin Rush reflected on changes that had taken place in his lifetime and noted that "taverns and beer-houses are much less frequented" than they had been in the 1760s, "and drunkenness is rarely seen in genteel life." Discreet quaffing could have led other people to conclude that drinkers were abstaining altogether since, in earlier times, many drinkers had partaken in visible public spaces and could become boisterous or combative under the influence. Rush warned readers, however, not to conclude that diminished visibility meant diminished usage. There was "still a good deal of secret drinking" among Philadelphians, he explained, and "a new species of intoxication from opium has found its way into our city." He knew of one person who had died from it.[134] Opium use, meanwhile, could go largely undetected, since habitués consumed it privately, and it could bring about repose or leave the user's behavior unaffected. Doctors, however, saw the trend. In *Directions for the Medicine Chest* (1811), Lewis Heermann, a surgeon in New Orleans, recommended medicines other than opium for the treatment of dysentery despite its effectiveness in treating diarrhea. This was because of "the too frequently habitual use of opium," he explained.[135]

By the 1820s, many Americans perceived laudanum as women's alcohol: a socially acceptable substance they took for restorative purposes—to ease their cares. It was considered inappropriate for women to drink, but society approved of women who took "a drug labeled a medicine and obtained through their physicians," as medical historians Sarah Tracy and Caroline Jean Acker have observed.[136] In the 1790s, actress Eliza Tuke Hallam took advantage of this distinction after she repeatedly appeared on stage while "in a State of partial

Intoxication," according to fellow thespian John Hodgkinson. A performance of hers in 1795 was "too disgustful to remember," he recalled, and he characterized the audience's response as "'she must insult us no more!'" As part of the damage control, Hodgkinson added, "a Report was industriously circulated that Laudanum was the Cause of Mrs. *Hallam's* frequent Incapability." Her husband Lewis, also an actor, was likely behind the report. Because laudanum was a medicine, the explanation could inspire sympathy, and it did. "The Public Voice turned," Hodgkinson continued, "and there was a Wish to see her again."[137] The story placed Hallam back within the confines of proper female behavior. In 1826, the Reverend Stephen Olin, in a letter to the wife of a colleague, summed up the popular practice. To "put trouble to death," he observed, "some of your sex use opium and many of mine use rum."[138] Although he acknowledged that drinking was more prevalent among men than opium with women, he saw a tendency among women—and almost exclusively women—to resort to opium to ease their cares.

Usage was especially widespread among elite women, a tendency that many attributed to their lifestyle. Because they attended late night gatherings, they were late to bed and late to rise. They also overate and indulged in rich, spicy foods. The conclusion was that they needed opiates to help them sleep and to treat their indigestion. In 1733, Scottish physician George Cheyne had dubbed this ailment "The English Malady." According to Cheyne, "nervous *Disorders*" were responsible for "*almost one* third *of the Complaints of the People of* Condition"—that is, members of the elite—"*in* England." The elite were so susceptible, he explained, because causes of the malady included "*the* Richness *and* Heaviness *of our Food*" and "*the* Inactivity *and* sedentary *Occupations of the better Sort (among whom this* Evil *mostly rages)*." Cheyne, meanwhile, believed that the only problem that could afflict the poor was laziness.[139] Later doctors would advance similar theories. By diagnosing an ailment to which only the elite were susceptible, they had a medical excuse to use opiates that others would have lacked.

Scottish physician Thomas Trotter maintained that a healthier lifestyle would cure these patients' ills. "Nervous people," he observed, tended to build their lives around their condition. They saw few people beyond their doctors and druggists, rarely went outside, and focused their conversation on "their own complaints." They should, he stated, abandon "luxurious living, depraved appetites, indolence of body or mind, or vicious indulgence of any kind inconsistent with health." If they exercised, worked hard, and sustained themselves with "plain fare," they would sleep soundly. Trotter expressed these concerns in *A View of the Nervous Temperament* (1808).[140]

Some in early America identified habitual opium use with elites. Dr. David Ramsay stated that some wealthy, idle southern men used opium to "rouse [their] senses." In his *History of South-Carolina* (1809), he explained that men needed "something to stimulate the senses, employ the body or occupy the mind." A man who had a "vacant mind" and "whose circumstances elevate him above bodily labor," therefore, focused on his senses. Although Ramsay identified "ardent spirits" as the most likely resort, he acknowledged that "tobacco, opium, and some other irritating substances" were alternatives.[141] In 1817, a writer for Baltimore's *Portico* depicted opiate users as "the nervous lady, who gains artificial vivacity from the secret use of the *aqua-vitæ*, or the depressed and morbid gentleman, who soothes his agitated mind by opium." The elite, however, would pay for their indulgence. Such usage "every moment inflicts torment," he wrote, and "threatens final gloom and annihilation."[142] Laudanum users included "the idle and luxurious man, who has lounged away his day in listlessness at home," according to a writer for the *Journal of Health*, and "the belle, whose pallid face and sunken eye show the exhaustion of the midnight assembly and dance."[143] The publication encouraged "cleanliness, regular exercise, [and] a moderate diet," as Thomas Horrocks has observed, and criticized tobacco and alcohol use.[144]

Americans who wrote on this topic tended to regard the lovers of luxuries as the white, urban upper class and to contrast them with virtuous, plain-living farming families. Consequently, many concluded that rural living was healthiest. In 1809, a writer for the *New York Medical and Philosophical Journal and Review* maintained that the "state of life most favourable to health" was one in which a person "ranges freely in the open air, leading a life of moderate labour, . . . and unused to enervating indulgences or excess." The life of a farmer's wife, he suggested, was ideal. He contrasted it with "the effeminacy of polished manners" and asserted that such practices not only eroded masculinity, but they also made people more susceptible to illness. "Too much refinement and luxurious indulgence," he explained, "bring on a train of nervous ailments." The remedy, he added, was "active occupations" in the outdoors.[145] Many believed that the healthiest diet was spare and simple. In 1817, General Henry Lee advised his son to adopt "the custom of fasting two or three days, living on bread and water, when disordered, rather than swallow drugs."[146]

In other cases, habituated men appeared to have lost the resolve and fortitude necessary to accomplish things. Some who made this observation characterized such men as having lost an integral part of what it meant to be a man. In 1830, a writer for the *Journal of Health* noted that prolonged laudanum use would change the user's "moral nature" by removing "all manly resolution." This enervation prevented him from addressing problems—specifically, deciding how to address them and then taking action. To "think is too great an effort," the writer explained, while "the sight of distress" elicited "childish grief" from the habitual user but nothing more—he would be saddened but lacked "sufficient incentive" to involve himself.[147]

Habitual opiate use, however, was not confined to cities. In more rural settings as in urban areas, many adherents were women. Fishermen's wives on Nantucket did not live luxurious lives, yet there were rumors of their opium use. In the early 1770s, French American writer J. Hector St. John de Crèvecoeur wrote that opium use was pervasive among women on the island. Many of them took "a dose of opium every morning," he wrote, and "would be at a loss how to live without this indulgence." In his *Letters from an American Farmer*, he added that the habit was "much more prevailing among the women than the men" and that the "harmless" habit was sustained "to preserve . . . cheerfulness." Crèvecoeur learned this information from the island's sheriff, Benjamin Tupper, who was a physician as well as a longtime opium user himself. Without it, Tupper told him, "he was not able to transact any business."[148]

Crèvecoeur was surprised that residents of Nantucket, hardworking people who lived modestly, would indulge in what he called an "Asiatic custom." He found it "hard to conceive how a people always happy and healthy, in consequence of the exercise and labour they undergo, never oppressed with the vapours of idleness" would need opium in order to feel content. While he found the women's usage surprising, however, he did not find it concerning. He considered Nantucket's society to be one of the finest he had seen.[149] Some have suggested that the women took opiates to endure a situation in which their husbands could be away for months at a time on whaling voyages and that they continued their use to avoid withdrawal or to treat the pains now recognized as withdrawal.[150]

Some Founders sought to discredit adversaries by suggesting that they used opium habitually. Statesman Gouverneur Morris, for example, was not pleased when James Madison was reelected president in 1812, both because Madison had defeated his friend, New York lieutenant governor DeWitt Clinton, and because Morris opposed the War of 1812.[151] In a letter to a friend, he reported that Madison "never goes sober to bed." Although he was not sure whether Madison consumed "opium or wine," he had heard that "pains in his teeth" the previous winter had led him "to use the former too freely."[152] Accusing an adversary of habitual opium use was effective, in part, because its impact on users varied and might not be noticeable at all. Other rumors derived from the notion that opium could make someone eloquent but that it was only an artificial eloquence. John Adams, for example, had heard that "Opium and liquid Laudanum . . . will produce Genius out of the coarsest Clay." Mentioning this in an 1821 letter to Dr. Benjamin Waterhouse, he then shared gossip he had heard about Alexander Hamilton. Though he would "not vouch for the truth of it," a parson had told him that Hamilton "never wrote or spoke at the bar, or elsewhere, in public, without a bit of Opium in his mouth."[153] This critique, although Adams himself would not endorse it, implied that Hamilton should not be applauded for his writings, no matter how impressive they were, because they were not authentic.

\* \* \*

Historian David Courtwright has cited 1830 as the year that medical publications began to focus increasingly on the issue of opium dependency, whereas they previously emphasized overdoses.[154] That year the editors of Philadelphia's *Journal of Health* pointed out, "We have repeatedly, in this Journal, entered our solemn protest against the sin of drunkenness." They then broached a different topic— habitual laudanum use—and characterized it as being as bad as intoxication from alcohol.[155] Around that time, reformer Sylvester Graham was including opium in his temperance lectures in New York. To his audiences, Graham condemned "Tea and Coffee, as well as Tobacco, Opium, and Alcoholic potables," as Horace Greeley later recalled.[156] And in 1830, the American Temperance Society awarded a prize to Edward Hitchcock for his *Essay on Alcoholic & Narcotic Substances, as Articles of Common Use.* Hitchcock justified addressing "spirit, wine, opium, and tobacco" collectively, explaining that all were "poisonous in their natures; unnecessary to the healthy; incapable of affording nourishment to the body; fascinating to diseased appetite, and destructive to property, health, and life."[157]

Just a few years later, medical authorities noted that opium use had become widespread among all classes. One of Dr. David Hosack's patients was a long-time opium eater, and he told Hosack that

> a vastly greater number of the people of this country, of both sexes and of all ranks, are slaves to the habitual use of it, than is generally supposed. Even among the very poor the practice of using it obtains in no small degree, and is daily becoming more prevalent.

Many were unaware of the problem, the recovering habitué went on, because most who used it "take it in a clandestine manner." He admitted that it would "perhaps" be better if doctors were aware of widespread dependency because, otherwise, they would not know why the treatments they recommended sometimes failed.[158] A writer for the *Journal of Health* agreed that laudanum use had become "fashionable." Many users were people in their prime rather than those who more typically overindulged—thoughtless youth and elderly people seeking pain relief. It also had a cachet that alcohol lacked, because it seemed "scientific." Although the writer insisted that nobody should envy habitual laudanum users, he admitted that many were members of the elite.[159]

As Americans learned of opium's role as a drug for pleasure-seekers, many considered it preferable to hard liquor. In his *Medical Inquiries and Observations,* Dr. Benjamin Rush noted that many people resorted to "strong drink" in order to deal with the "pressure of debt, disappointments in worldly pursuits, and guilt." He maintained that religion provided the only true cure. If a person did not pursue a religiously oriented solution, Rush continued, he insisted that "wine and opium should always be preferred to ardent spirits," because he believed they did less damage to the user and that "the habits of attachment to them are easily broken."[160]

The nonmedical consumption of opiates was, nonetheless, suspect in early American society in a way that alcohol was not, because people partook secretly and did not recognize the dangers until it was too late. Alcohol use was identified with sociability, while opium was not. Drinkers would buy rounds of drinks and offer toasts. An opium eater or laudanum habitué, however, after buying the drug, would likely consume it at home alone.[161] Drinkers' behavior could give them away, but this was less likely with those who took opiates. And while opiate use was often hidden, its hazards were, as well. In 1826, a writer for the *New-York Mirror* stated that "immoderate drinking" was much more "deadly" than opium use, but he warned that opium use would lead people to what would later be called tolerance and dependency. Without the drug, the user would become "keenly aware of the deprivation, and he would need larger and larger doses." A person who tried to quit would experience "the acme of human misery." For this reason, he advocated using opium only to treat "severe pain," not "to raise the spirits."[162]

Many writers warned their audiences that opiate use would lead to an early death. Temperance advocate Edward Hitchcock, for example, cautioned that the years of a laudanum habitué "will be but few and miserable" and insisted that the user "is destroying himself as surely as if he were swallowing arsenic, or had the pistol applied to his head."[163] Part of this perception derived from the widespread but mistaken notion that opium was a stimulant.[164] At the time, many believed that a stimulant, by making a person's system work faster, would hasten death. In 1817, British physician John Reid explained this theory in a series of essays republished in Philadelphia. He likened human arteries to the "wheel of a carriage" that would travel a certain distance—the distance representing the length of a person's life. Just as the wheel would perform only "a certain number of rotations," he explained, the arteries were "allotted only a certain number of pulsations before their vital energy is entirely exhausted."[165] Therefore, stimulation would bring the carriage more speedily to its destination. And, so the theory went, a drug would move users toward their fate by the same pace that it stimulated them. Such beliefs help to explain why so many believed that few opium eaters would reach old age.

* * *

The secrecy of opium habitués born of shame further delayed medical progress and, thus, the discovery of an effective treatment. In 1832, a doctor admitted that the medical community did not know the nature or extent of opium's negative effects on users. He added that learning the answer would be difficult, because "the unhappy victims of this habit labor even more sedulously than those addicted to the use of ardent spirit, to conceal the fact from notice."[166] In the 1830s, however, medical journals devoted an increasing amount of attention to the problem of drug dependency and the search for effective treatment. In 1833, for example, writers for the *Boston Medical and Surgical Journal* asked readers whether there was "any sure and safe method of curing a person of the habit of opium eating, when that habit is confirmed by many years' use of the article." They acknowledged that "not many" Americans were "addicted to the free and constant use of opium" but insisted that people in this situation were eager "to be rid of so dreadful an evil." As an example, they referred to one woman who pled with her doctor for some treatment "to break up this habit to which she has been many years a bound and servile slave."[167] Dr. Carl Ludwig Seeger of Northampton, Massachusetts, responded and stated that he had "cured a vast many." He recommended giving a habitual opium user smaller and smaller doses of the drug, without letting her know what he was doing. Meanwhile, the patient should have a "warm, well ventilated" room, "simple . . . but nourishing" food, daily exercise, frequent baths, and pleasant conversation.[168]

Some assumed that laudanum users should be able to end their use with willpower alone, but doctors responded that the drug's hold was more tenacious than anyone would expect. Seeger, for example, stated that opium dependency was a "real and complicated disease" and that he had "feelings for the miseries of my fellow beings" and was thus eager to help them.[169] In the *Boston Medical and Surgical Journal*, a doctor described his patient's agony when he tried to reduce her use of the drug. She was "convulsed for hour after hour in every muscle, and vomiting almost without intermission," he wrote. She "insisted on bearing it all," her doctor wrote, and to do so "more by far than we ventured to advise."[170]

This did not mean that American doctors sympathized with all habitués; they distinguished those whose use began as an indulgence from those who began taking an opiate for medical purposes, and they tended to sympathize only with the latter. As one doctor explained:

> When we allude to opium eaters, we mean those only who took it originally as a medicine for some nervous affection, and continue it from necessity, rather than from choice;—who take it, not to intoxicate, but to . . . enable them to attend to business, and to appear like other people.

Of those who take opium for the purposes of unnatural excitement and inebriation, we have no knowledge. They need less of our sympathy, and would excite us less to exertions in their behalf.[171]

The doctor sympathized with those who took the drug to remain productive and who wanted to fit in with everybody else. Those who wanted to feel better than normal, however—who pursued "unnatural excitement"—were not interested in fitting in or meeting their obligations. Because they were not concerned with the social good, they attracted little sympathy.

* * *

Americans who wrote about domestic drug use in the early nineteenth century tended to approve of the use of narcotics for medical purposes but to criticize what they regarded as pleasure-seeking use. They objected to users' lack of productivity, but many misunderstood compulsive drug use, as they concluded that habitués continued to use drugs because they chose not to exercise self-control. Usage was widespread, however, and as the century progressed it would escalate, largely due to doctors' extensive use of opiates and the solace that they brought to users. Domestic habituation, however, would long receive only occasional mentions in the popular press.

# American Drug Use Quietly Escalates, 1842–1867

As he reviewed the accumulated information about narcotics, Dr. David Cheever concluded that many white and "civilized" people were developing an appetite for the stronger substances. He divided drugs into two categories. Some, such as coffee and tobacco, were widely used, their use was socially accepted, and those who partook of them did so openly. Other substances, such as opium and hashish, produced a more noticeable effect, and those who used them did so secretly. In the early 1860s, Cheever saw a growing inclination among white users toward drugs in the latter group. The "Caucasian races," he wrote, were "no longer content with tobacco, coffee, and tea." Instead, they were "beginning to crave and use the stronger narcotics." He saw this in the United States and Europe. The "majority of civilized men," he asserted, used tobacco and did so publicly. "Opium and hemp," however, "if indulged in, are concealed by the Western nations."[1] The tendency to obscure such use suggested that society would have disapproved of it. The disapproval could have derived from the substances' potency and their effects and because their nonmedical use was associated with the non-Western world. Even so, these substances were growing in popularity, a fact that some other commentators also acknowledged.

\* \* \*

In 1857, a writer for *Harper's Weekly* stated that "whoever has sojourned for a season among Chinese or Hindoos" and observed their "sensual vices" would recognize "the confirmed opium sot." These habitués had bloodshot eyes and bewildered expressions, and they sniffled "as with an incipient influenza." Observers could find them "stretching their lazy lengths on paper mattresses" in Hong Kong, smoking cigars in Calcutta, or shivering aboard a steamer in the Bay of Bengal.[2]

*Habit Forming*. Elizabeth Kelly Gray, Oxford University Press. © Oxford University Press 2023.
DOI: 10.1093/oso/9780190073121.003.0003

A person did not have to be among the "Chinese or Hindoos" to see opium's impact, he continued, because the practice had grown popular in New York City among all classes. American habitués were "in workshops and behind counters," he insisted, "in doctors' offices, and in the pulpit," "in Fifth-Avenue drawing rooms and opera-stalls, as well as at firemen's halls and the third tier of Purdy's National Theatre." Customs-house statistics revealed that the United States was importing opium at a rate that greatly exceeded its population growth and medical need. The writer attributed the growing nonmedical use to the fact that many Americans led fast-paced lives and reached for opium as a restorative. In America, he wrote, the "mind is so intense, and so early burns itself down to a socket." As a result, "it calls to be fed with opium, as the only seeming alternative to extinction." Yet the drug's effects were inconsistent. For example, it could lead to a newspaper editor's "electrifying brilliancy yesterday and somniferous dullness to-day." He added that many opiate habitués wanted to end their use but did not know how. When a New York paper ran an article about "the use and abuse of a powerful narcotic," the writer recalled, "a number of persons" wrote to the journalist, "confessing their bondage to the unsparing fiend of opium . . . and imploring" the writer "to help and save them."[3] Articles like this one, however, would appear rarely before the late 1860s.

Between 1842 and 1867, nonmedical opiate use and drug dependency in America rose sharply, but few discussed domestic habituation publicly. The increase in habitual use resulted, in part, from the temperance movement. As the pressure to stop drinking increased, many imbibers gave up alcohol and switched to opium. Because it was a medicine, its use was socially acceptable. The Civil War also increased habitual use, as doctors used opiates to treat soldiers' ailments and injuries. Decades later, some veterans were still using them. The greatest impact, though, came from doctors' use of opiates in treating other patients, especially affluent women. Many well-to-do women found solace in opiates, and they were more likely than men, or poorer women, to seek medical attention. Also, many regarded frail health as a mark of gentility. The paucity of public discussion made it easy for people to hide their habit. It also meant that there was little effort to warn the public about the risk of dependency or to end the medical practices that led to it. Meanwhile, habitués continued to suffer, as there was little discussion of effective treatments.

Of the articles that were published on the topic, many were compassionate accounts of the effect of habituation on members of the white middle class while others were critiques of drug use by the elite and the poor. Commentators tended to suggest that middle-class habitués turned to opiates to restore health and productivity and that others used them self-indulgently and were uninterested in meeting their obligations. Poorer users seemed to receive attention from the press only if they used deceit or committed crimes to get drugs, which rendered them unworthy of sympathy. The origin of their use received almost no consideration, and the same was true for any people of color who became habituated. Some suggested that black people would not need opiates for medical reasons, thus depriving them of any accepted reason for their use. A popular theory, for example, held that African Americans, unlike white people, rarely became ill. Meanwhile, it was possible to posit a flattering and popular explanation as to why opiates seemed to affect one group disproportionately. Some contended that opiates affected people's minds and that people who used their minds the most, understood to be white, were therefore most affected by the drugs.

\* \* \*

The discovery of morphine, early in the nineteenth century, revolutionized the field of pain management. Chemist Friedrich Sertürner isolated the drug, which is the main alkaloid of opium, in Paderborn, Germany, around 1804. He named it for Morpheus, the Greek god of dreams.[4] With morphine, a doctor could administer precise doses of painkillers and soporifics that would have "predictable therapeutic action," as David Courtwright has noted.[5] The doses were much more precise than a quantity of opium or laudanum could be, as the strength of the latter substances could not be ascertained. Opium was "a complex plant extract with wide variations in potency," as historians Caroline Jean Acker and Sarah W. Tracy have noted. Morphine, on the other hand, was "a single compound."[6] Rosengarten and Company, a pharmaceutical firm in Philadelphia, began to extract morphine from crude opium in 1832.[7]

American consumption of opiates increased sharply between 1842 and 1867, as opium imports rose much faster than population growth in this period. In 1865, a writer for the New York Journal of Commerce reported that the value of opium imported into the United States between 1840 and 1862 had grown more than twentyfold. Although he acknowledged that wartime demands had played a role, he pointed out that most of the increase predated the Civil War and owed to the demand from habitual users.[8] The actual increase almost certainly exceeded what these figures suggest. As David Courtwright has noted, the nation had no duty on opium until 1842. Once the duty was imposed, there was an incentive to smuggle, to avoid the expense. Therefore, the figures after 1842 likely underestimate the amount brought into the country.[9]

Longtime druggists witnessed this growing demand firsthand. By 1870, "Dr. S. S." had been working for twenty years as a doctor and druggist in a New England city of ten thousand inhabitants. Although the population had grown "only inconsiderably," he wrote, his sales had increased "from 50 pounds of opium the first year to 300 pounds now; and of laudanum four times upon what was formerly required." He added that about fifty people bought opiates

from him on a regular basis. Alonzo Calkins, who wrote extensively about habitual opium use, included the doctor's account in his 1871 book *Opium and
the Opium-Appetite* and added that there were many similar stories: "Such is no
solitary record."[10]

At mid-century, opiates remained medically invaluable. The demand for them
was great. A writer in 1846 suggested that, in a family's medicine chest, bottles
"labeled 'paregoric' and 'laudanum,' were exhausted three times as often as the
others."[11] Half the prescription drugs provided by two druggists in Virginia City,
Nevada, in 1862 and 1863 were opiates.[12] Granted, all these drugs cannot be
assumed to have been used for medical purposes, even though they were provided in a medical context, but opiates were crucial as pain relievers and sleep
agents. Although Dr. Oliver Wendell Holmes said in 1860 that it would be best
for humanity if all the medicines "as now used, could be sunk to the bottom of
the sea," he made an exception for opium.[13]

Part of the domestic increase in use owed to a series of epidemics. Americans
endured attacks of cholera in 1832 and 1849 and a lengthy epidemic of dysentery
in the late 1840s. Doctors used opiates to treat both ailments, because opium
has a constipating effect.[14] Opium and laudanum were "sovereign remedies and
preventatives for cholera," according to medical historian Charles Rosenberg,
and many apothecaries advertised the drugs.[15]

There was opposition to giving opiates to children, due to the risks, but
the practice continued. Some doctors maintained that the medicines could be
administered safely to infants in the recommended doses if they were given infre-
quently.[16] In her 1842 medical guide for women, however, Mary Gove deemed
the use of Godfrey's Cordial and similar preparations to be the "dreadful practice" of "ignorant" parents.[17] Overdoses were one risk, while other consequences
appeared over time. Some parents unwittingly habituated their babies. One
woman gave her daughter Mrs. Winslow's Soothing Syrup. The doses grew larger
and larger over a period of months and, according to the mother, the baby would
"scream and kick all the morning" until she received it. The mother saw no ur-
gency in heeding the doctor's advice to wean her child from the drug.[18] In 1833,
Dr. William Alcott wrote about a woman who "gave her infants laudanum to
keep them quiet, while she could labor." As a result of the practice, he added,
almost all the children had "inferior intellects," and many had "little energy of
character."[19]

Some parents did give opiates to babies and then leave them unattended,
either to go to work or simply to go out. In 1859, an illustrator for *Harper's
Weekly* captured this in the image "Opium—The Poor Child's Nurse." In it, a
baby lies in a cradle, alone at home. He rubs his eyes as he awakens in a room
with crumbling plaster, a broken chair, and a bottle marked "Opium" on a table.
The illustrator laments the fact that administering the drug was the practice of

some impoverished parents who could not stay at home with their babies yet lacked the means to hire someone to mind them.[20] Babies in more affluent households were also often lulled to sleep with opiates. In the early 1840s, a dentist in Grafton, Massachusetts, saved the life of a baby who had been given laudanum instead of paregoric. The family's affluence is indicated by the facts that they lived in a "good looking house" and the appreciative mother gave him a gold necklace.[21]

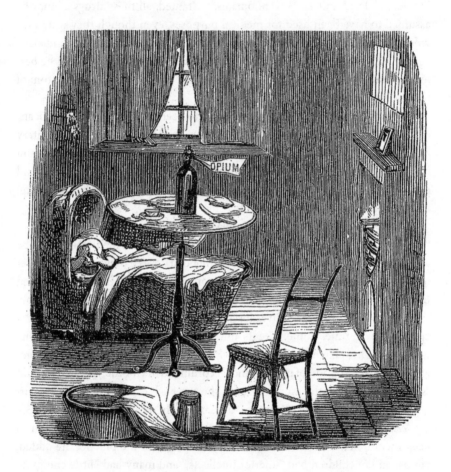

OPIUM—THE POOR CHILD'S NURSE.

*Figure 2.1.* "Opium—The Poor Child's Nurse," *Harper's Weekly,* January 29, 1859. Before the popular press focused on domestic drug habituation it reported on other problematic aspects of American opiate use, such as the excessive use of "soothing syrups" to lull babies to sleep. Some mothers would leave their slumbering charges unattended. This artist focused on a poor family, but well-to-do parents also used these elixirs. Courtesy of Harpweek.com.

In part, the increase in opiate use was an unintended consequence of the temperance movement. This movement, the century's "longest, most popular social cause," as writer Catherine Gilbert Murdock has noted, was focused on ending alcohol consumption. It began early in the century and continued until the passage of the Prohibition amendment.[22] Many temperance advocates hoped that people would find alternate ways to relax or to cope with life's challenges. Dr. John Stainback Wilson, for example, insisted that a bath or shower was more pleasant than the effects of wine, opium, or snuff.[23] Public pressure could stop many people from drinking alcohol but, in many cases, it did not end their use of intoxicants altogether. Many chastened drinkers found opiates to be an appealing alternative. Because they were medicines, a person could buy and consume them without garnering suspicion or criticism. New Yorker George Templeton Strong noted the trend in the spring of 1843: "Opium chewing prevails here extensively, much more so than people think," he wrote. He saw the usage as having "greatly increased" as a response to "the blessed Temperance Movement." To him the correlation was understandable, given human nature. A "'movement' of that sort never moved away from the *principle* of any vice," he insisted. At most, it could only "drive this or that development of it into the background for a while."[24] Along similar lines, in 1849 Dr. Joel Shew stated that the "Washington temperance movement" in New England was "immediately" followed by an escalation of opium consumption. To him, the cause and effect were clear and would be "a hard lesson for temperance men."[25]

While the temperance movement inclined people more toward opiates and other drugs, the prohibitory Maine Laws likely hastened the switch. In 1851, the state of Maine banned the "manufacture, sale, keeping or depositing for sale of intoxicating liquors," with limited exceptions, and thirteen other states followed over the next few years.[26] Some New Yorkers warned against adopting the "Maine Law." "The use of other stimulants will be very greatly increased," a writer for the *New York Evening Post* cautioned in 1855. An increase in opium use bothered him acutely, as he considered the habit both dangerous and easy to hide. It was "one of the . . . most dreadful forms of intemperance," he wrote, yet one that could "be indulged with most secresy [*sic*]."[27] Art critic Clarence Cook stated that opium sales in Boston had "increased to an alarming extent" following Massachusetts's adoption of the Maine Law.[28] In 1869, the Medical Society of the State of Pennsylvania agreed that "the opium habit is greatly on the increase" and that it was "especially . . . increasing in those communities and states where the sale of intoxicating liquors is prohibited by law."[29] Maine's governor, Dr. Alonzo Garcelon, also saw the effects. In an 1879 address to the Maine Temperance Convention, he stated that opiate use had "increased to an alarming extent." Even some temperance advocates indulged in laudanum, while ladies moistened their handkerchiefs with "chloroform and ether . . . to allay nervous excitement."[30] These sweet liquids were medically used as anesthetics.[31]

Part of the increase in opiate use resulted from doctors' widespread dispensing of them in the Civil War. In addition to their efficacy as painkillers, these drugs helped to prevent malaria and to treat diarrhea and dysentery.[32] There is evidence that doctors distributed them indiscriminately. One Confederate doctor, for example, gave opium to every soldier who had diarrhea.[33] Some physicians sprinkled powdered morphine into wounds, rarely measuring the amount. Doctors also used laudanum to diminish the pain associated with amputations. Historian Jonathan Lewy estimates that the Union side administered "over 80 tons of opium powder and tinctures" during the war.[34] The demand for medicine during the war was a boon to the pharmaceutical industry. Over the decade of the 1860s, the number of American chemical manufacturers increased from eighty-four to three hundred.[35]

Doctors also used opiates to treat chronic disorders; their effects became more noticeable years after the fact, as habituation resulted. In 1871, Boston druggists attested that their customers included habituated veterans.[36] In 1876, a Union veteran blamed his dependency on the doctor who had given him morphine. Although he recognized that it might have saved his life, he also believed the "blundering" doctor was guilty of malpractice.[37] Another soldier was wounded in battle and endured a series of amputations to one arm. In 1877, his doctor reported that the man "formed the morphia habit" when trying to treat his pain.[38] Many habits endured for decades. Between 1885 and 1900, doctors at the National Home for Disabled Volunteer Soldiers treated thousands of cases of morphine addiction.[39] In 1919, the patients at a morphine maintenance clinic in Shreveport, Louisiana, included an eighty-two-year-old Confederate veteran who had been given morphine during the war after he was shot in the head. By the time he visited the clinic, he had been addicted for fifty-five years.[40]

Many veterans hid their habituation, fearing that their dependency could jeopardize their pensions.[41] In 1902, Dr. T. D. Crothers, who worked with habitués, stated that this was an issue for many veterans who used morphine to treat the "pain and suffering" associated with war-related injuries.[42] In 1893, his group, the American Association for the Study and Cure of Inebriety, had advocated that the pension bureau recognize that opium use was a "natural sequence and entailment" following the contraction of a disease or injury while in military service.[43]

While some held veterans blameless for addictions that resulted from war-related injuries, others censured them for not bearing their pain stoically. Indianan Clinton Smith, for example, was shot in the arm in the Battle of Chickamauga. He took morphine to control his chronic pain, became addicted, and died of a morphine overdose in 1884. Congress approved a pension for Smith's widow, but President Grover Cleveland vetoed the measure. He attributed Smith's death to "intemperate" behavior, not to his injury. For this reason, Cleveland concluded that granting the pension would "establish a very bad precedent."[44] The staff of the *Indianapolis Journal* decried the veto as "unwarranted and outrageous" and emphasized that Smith's morphine use had not been an indulgence. "A braver boy never went forth to do battle," they asserted, and they pointed out that Smith's wound never healed properly. This had caused excruciating pain that only morphine could relieve. They implied that it was not Smith but his detractors who were intemperate. The only person in town who defended the president, they wrote, was "one old copperhead, whose hide is constantly soaked with bad whisky."[45] Although some "fellow veterans, relatives, friends, and even some doctors" defended habituated veterans and deemed them blameless, these advocates were in the minority, as historian Jonathan Jones points out. Many instead attributed their continued use to poor character and a lack of self-control.[46]

For these veterans, their addiction—and, for some, their consequent inability to earn a living—caused them to appear unmasculine to others and, sometimes, to themselves. Many people equated manliness with independence, self-control, and moral behavior. Addicted veterans, however, depended on their drugs. Opiate dependency often led to financial difficulty, as many habituated veterans could no longer support their families and the cost of opiates added a new and potentially significant expense. Some turned to family and friends for financial help. Meanwhile, critics came from all corners, and some habitués agreed with their critics. "Most doctors, military officials, and even addicted veterans themselves decried opiate addicts as unmanly and immoral," Jones observed.[47]

The war's impact on rates of habitual opium use becomes greater, of course, when everyone who turned to opiates as a consequence of the conflict is counted. Louisa May Alcott, for example, tended to Union soldiers as a nurse and contracted typhoid fever. Dangerous treatments weakened her further, and she used opiates for a long time to cope with chills and sleeplessness. In an 1870 letter, she indicated that her usage had become habitual, though she diminished her doses: "My bones are so much better," she wrote to her family from France, "that I slept without any opium or anything,—a feat I have not performed for some time."[48] In his 1868 work *The Opium Habit*, Horace Day pointed out that soldiers' "anguished and hopeless wives and mothers" took opium to find "temporary relief from their sufferings."[49]

Habitual use was more extensive in the South, partly due to the war's outcome, but also because of the scarcity of good medical care as well as the region's endemic diseases. In 1877, an opium dealer reported that men who had been "impoverished by the rebellion, have taken to eating and drinking opium to drown their sorrows."[50] Dr. Leslie Keeley reported that "some districts in the South are almost devastated by the opium disease." He believed that the protracted use did not derive wholly from financial losses. The "devastation," he wrote in 1892, "has continued long after wrecked plantations have been restored."[51] Also, many southerners suffered from diarrhea, dysentery, and malaria and consequently kept opiates on hand.[52]

The war is not totally responsible for the overall increase in drug use. As public health specialist Mark Quinones has noted, Americans were using drugs "at alarming rates" long before the firing on Fort Sumter.[53] Although the war contributed to the national addiction rate, habitués after the conflict were disproportionately women.[54] Also, the number of habitués emerging from the war was tempered by the fact that, during the conflict, the use of syringes was not yet widespread. Therefore, most morphine would not have been administered by injection, the method most likely to lead to addiction.[55] While the war contributed to the growth of drug dependency in nineteenth-century America, and the consequences of that use endured for many decades, it was one of many factors, and not the most significant one.

Most of the increase in opiate habituation in the middle third of the nineteenth century originated with medical use by middle-class women who were following a doctor's advice or who were self-administering it. The use of opiates as painkillers appealed to patients who sought comfort and to young doctors who wanted the alleviation of pain to be a hallmark of modern medicine.[56] Women were more likely than men to receive a prescription for an opiate due to the widespread belief that they were less able than men "to bear pain and psychic discomfort," as Dr. Stephen Kandall noted. Also, much of women's physical pain at the time derived from gynecological ailments for which no cures existed.[57]

There was, at the time, a correlation between opiate use and white, female lassitude. Many middle-class female habitués were invalids, but this attracted little curiosity, as many regarded poor health as a lady's natural state. It was "fashionable" for a woman to be ill, literary scholar Ann Douglas Wood has noted, because many regarded ill health as a sign of gentility.[58] In reality, their weakness and "predisposition to illness" partly resulted from social mores regarding how they should dress and eat. Long skirts, petticoats, and corsets impeded their movement and constricted their breathing. Also, doctors and parents discouraged women's physical activity and their consumption of protein, even though avoiding both led to anemia. Many Americans, however, both male and female, concluded that "frailty and delicacy" and "unhealthiness" were middle-class women's lot, according to Diane Price Herndl, a scholar in women's and gender studies.[59] Historian Mara Keire has suggested that some doctors may have not minded having such patients, as opiates would have turned "the willful hysteric into a manageable invalid," lethargic and quiet.[60] It was probably easy for these women to hide their habituation, since the passive behavior that resulted from drug addiction would have resembled the behavior that was expected of them.[61]

Some objected to the fashionableness of invalidism. In the introduction to his 1849 volume *Matron's Manual of Midwifery*, Dr. Frederick Hollick lamented that it had become popular. "Custom and false notions have given this melancholy state the stamp of propriety, and thrown around it the charm of fashion," he explained. While invalidism was deemed *"genteel,"* he rued, "robust health and physical capability is termed *coarseness* and *vulgarity."*[62] And in *Woman in American Society* (1873), Abba Goold Woolson criticized the fact that the "accepted type of female loveliness" was a "sweet-tempered dyspeptic" who was *"petite* and fragile, with lily fingers and taper waists."[63] But within the middle class, fragility was in vogue. In 1866 Catharine Beecher, an advocate for women's education, asked friends in various cities to rank the health of ten women they knew. Some of them reported not knowing a single woman who was truly healthy.[64]

Many middle-class women were complicit with this. They were "willing to think of themselves as ill and to accept the role of invalid," Herndl has noted.[65] Some might have delayed recovery from an illness in order to appear genteel, while others likely did so to avoid household responsibilities and expectations or to take more control of marital decisions. Illness enabled a woman to "escape from the too pressing demands of bedroom and kitchen," Ann Douglas Wood writes.[66] Historian Carroll Smith-Rosenberg agrees that "taking to one's bed" could have been "a mode of passive aggression."[67] For some, insisting that they didn't feel well could have been their only way either to get rest or to avoid another pregnancy. While many people sympathized with invalids, others perceived them as manipulative.[68]

Many women who initially used opiates for medical purposes then discovered their effectiveness as sedatives and kept taking them. In 1855, writers for the *New-York Observer* stated that many women took them because the drugs gave them "a dreamy sensation" that released them from "the pressure of ordinary cares and perplexities."[69] This quality was valuable to women who were weakened by grief or other personal challenges. Such events could include deaths in the family, miscarriages, financial setbacks, or the despondency that could result from overwork and an "unsatisfying life situation," according to Smith-Rosenberg.[70] In 1856, a woman admitted to her cousin that she became a habitual morphine user in the months following her daughter's death. In a letter, she recalled of those months, "If I ever slept, I did not know it, my mind in a complete wreck."[71] Later in the century, a Vermont woman found that opium helped her to endure living with her drunken, violent spouse. "Her husband was dissipated, and as he made night hideous, she wanted something to give her rest," Dr. E. W. Shipman explained in 1890.[72] While doctors sometimes prescribed narcotics for their tranquilizing effects, it was more common for women to use drugs that doctors had prescribed to them to treat something else.[73]

Many members of the upper class, especially women, found that opiates helped them socially by enhancing their wit. In 1840 James Gordon Bennett Sr., editor of the *New York Herald*, noted that the upper classes were increasingly indulging in opium and laudanum. This included people who were "fashionable and intellectual," as a writer for New Orleans's *Times-Picayune* summarized, "particularly the gay women who shine in society, and the cavaliers who are distinguished for their refinement and literature." If someone at a soiree was "particularly brilliant," the journalist reported, "ten to one they are opium eaters."[74] In 1855, a woman wrote to the *New York Times* to report that laudanum use had become prevalent among New York's women. She had discovered, for example, that she had five wealthy, female acquaintances who were habitués.[75] And Alonzo Calkins wrote of a "New York lady" who drank a pint of paregoric each day in the early 1850s. Under its influence, she "shone amid the throng from eight o'clock in the evening to midnight and past," he wrote, "often seeing the grey morning ere she retired for bed."[76]

Others identified men in the professions as opiate users. In 1857, a writer for the *Flag of Our Union* stated that "the vice of opium-eating" had become a problem among "ladies" and "members of the learned professions." Such reports, he added, "cause us to sigh for the degeneracy of the Anglo-American race."[77] In 1862, a writer for *Hall's Journal of Health* reported that only a tenth of the nation's imported opium was used "for medicinal purposes." The rest was used by habitués in the elite and professional classes—"lawyers, physicians, literary men, and ladies, who move in the higher circles of society."[78] The problem was of long duration, especially among doctors. Dr. J. B. Mattison asserted that "physicians form a large proportion of opium habitués," and he had treated several of them himself. In 1883 he stated that in one New England city, more than 30 percent of the doctors were "addicted to some form of opium."[79] Dr. Thomas Blair recalled a group of physicians who had worked at a hospital around 1890. Of those fourteen men, he noted thirty years later, "twelve had died drug addicts or drunkards." Although the high rate was exceptional, he saw it as a good example of how little thought doctors had given at the time regarding the use of narcotics.[80] The proportion of medical habitués varied from place to place, but their rate of habituation was noteworthy.[81]

Americans at mid-century were also using an increasingly wide variety of drugs, including ether and chloroform. Dentists used them when pulling teeth, and doctors used them before delivering a baby, performing an operation, or treating respiratory problems.[82] Many people became aware of the drugs' hallucinatory properties when receiving medical treatment. A dentist, for example, gave Henry David Thoreau ether in 1851. Under its influence, Thoreau wrote, "You are a sane mind without organs."[83] Stories about its effects sparked curiosity. When Margaret Fuller sought out a dentist for a toothache, she admitted that she looked forward to experiencing the anesthetic, "after all the marvellous stories I had heard." She inhaled it and dreamed she was "wandering in long garden-walks, and through many alleys of trees."[84] An elderly woman who used chloroform as a medicine enjoyed it so much that she thought "every poor man ought to possess a bottle" of it.[85] Some youth used the anesthetics for amusement. In the 1830s and 1840s, many engaged in "frolics," where they would inhale ether, chloroform, or laughing gas and enjoy the effects.[86]

In the late 1860s, many women used chloroform to intoxicate themselves because it was effective and easy to hide, and users were often unaware of its dangers. In 1869, the *Cincinnati Enquirer* reported that, in New York, "all classes of women, from the inmates of the shameless haunts of Greene street to the belles of the Fifth avenue and the pupils of fashionable boarding-schools" used it. It produced "dreamy intoxication" while leaving behind "few apparent traces." The writer was concerned, however, that many women were unfamiliar with its ill effects, which could be "subtle and sudden." Use could prove fatal, for example, even if the user did not increase the dose.[87] Around the same time, Dr. Alonzo Calkins reported that ether and chloroform were becoming more popular than opiates "among the ladies of the favored classes in Boston."[88] Some doctors did not warn their patients or their patients' families of chloroform's hazards, instead encouraging its liberal use. In the early 1880s, a doctor visited a female patient and, just before leaving her home, instructed her husband "to give her chloroform freely, and not to be afraid of it."[89]

The dangers included habituation. In 1849, John C. Warren asked doctors to avoid recommending it as a painkiller, because some patients would use it habitually.[90] One man's chloroform habit began right after he had a tooth pulled. He decided to inhale some before going to sleep and then felt "the delightful sensation of being wafted through an enchanted land into Nirvana." His experience was not like drunkenness—his "blissful" state seemed far different from that of "the wretches I had sometimes seen staggering through the streets." Continued use, though, brought on nausea and diarrhea. Ultimately, he ended his use through "sheer force of will."[91] In part, however, the popularity of ether and chloroform would be limited because hypodermic injections of morphine were more convenient.[92]

\* \* \*

For the most part, habitués could hide their habit, so long as they had their drug. Their behavior would not betray them, as often happened with heavy drinkers, and except for those who were regarded as invalids, they did not appear to be ill. Dr. Nathan Allen pointed out that opium's "pernicious effects . . . are far more easy to be concealed than those of alcohol."[93] Of course, these users had to maintain their habit in order to appear "normal." William Wood wasn't trying to end his opium use one spring day in 1852 when he accidentally left home without some of his drug. Authorities found him "raving like a maniac" that evening, and he explained—as the *New-York Daily Times* reported—that he was "in the habit of eating opium" and, deprived of his drug, became delirious.[94]

Some habitués had friends and family who sought to hide the dependency and to limit its damage. In the 1840s, rumors circulated of Edgar Allan Poe's habituation, which his cousin Elizabeth Poe Herring later confirmed. She had visited Poe and his wife in Philadelphia in the early 1840s. She rarely saw him drink. Instead, as she later recalled, "for the most part, his periods of excess were occasioned by a free use of opium."[95] She admitted that she "had the misfortune to see him often" under the drug's influence. Those close to him tried to hide his habit and to limit his ability to get opium. They "did all possible to conceal his faults & failures," she recalled, and when he would go out, they would "follow him to the gate and take his money & watch away from him." Poe apparently regretted his condition and his behavior, but he could not change. His "penitence was genuine," Herring recalled, but "he made good resolutions only to be broken."[96]

The general silence on the topic, of course, meant that users who wanted to end their use had to navigate the process on their own, a tortuous journey that often included relapses. In 1853, for example, an opium habitué described his efforts in this regard to readers of the *New York Medical Times*. When he stopped using opiates, he went for ten days and nights without sleep, and his blood "felt like boiling water." After four weeks he felt better, but weak. For "a whole year," he recalled, "I was feeble as a child, and one walking repository of aches and distressing sensations." He did not remain free of the drug. When he visited doctors to treat his neuralgia, they gave him morphine, and he returned to his habit.[97]

Some habitués found it difficult to hide their dependency when they tried to quit. The typical user wanted to keep his habit a secret and therefore sought "to cure himself, without seeking the assistance of medicine," according to Dr. Leslie Keeley.[98] When Horace Day decided to end his use, he was glad that his house was situated in such a way that no neighbors would notice any "outcry of pain" or "eccentricity of conduct."[99] And in 1876, a clerk who tried to end his morphine use found it impossible to do his job and end his use without revealing his condition. "I was suffering in secret, my employer knowing nothing of my thraldom, and I could not work with the accursed appetite raging within me," he explained. Unable to resist, he took more of the drug—and then regretted it.[100] Dr. Joseph Parrish, who ran a clinic in Media, Pennsylvania, in the 1860s, lamented that many compulsive opium users had no support as they tried to end their usage.[101] The "doomed victims," he wrote, "grope their way by thousands through their life of semi-oblivion, ... without one welcome voice to inspire any earnest resolutions towards resistance and self-conquest."[102]

This loneliness was aggravated by non-users' belief that ending drug use required only willpower. Therefore, such people often concluded that merely ordering someone to stop using should suffice. Instead, such requests often pushed the habit behind closed doors, due to the intensity of the habituation. In the early 1850s, for example, Brooklyn resident John Titus confronted his wife, Rosanna, about her laudanum use and forbade her from taking the drug. She sustained the habit secretly for two years, at which point she died from an overdose.[103] Similar episodes underscored the intractable nature of drug dependency. According to H. Wayne Morgan, "every addict-memoirist" insisted that "their addiction and relapse resulted not from lack of will or the desire for normality, but because of processes beyond the control of even normal people."[104]

Some people tried to end their use with help, but few appreciated how intense the habitué's craving could be. In the late 1830s and 1840s, poet John Lofland's friends strove to break him from his laudanum use, for example, but the challenge was herculean. He experienced "intense suffering" as a result of his withdrawal, he later explained, and therefore sought "every opportunity to obtain" the drug. When his friends were asleep, he went to the home of his cousin, a doctor. "I knew where the laudanum bottle was," he explained, "and with delirious joy I seized it, and drank four or five ounces." On another occasion, his friends took him to the hospital to try to end his usage, but he left when nobody was watching him and found a druggist. After consuming the laudanum he chose not to return home, "lest my friends should send me back to the Hospital." He later returned there, however, and he begged the doctor "to give me laudanum enough to calm my system, but all in vain," the poet lamented. After a restless night, he bribed a carriage driver to bring him opium. His usage did not end until his physician warned every druggist in Baltimore not to sell opium to him and ensured that nobody who visited Lofland gave him any. "I tried to obtain it," Lofland recalled, "but as they say in Baltimore, '*I couldn't come it.*' "[105]

Those who were determined to end their opium use found the experience agonizing, and some placed themselves beyond reach of the drug in hopes of guaranteeing success. One anonymous habitué insisted that when a person who was addicted went for twenty-four hours without the drug, he would perspire and experience pain as well as a "floodgate" from the stomach and bowels. An "acrid and fiery diarrhoea sets in, which nothing but opium can check," he explained. His body would become "as limp as a dish-rag, and as lifeless." The attraction of taking more opium was intense: it would "brace the man right up."[106] As a consequence, many attempts failed. Some literally chose to imprison themselves. In 1841, a woman was remanded to Boston's House of Correction, at her request, to end her opium habit.[107] Others thought the answer was to move to a rural setting. James McCune Smith, the first African American physician, recalled a patient of his who wanted to end her laudanum use. In the spring of 1843, "she went into the country . . . where she could not obtain any laudanum." Upon returning to the city, she resumed a moderate use of it. And in 1851, a doctor in New York treated a patient who had become a habitual opium user following the amputation of his leg. "I propose to send him into the country for a few weeks," the doctor wrote, "to confirm his cure."[108]

Many physicians and people who were addicted described habitual drug users as "slaves," since they were beholden to their drug and therefore lacked full autonomy. The analogies were often overt. Two books about drug dependency— Leslie E. Keeley's *The Morphine Eater* (1881) and Henry G. Cole's memoir, *Confessions of an American Opium Eater* (1895)—shared the subtitle *From Bondage to Freedom*, which borrowed from the title of Frederick Douglass's 1855 autobiography.[109] Keeley asserted that being "slaves of a 'drug!'" was "the most damnable" form of slavery "on earth; a bondage to a soulless, merciless tyrant; a captivity whose daylight is Despair and whose Hope is Death."[110] In recalling his successful attempt to end his morphine use, Cole compared his own "early days of his deliverance" from opium habituation with how a "black slave" would have felt during his "first few months of his liberation from a life of slavery's curse."[111]

Meanwhile, some habitués felt a sense of shame for their condition that rendered them morose and even suicidal, while those around them did not realize the extent of their anguish. The Reverend G. W. Brush of Delaware, Ohio, for example, began taking morphine around 1850 for medicinal purposes and became habituated. An attempt to quit led to acute diarrhea, and he abandoned a second attempt when he had to take care of some work that he could not complete in his "shattered state." After sixteen years of dependency, he sought medical help. The forty-year-old minister feared "that his life was a failure," Dr. Lewis Barnes recalled, given his apparently intractable condition. Brush also believed that "every one was ready to despise him," Barnes added, "and that his usefulness was therefore at an end."[112] A third attempt to quit appeared to succeed, but when Barnes went to hear Brush preach, the doctor could tell "from his manner, that he was returning to his habit." A week later, the preacher hanged himself in his barn. Dr. Barnes insisted that nobody could understand the suffering of drug dependency without witnessing it or enduring it firsthand. "Let no man judge him," he insisted, "and least of all, those who are strangers to the fascinating and infernal strength of his enemy."[113]

Those who studied habituation or experienced it themselves tended to be compassionate. Moses Clark White, who conducted research about opium while attending Yale's medical school in the 1850s, had nothing but sympathy for habitués. The "poor enslaved victim," he wrote in his dissertation, lacks the "energy or resolution to break away from the chains which bind him."[114] Sophia Hawthorne, a painter and the wife of writer Nathaniel Hawthorne, developed morphine dependency following her medical use of it as a girl. That experience, she later stated, "has given me infinite sympathy and charity for persons liable to such a habit."[115]

Those who did end their use would presumably be exuberant, but some looked back on opium's effects wistfully. When novelist Sylvanus Cobb Jr. stopped using opium, he did look healthier, but he was dissatisfied. In the spring of 1869, he told Boston drug merchant Charles Edward French that he had given up the drug. That evening in his diary, French noted that when he had seen Cobb on an earlier occasion, he "looked like a corpse." The writer was, however, "now healthy & happy."[116] But years earlier, in another period without the drug, Cobb had found life unsatisfying. He had deemed abstinence "tedious" and could not rediscover the focus that opium had provided. In nine years without opium, he admitted that he "never . . . felt a real natural, vimmy, ambition to labor." He had then resumed his use.[117]

\* \* \*

Impoverished people who were drug dependent were often blamed for their condition, in part because their habit came at a cost to society, such as when they broke the law by stealing to support it. One woman, for example, ended up in New York's St. Lawrence County jail in 1834 because she had "committed a number of forgeries in order to obtain *opium*," noted the sheriff, Lemuel Buck. "Previous to her contracting this habit," he added, she had been "a woman of fair character and respectability."[118] They were not always given the courtesy of anonymity. In 1860, the *New York Times* reported that "a female opium-eater, Julia Parsons, died recently in the Pittsburgh Jail. She had been for some years a confirmed vagrant."[119]

Indigent drug users tended to garner attention from the press when they were caught trying to acquire a drug through theft, fraud, or other deceptive means. Typically, the people who relayed these stories were unsympathetic toward them—focusing on their crime, not on their dependence. For several reasons, these habitués became objects of derision: they were dependent and were not trying to end their use, they broke the law to get the drug, and their scheme was so poor that they had been caught. Meanwhile, such accounts rarely addressed how their use originated, leaving open the possibility that it had always been an indulgence. The degree to which they wished to end their habit was rarely mentioned, and even if they ardently wished to do so, they would have lacked the means to engage a doctor. The stories tended to focus on lies or other forms of deceit. In 1881, for example, a "haggard, weather-beaten tramp" asked a man for money for bread but later admitted, as Dr. D. W. Nolan wrote, "that it was opium, not bread, he craved."[120]

One woman whose ruse was exposed had played on abolitionists' goodwill. When "Mary Smith" met anti-slavery activists early in 1852, she presented herself as having escaped from slavery and as being an acquaintance of abolitionist Lucretia Mott. Abby Kelley Foster, however, another abolitionist, found her story unconvincing. She suspected from Smith's "manner and story" that she was lying and then confirmed that Mott had never heard of her. Smith disappeared, but the next year she imposed on a couple who frequently housed fugitives from slavery. Foster confronted Smith, but her hoax had been effective. She had stayed with many abolitionists and used multiple aliases. She told Foster that she could consume huge amounts of opium, and Foster concluded that the woman made up her story of being a fugitive "to obtain the means of gratifying her depraved appetites" for opium and tobacco. Foster wrote to the *Liberator* and implored editors of other anti-slavery papers to reprint her account, to prevent readers from assisting the "most hardened imposter I have ever seen."[121]

While abolitionists understandably took umbrage that a habitual opium user had taken advantage of their kindness, accounts of impoverished drug users' failed schemes created a negative perception of all of them, especially as the stories did not address the origin of their use or whether they wanted to stop, and stories of poor-but-honest users were rare. Meanwhile, the humiliating lengths that some went to in order to acquire it underscore just how intense their addiction was. In 1860, Ohio medical student William Brown sent the *Medical and Surgical Reporter* his account of a Morgan County mendicant. For at least ten years "A. C." appeared to suffer from convulsions, a result of "black balls" in her vagina that needed to be removed. For a while, a doctor gave her opiates as a painkiller and did not closely examine her. Later, though, another doctor studied one of the balls and concluded that it was a ball of dough painted black and that the woman had concocted the ruse to obtain opium. When they confronted her on the matter, according to Brown, "she cried, and swore, and stoutly denied the accusation" and was confronted again when she tried a similar ploy. Brown presented the story as humorous, noting that "the mind wearies . . . of fevers and inflammations, and delights occasionally to dip into the wonderful and strange." He likely justified his tone on the grounds that, according to him, the story ended happily. When the woman was confronted the second time, she promised to give up the drug. The doctors gave her "diminished doses," Brown reported, and ultimately "I believe, succeeded in breaking up her bad habit."[122] It is unconfirmed that this method worked with her, and Brown admitted that he was uncertain. Nonetheless, such accounts suggested that the poor could be cured easily and that their situations could therefore be a source of amusement.

Those who stole or deceived to sustain their habits were repeatedly treated with amusement and derision, with no consideration for their plight. In the mid-1840s, for example, a former minister who had "abandoned himself to drink and opium eating" was pressured to try a "sweating and steaming" process, which was supposed to end his use. In the midst of it, however, there was a strong smell of laudanum. The minister had concealed a small vial of it "about his person," and during the treatment, it broke. The writer for the *Boston Medical and Surgical Journal* considered the story "amusing" but mentioned that the man soon thereafter entered the Worcester Insane Asylum.[123] Around 1840, some medical students in Syracuse, New York, poisoned a man who stole to support his habit. The morphine habitué frequently pilfered the drug from a doctor's office. The students, aware of his pattern, "put strychnine into a morphine bottle," Dr. A. B. Shipman recalled. When the man consumed it, he endured "spasms" and "terror," which gave the students "amusement." The students might have felt justified in poisoning the thief, but Shipman regarded the students as "wicked wags who were . . . uncharitable and heartless."[124]

Although there were accounts of habitués stealing the drug or lying to get it, many poor users bought it legally or did without. In 1842, the proprietor of a Philadelphia drugstore told a reporter that some "needy and unfortunate" people began using opium to treat "sickness and pain" and then "found it impossible to abandon the habit." That is, they became habitual users in the same way that many members of the middle class did. Miserable without the drug and sometimes unable to purchase it, the writer continued, they were "indeed to be pitied." If habitués went for a while without it, he added, they would be "trembling in every limb." Frequently, they would pawn clothes and furniture to get money for opium.[125]

Being well connected, meanwhile, could help someone who committed a crime while under the influence of a narcotic. Charles Weston, for example, was arrested in New York City in the fall of 1866, charged with indecent exposure. While Isabella Calkins had been working in a store window, Weston walked past multiple times. His clothes were "very much disarranged," a writer for the *New-York Times* reported. He was "indecently exposed" to Calkins, who had him arrested. In court, Weston explained that he suffered from neuralgia and was "in the habit of taking opium, laud[a]num, hasheesh and other narcotics" as painkillers. On the day in question, he maintained, he was "overcome by these drugs" and was therefore "unconscious" of his actions. He was convicted, but three days later he received a suspended sentence, as the judge believed he was not responsible for his actions. The well-connected man avoided a sentence thanks to "several well-known gentlemen," but the reporter suggested it would have been better had he gone to jail for six months, as perhaps he could then have emerged "a healthy, vigorous man."[126]

There was broader support for nonmedical opiate use when it appeared to enhance users' productivity—helping them to make discoveries or to improve the quality or quantity of their work. In 1860, for example, physicians Félix Frédault and Marx E. Lazarus wrote in a Transcendentalist publication that people with "cultivated and highly susceptible minds" were most likely to use opium and hashish. These people, they explained, were interested in learning "the profound mysteries of the human soul, which [those drugs] alone can give."[127] And in 1875, Dr. C. C. Cranmer asserted that opium enabled some lawyers to make their "finest flights at the bar."[128] It could also enhance productivity. In the 1840s, Sylvanus Cobb Jr. had begun using laudanum medicinally, and he later took opium to aid him in his work. A "small pill of gum opium" he explained in a letter to a confidante, enabled him to write with "a concentration of thought that was never to be experienced otherwise."[129] We cannot establish the extent of opium's impact on his career, but Cobb was prolific. "The first writer to mass-produce popular romances," he was a successful novelist, if not always a respected one.[130]

\* \* \*

In the mid-nineteenth century, racist beliefs shaped widely held understandings of opiates' effects on users. Dr. Nathan Allen, for example, asserted that members of different races had different "temperaments," or constitutions, and that their constitutions determined how opium would affect them. He stated that many white people had a nervous temperament, which Scottish phrenologist George Combe associated with intense brainwork, paleness, and "delicate health." Allen maintained that when such people took an opiate, the drug operated "directly and effectively on the mind," though it also damaged them physically. On the other hand, opium use by those who had less "development and activity of the brain"—here he referred to the "Indian and Negro"—would produce effects that were "more of an animal nature."[131]

Some suggested that opium use could make people of color violent and that extra surveillance of them was, therefore, justified. In 1855, the *Ladies' Repository* reprinted a British account that opium's effect "varies, to a great extent, according to the temperament and race of the individual." People who were "sluggish" would become "active and conversable." The writer added that opium would make "excitable people, like the Javanese, the Negro, [and] the Malay . . . perfectly frantic."[132] Dr. Alonzo Calkins agreed that opium use made "*The Malay race* . . . impetuous and irascible, vindictive in their dispositions and reckless of consequences." He reported that "armed sentinels" stood near where Javanese would gather to use opium to combat "any attempted violence," and the sentinels could kill "any dangerously-turbulent person."[133]

Prejudiced views also shaped understanding of the degree to which people would need the drugs. Some white Americans incorrectly believed that African Americans had an inborn heartiness that whites lacked and that, as a result, black Americans would never need opiates as medicine. One Virginia slave owner, for example, disdained suggestions that an enslaved woman could ever be ill. Such a woman "plays the lady at your expense," he insisted, thus reinforcing a perceived correlation between class and health. Some whites concluded "that black women never suffered any illness at all," as women's studies scholar Diane Price Herndl has observed. In reality, people who were enslaved were frequently unhealthy, given their poor diet and the poor conditions in which they lived and worked. All these circumstances made them susceptible to disease. Yet the notion of African American haleness and white weakness provided a way to justify drug use by whites and by whites alone.[134]

Racism in the Civil War era made medical care inaccessible to most African Americans but, ironically, consequently spared most of them from the risk of opiate dependency. Time and again, white authorities found reasons to deny health care to black people. Many Union doctors, for example, erroneously believed that white and black Americans were physiologically different. This provided them with a reason, or an excuse, to refuse to attend to black patients. Soon after the war, the federal government maintained that freedpeople's health should be handled at the state or local level. State and municipal institutions, however, asserted that they would only treat "citizens," whom they defined as white. Thus, freedpeople could not receive treatment.[135] Even freedpeople who had the money to visit a doctor could have trouble finding someone who would treat them.[136] Meanwhile, most addictions resulted from a doctor's prescription, and thus contracting a habit in this manner became less likely for African Americans. Also, white southerners tended to live longer than their black counterparts. As a result, African Americans were less likely than whites to contract diseases associated with old age for which narcotics could be beneficial. In this respect, their shortened life spans also diminished their likelihood of contracting a drug habit.[137]

Some doctors, however, perceived the low level of habituation among African Americans as a sign of inferiority by suggesting that genteel people had delicate health, which was why they had used opiates in the first place. In 1885, a doctor would state in the *North Carolina Medical Journal* that "the colored man is not as susceptible to the habit as the white" because he lacked "the same delicate nervous organization, and does not demand the form of stimulant conveyed in opium." He added that most cases of opium addiction began because the user sought to cure nerve pain. He asserted that "the negro, owing to his lower nervous development, is not liable to diseases of this character."[138] Although this doctor was explaining why a racial disparity existed in cases of addiction, he was also implying that society would only sanction white people's use of opium.

Many white, middle-class Americans focused on apparent differences along lines of race and class when they regarded drug use and habituation rather than seeing similarities. Some African Americans used opiates for the same reason that many white people used them—to alleviate cares. Sometimes, they developed a tolerance. In the 1840s, an eighteen-year-old black woman in Pennsylvania took laudanum in increasing doses and told friends that it made her "merry and so strong." She bought some midday on a Saturday and told them that she planned to have "a right happy afternoon." She took an excessive dose, her friends summoned a doctor, and he revived her and wrote about the encounter.[139] From his account, one can glean that she acquired the drug legally, took it to enjoy a respite from daily life, and her ongoing use of the drug had not led her to become violent. In the writings of the era, however, there was little inclination to highlight the ways in which opiate use by African Americans resembled that of white habitués.

\*\*\*

Few advocated laws restricting opiate use; while some encouraged the use of moral suasion, even those who wanted legislation doubted that anything would be passed. In 1850, the staff of Pittsburgh's *Daily Morning Post* stated that there were "hundreds, perhaps thousands of ladies in this neighborhood, who are habitual opium eaters. Horrible!" They recommended the encouragement of public pressure to curtail usage: "We think some societies should be formed," they wrote, "for the purpose of suppressing the practice."[140] In 1852, Dr. J. S. Scofield in the *New-York Daily Times* called for legislation to limit access to opiates and endorsed committing opium eaters to asylums. He explained that an "alarming" amount of opium was sold in the city and deemed the habit the "worst species of intemperance." He admitted that morphine could soothe the "desponding mind" and give the user "pleasurable sleep," but he warned that this was "a brief calm before a terrible hurricane." He believed the only solution was "some special legislative enactment, limiting or regulating the sale of opium," but he was pessimistic about this path because the process was slow and there would be "serious opposition," as there had been with the Maine Law. Short of legislation, he recommended moral pressure and placing habitués in asylums—against their will, if need be.[141]

\*\*\*

In the mid-nineteenth century, many Americans were using a variety of drugs, including chloroform, ether, and opiates, to allay pain, impart calm, and promote rest, at a time when the temperance movement deemed alcohol use to be unseemly. At this time, some were also intrigued by cannabis, which was available as a medicine. It played only a minor role in the American pharmacopeia, but its reported hallucinatory effects led to use, primarily by members of the white middle class. The varied uses of hemp and hashish, meanwhile, would reinforce the perception that there was a correlation between drug use and productivity at both the individual and the national levels.

# The Vogue for Hashish, 1832–1884

As drug habituation increased in the mid-nineteenth century, some Americans experimented with cannabis, a drug whose pleasure-seeking use had been associated primarily with the non-Western world. Geography appeared to determine how psychoactive the plant would be. In his essay on "Narcotics," Dr. David Cheever stated that *Cannabis sativa* and *Cannabis indica* were "essentially the same plant" but that the climate in which it was grown determined how "narcotic" it would be. In the United States and Europe, the plant's fibers would "harden into flax and cordage," while elsewhere it would exude "a fragrant green resin, which is powerfully narcotic." According to the doctor, none of the populations who used cannabis for its psychoactive effects were Westerners. Its consumers included people "on the plains of India; on the slopes of the Himalayas; in Persia; in Turkey; in Northern Africa among the Moors; in Central and Southern Africa, even by the Hottentots; and . . . the native Indians of Brazil."[1]

Cheever included accounts of hashish's positive and negative effects. He quoted Jacques-Joseph Moreau, the author of *Hashish and Mental Illness*, who had stated in 1845 that small doses of the drug produced a feeling akin to what a person experiences upon hearing "tidings which fill him with joy." The doctor, however, repeated the inaccurate belief that hashish use spurred violence and that it removed the fear of death for the so-called Assassins in the twelfth century. He also stated that "Javanese hasheesh-eaters . . . when mad with hemp, sometimes plunge into the streets, and *run amok . . .* killing all whom they meet."[2] Cheever was mistaken. In *The Seven Sisters of Sleep*, Mordecai Cooke told of the residents of Java—an island in Indonesia, then part of the Dutch East Indies— consuming a drug and "running amok." Cheever reviewed this book, but Cooke said that it was opium, not hashish, that led to this behavior. Cooke also stated that this was only the behavior of "*certain* Javanese."[3] Furthermore, the widely accepted definition of "running amok" was itself a colonial construction.

Cheever was glad that the author of 1857's *The Hasheesh Eater* had provided a firsthand account of habitual use of the drug, and he hoped it would serve as

*Habit Forming.* Elizabeth Kelly Gray, Oxford University Press. © Oxford University Press 2023.
DOI: 10.1093/oso/9780190073121.003.0004

a warning to readers. He thought the work paled in comparison to *Confessions of an English Opium-Eater*, but he was glad to have "the only English treatise on Hasheesh," in which the author recalled the "painful visions and apparitions in his dreams long after he had renounced the drug."[4]

* * *

Dr. George Wheelock Grover was walking in Baltimore's business district when a sign for "Gungawalla Candy, Hashish Candy" caught his eye, and he wondered how powerful it was. The product was a popular confection in the 1860s. Advertisements promoted it as imparting strength and "exhilaration." Exotic Eastern imagery was central in the promotions. One brand was sold in "beautiful gold, silver and ivory boxes," which suggested Eastern opulence. A Gunjah Wallah Company ad played on perceptions of Middle Eastern culture as sumptuous and imaginative. "Arabs use Hasheesh every day of their lives," it stated, and they were admired for "the luxuriance of their imagery" and their "harmony and expressiveness of language." Grover bought a box of it and took some around 11 A.M., while sitting with fellow doctors at the Eutaw House hotel.[5] Advertisements for the candy did not indicate what it contained, besides hashish. It could have been akin to a preparation of hashish that was popular in the Ottoman Empire. "The leaves of this plant are sometimes fried in honey and butter to extract the active resinous portion," a writer for *Scientific American* explained, "and this they eat, as we should, gum drops."[6]

Grover did not feel the candy's "thrillingly pleasant" effects until three hours later, by which time he was dining with friends. He told them that it must be "a day of jubilee" or some other celebration, based on his distorted perceptions. He pointed out that the tables were "set with golden plate," waiters appeared to wear "velvet costumes," hundreds of canaries sang in cages, and bands played. Meanwhile, he experienced what he called "double consciousness." When he reached for a glass of water, for example, it seemed as if someone else's hand was grasping the glass. And when it was time to leave, he told his friends that he would need "servants with a Sedan chair" to help him do so. The room appeared to be miles long, and he could not reach the exit "without frequent spells of resting."[7]

In the 1860s, hashish became popular with America's white middle class, many of whom tried it either for a lark or as a medical experiment. They tended to regard their use as amusing, perhaps because the practice was not widespread domestically but also because they regarded themselves as responsible users. Many Americans learned about hashish use and its effects by reading Alexandre Dumas's *The Count of Monte Cristo* or the firsthand accounts of American users Bayard Taylor and Fitz Hugh Ludlow.

Many, however, associated the widespread pleasure-seeking use of the drug with non-Western societies, where the people appeared to be unproductive. Some saw *Cannabis sativa,* known as hemp, and *Cannabis indica,* which had more narcotic resin, as epitomizing a difference between an industrious, productive West and a lethargic, dreamy East. There was also a persistent belief that hashish use made some non-Western people violent. Most of these stories were inaccurate accounts from partisan observers; others were not typical but were perhaps more interesting than actual representative accounts of sedate use. At this point, American enthrallment with hashish was ephemeral. Opposition to its use would increase early in the twentieth century, when it was associated with Mexican immigrants and, not coincidentally, renamed "marijuana," to reinforce the perception of it as a foreign substance.

\* \* \*

Cannabis use originated in Central Asia many millennia ago, and merchants and others spread it throughout the world, to be used both as hemp and as a psychoactive drug. There is evidence of its use in Siberia from around 3000 B.C.E. Around 2000 B.C.E., traders along the Silk Road carried it to parts of East Asia and what would become the Middle East and Eastern Europe. It also reached India around that time, where there would be "a long and continuing tradition of psychoactive cannabis cultivation," as geographer Barney Warf has noted. Teutonic tribes brought it to Germany during the Early Iron Age, and it reached Great Britain in the fifth century C.E. By the mid-twelfth century, cannabis had reached Egypt, from India and Persia. By the thirteenth century, Arab merchants had introduced it in Eastern Africa. Archaeological evidence suggests that Africans in Lalibela—what is now northern Ethiopia—were smoking cannabis from water pipes by the fourteenth century. Arab traders spread cannabis down Africa's east coast, after which it spread to central and southern Africa. Cannabis reached Latin America in the sixteenth century.[8] In the seventeenth century, King James made hemp cultivation mandatory in the Jamestown colony in North America.[9]

Nineteenth-century Europeans and Americans would perceive two distinct types of cannabis plant, but the reality is more complex. Carolus Linnaeus had considered there to be only one species of hemp. In 1753, he classified it as *Cannabis sativa.* Thirty years later, French naturalist Jean-Baptiste Lamarck concluded that there were two species, and he added *Cannabis indica,* which referred to cannabis that affected users in a psychoactive way.[10] The distinction was based on the observation that the Indian version "contained far more resin than the European plant," as Dr. Ernest Abel has observed.[11] Even so, botanical taxonomists remain divided regarding the number of cannabis species. While there are "biochemically different strains" of cannabis, as Dr. Ethan Russo explains, all types of it can interbreed. He has concluded that cannabis's effects are too complex for the plant to be neatly divided into a couple of categories, and he considers the assertion that there is a clear distinction between *Cannabis sativa* and *Cannabis indica* to be "nonsense."[12] This chapter, however, will refer to *Cannabis sativa* and *Cannabis indica,* because these classifications were used by mid-nineteenth-century Americans and are central to their perceptions.

As Lamarck observed, some supplies of cannabis produce more extensive psychoactive effects than do others, and terms that relate to the level of intensity are sometimes confused. The plant's effects are determined by where it is grown and how it is consumed. In terms of producing a psychoactive effect, its most important cannabinoid is tetrahydrocannabinol, better known as THC, which was first isolated in 1964. Cannabis that is cultivated in locations with milder temperatures has less THC than does cannabis grown in hotter locales. Meanwhile, the flowering tops of the cannabis plant have more THC than do other parts of the plant. "Hemp" is another name for *Cannabis sativa,* and it has less than 1 percent THC. Hemp fibers are used to make rope, sails, and canvas; the word "canvas" comes from the Greek word "kannabis." "Hashish" refers to the sticky resin from the flowering tops of the plants. It has a much higher percentage of THC than does hemp, reaching somewhere between 4 and 20 percent, though nineteenth-century varieties did not reach the latter figure.[13] "Cannabis" can refer both to the cannabis plant and to the parts that produce psychoactive effects.

The variety known as *Cannabis indica* was consumed in a variety of ways in the nineteenth century, and some terms related to these forms have been defined varyingly over the years. Mordecai Cooke listed some of the options in *The Seven Sisters of Sleep* (1860). Hashish could be "boiled in fat, butter, or oil, with a little water," and then made into a pastry; powdered or formed "into pastiles," for smoking; or made into an "electuary"—a medicine combined with something sweet, such as honey or spices.[14] The terms, however, were not used consistently. "Hashish" was also used to refer to the process where the leaves and flowers were boiled and then combined with butter and spices.[15] And as a writer for *Beadle's Monthly* observed in 1866, "hasheesh or hashish, appears to be the general name given to all the preparations derived from the hemp-plant."[16] Bhang, which is also derived from cannabis, was the least potent of the substances derived from cannabis.[17] It is made of the dried "leaves, seeds, and stems" according to David Courtwright, and it is "often mixed with sugar, black pepper, and water or milk."[18] Again, use of the term varied. European travelers in India used the word "bhang" to refer to "all the forms of cannabis they came across," according to writer Martin Booth. The practice of smoking hashish began in the early seventeenth century, when Europeans and people in the Ottoman Empire were caught up in the tobacco-smoking craze.[19]

Those who smoke hashish experience its effects more quickly than those who eat it, and they are better able to control their intake, but those who eat it experience a longer psychoactive effect than do smokers, although the reactions, including side effects, could be stronger. Hashish that is eaten is as much as three times stronger than that which is smoked, because burning it causes at least half of the active ingredient, perhaps as much as 90 percent, to disintegrate or oxidize.[20]

Some Westerners presented hashish as the Eastern alternative to alcohol, an analogy that made the substance seem familiar and that did not disparage its consumers. In 1804, for example, Scottish physician Thomas Trotter—in a book that was reprinted in Philadelphia—asserted that "bang" affected users in much the same way that alcohol did. Those effects were not wholly positive; "habitual use" of either one, he wrote, caused "almost the same diseases." He suggested, however, that those who consumed bhang did so for the same reasons that Westerners drank. Muslims drank bhang "to rouse their spirits," he explained, and favored it only because their religion forbade the consumption of wine.[21]

Other writers also characterized hashish as a strong Eastern intoxicant but acknowledged its benefits. In 1832, an article in North Carolina's *Roanoke Advocate* characterized bhang as a "powerful and peculiar inebriant" that was used "throughout Egypt, Persia, Arabia, and Hindoostan." Although the writer stated that hashish "excites sensual propensities," none of its other effects would have raised great concerns. "It produces tranquility of mind, and a singular kind of exhilaration," he explained, "during which the person laughs involuntarily, speaks incoherently and sings and dances without staggering or giddiness." It also "stimulates courage," he added. And while the person was asleep, "it promotes agreable [*sic*] dreams."[22] In 1855, several publications reported that *Cannabis indica* provided users with "a delightful exhilaration of mind" and that it was "much celebrated by travelers in Persia."[23]

Hashish also had apparent medical value, though its effects could be unpredictable. In 1839, William Brooke O'Shaughnessy, an Irish physician working at the Medical College of Calcutta, reported that it had value as an anti-convulsive treatment. He detailed his use of it to cure patients with rabies infections, tetanus, and delirium tremens.[24] Although hashish was, for some patients, a better sleeping aid than opium, it often had little or no effect. In the 1850s, German physician Bernhard Fronmüller gave *Cannabis indica* to about a thousand patients. He concluded that its effects were inconsistent. One limitation to cannabis's medical usefulness was the fact that chemists could not isolate its psychoactive component, as had been done with opium. As a consequence, its effects varied widely.[25] In 1891, Dr. E. H. Squibb, a founder of the pharmaceutical company now known as Bristol-Myers Squibb, stated that "*Cannabis Indica* has fallen considerably in the estimation of the profession, both in the old and this country," due to "its variability and often noticeable uncertainty of action."[26]

\* \* \*

Some nineteenth-century Americans linked the apparent lack of productivity in some Eastern nations to the widespread use of psychoactive substances, such as *Cannabis indica,* and the acceptance of their use. In 1859, for example, David O. Allen, an American missionary in India, suggested that the subcontinent's natives had great potential but had attained a "compromise between a career of intellectual advancement and a lapse into imbecility." They had not achieved more, he maintained, due to "climatic enervation," which owed in part to the availability of cannabis. "Here in India is the paradise of your genuine Hasheesh-eaters!" he wrote. He pointed out that Indians who wanted to partake would not face social censure; they did not have to "steal like a culprit into the druggist's" to buy it. Instead, "the sky rains it upon you; the air surfs it against you; the flowers breathe it up to you."[27] Others agreed. In 1858, a writer for *Scientific American* attributed the "drowsy appearance and indolent character of Eastern nations" to their climate, their natural bounty, and the people's "use of powerful narcotic drugs," whether opium consumption in China or "hasheesh" among the Ottomans and in "the north of Africa, the southwest of Asia and a portion of Europe."[28] And in 1882, a writer for *Frank Leslie's Popular Monthly* asserted that hashish was consumed in much of Asia "in immense proportions by people of all classes." These people apparently thought only of their own gratification. "Free from care or thought," he wrote, "these fiery sons of the South give themselves up to the enjoyment of their dream, forgetting everything save the pleasure of the moment."[29]

Perceptions of cannabis's main two subspecies reinforced a notion, popular in the West, that contrasted Western industry and ambition with Eastern lassitude and indulgence: that people in the West used cannabis for constructive purposes while it made users in the East unproductive. Consequently, so the theory went, the plants shaped the lives of their users in strikingly different ways. Westerners used hemp to make rope. It helped them to build ships and travel the world for exploration, trade, and conquest.[30] *Cannabis indica,* meanwhile, made users less productive, by inspiring hours of reverie.[31]

Hemp had been cultivated in America since the early colonial period. Settlers of the Jamestown colony grew hemp to make clothing and rope. Following England's defeat of the Spanish Armada, the nation's power rested largely on its maritime supremacy. Consequently, the government had a great need for hemp, used in ropes for ships. Beginning in 1619, the cultivation of hemp was mandatory in Jamestown. In the 1630s, however, England was getting almost all its hemp from Russian merchants. The king encouraged production in America to avoid depending on a foreign provider. Demand for hemp was also strong in New England because of the region's shipbuilding industry.[32] The profits could be significant. By 1750, the value of hemp produced in Virginia was about 22 percent of the value of the colony's tobacco production.[33]

Some have suggested that the enslaved population in colonial America or the early United States would have used cannabis as an intoxicant, since it was used for that purpose in parts of Africa, but there is little evidence to support this theory. Eugene Genovese, in his landmark study of American slavery, found no evidence that enslaved people "acted on their knowledge of the narcotic effects of hemp."[34] Many may not have had such knowledge. Thomas Jefferson's writings, for example, suggest that the people he enslaved were not indulging in cannabis. In 1815, he decided to give them clothes made of cotton rather than hemp, because hemp cultivation was "so slow, so laborious, and so much complained of by our laborers," as he explained in a letter.[35] It is difficult to conclude that the bondspeople were enjoying the plant's narcotic effects if they were criticizing the requirement that they cultivate it. Elsewhere, enslaved people's use of cannabis was evident. David Courtwright points out that enslaved Angolans used cannabis in Brazil, where it was regarded as "the opium of the poor." No parallel in colonial North America, however, has been found. Courtwright explains this by noting that Africans in the British colonies came from parts of west Africa where cannabis use was not widespread and that European colonists, content with alcohol and tobacco, sought nothing else.[36] Geographer Chris Duvall, who has studied cannabis use in Africa and in a global context, has concluded that "there is no evidence or suggestion that slaves introduced cannabis to the United States."[37]

\* \* \*

False assertions regarding a Muslim sect called the Nizārī Ismaili in the Middle Ages resulted in a widely held belief that hashish use caused members of the group to commit assassinations. In the early nineteenth century, Antoine-Isaac Silvestre de Sacy, a French professor of Arabic and Persian and a well-respected scholar of Asia, propagated the untrue notion that hashish use caused Ismailis to become both murderers and unreservedly obedient followers. In 1809, he stated that Arabic manuscripts referred to the Ismailis as "*al-Hashishiyya*"— "hashish-eaters," essentially—and that this was because of their use of the drug. He asserted that hashish use caused "violent delirium," that some Ismailis were "raised to kill," and that, due to hashish use, they demonstrated "absolute resignation to the will of their leader." He also concluded that the word "assassin" derived from the Arabic word for "hashish."[38]

There is no credible evidence that the Ismailis were assassins or hashish users, and scholars have traced the claims back to disparaging accounts that their adversaries promoted.[39] The Nizārī Ismaili, Shia Muslims, were living in Persia and Syria. In 1090, they had taken a mountain fortress in northern Persia. They worked to create a Nizārī Ismaili state and, in the twelfth century, they acquired castles in Syria's mountains to establish a base there. The Ismailis, however, faced opposition from Sunni Muslims and from crusaders, and the Nizārī Ismaili state would collapse in 1256 due to Mongol attacks.[40] Travelers and historians misrepresented the group's actions and motivations, omitting important context. While Ismailis sometimes resorted to violence, so did non-Ismailis. Some Ismailis were willing to sacrifice their lives for their cause, but that pertained to fighting in battles, not to the use of assassination tactics. The myth, meanwhile, developed because people who opposed them spread the most pronounced stories about them. Muslims outside the Ismaili sect tended to regard them as heretics and to treat them as outcasts, and crusaders spread stories about them in Europe.[41] Because they endured persecution, Ismailis were reluctant to push back against negative accounts. Farhad Daftary, a scholar of Ismaili studies, explains that the "Assassin legends" took hold in Europe because most Europeans knew little about Islam and were fascinated by the crusaders' "romantic and fascinating" tales.[42] In his fourteenth-century travel account, Marco Polo stated that the Ismailis' leader gave his followers an "intoxicating potion" to turn them into obedient assassins. His account was based on "black legends," according to historian David Guba Jr., but the work further popularized the story in Europe.[43]

Meanwhile, Sacy misunderstood the era's texts. He relied on the writings of Sunni Muslims who opposed the Ismailis, and rather than focusing on nuances in their writings, he read them literally. When they referred to the Ismailis as "hashīshīs," they used the term figuratively, to deride them as "'low-class rabble' and 'irreligious social outcasts'" rather than actually stating that they used hashish, according to Guba.[44] Philosopher Mirt Komel adds that "Assassins" was "a scornful term employed by the Sunni majority of Muslims in order to disqualify the Nizaris."[45] There are no direct references to hashish use by the Ismailis in contemporary sources. The association of Ismaili assassins and hashish, however, endured. Guba attributes the myth's longevity to a popular perception in the West that drugs were "stereotypical markers of Oriental barbarism."[46]

These inaccurate reports tarnished nineteenth-century Americans' perceptions of the Ismailis and of hashish. In the 1820s, several American journals published a review of Austrian Orientalist Joseph Von Hammer's *The History of the Assassins: Derived from Oriental Sources*. The review stated that the word "Assassin" derived from "*Hashish*, which signifies the bang or opiate of hemp-leaves," and that murder was "the use they made of the opiate prepared from that plant."[47] In *The Lands of the Saracen* (1855), Pennsylvanian Bayard

Taylor stated that hashish had been used in "the East for many centuries" and that "Saracen warriors" used it during the Crusades "to stimulate them to the work of slaughter."[48] And in 1862, a writer for the Quaker periodical *The Friend* stated that the "intoxicating influences of this drug" gave its users "contempt of death."[49]

\* \* \*

Western use of hashish as an intoxicant increased in the early nineteenth century, when Napoleon Bonaparte's soldiers brought the practice from Egypt to France. In 1798, Napoleon led forty thousand French soldiers on an expedition to Egypt to gain control of the country's commodities and put him in a position to attack British India. When Great Britain destroyed France's fleet and imposed a blockade, the soldiers were marooned in Egypt for a year, and they had limited access to alcohol.[50] Many of them adopted the native practice of consuming cannabis in various ways, including smoking it, inhaling its vapors, and eating and drinking products made from hashish. Napoleon prohibited use of the drug in 1800, because it was undermining the soldiers' effectiveness. When they returned to France in 1801, however, they brought the practice with them.[51]

Some Western hashish users were Romantics, celebrating emotion and nature, in a movement that would criticize the Industrial Revolution and other aspects of modernity.[52] In the 1840s, some French writers who ate hashish formed a social club, Le Club des Haschischins. They believed that the drug, which they ate as a kind of jam, either from a spoon or on bread, could help them to reach "the subconscious source of emotion which they were convinced was only viewed in dreams," according to Martin Booth. Members of the club included novelist Alexandre Dumas and poet Théophile Gautier, who coined the term "Art for Art's sake."[53]

Many Americans could have first learned about hashish's intoxicating properties on reading Dumas's popular *The Count of Monte-Cristo* (1844). Five years after its publication, a reviewer for *Godey's Magazine and Lady's Book* insisted that "everybody read 'Monte-Cristo.'"[54] In the novel, a seaman named Edmond Dantès is wrongly imprisoned. He escapes, grows wealthy, and seeks revenge on his accusers. Dantès develops a taste for hashish and introduces it to others. At one point, a man named Franz dines with Dantès, who presents him with an unfamiliar "greenish paste." It is "the purest and most unadulterated hashish of Alexandria," Dantès says, and he describes its potential:

> Are you a man of positive facts, and is gold your god? taste this, and the
> mines of Peru, Guzerat, and Golconda are opened to you. Are you a man
> of imagination—a poet? taste this, and the boundaries of possibility

disappear; the fields of infinite space open to you, you advance free in heart, free in mind, into the boundless realms of reverie. Are you ambitious, and do you seek after the greatness of the earth? taste this, and in an hour you will be a king, not a king of a petty kingdom hidden in some corner of Europe, like France, Spain, or England, but king of the world, king of the universe, king of creation.

Dantès states that "those Orientals; they are the only men who know how to live." Upon trying it, Franz is as impressed as Dantès. He realizes that "all the bodily fatigue of the day . . . disappeared." As the chapter closes, Franz sinks "back, breathless and exhausted, under the painful yet delicious enthrallment produced by the hashish."[55]

Soon after the publication of Dumas's work, a Vermont newspaper published Gautier's account of the effects of hashish use. His narrative could have heightened American interest in the drug. To Gautier, while he was under the influence it appeared "that his body was dissolved. . . . He clearly saw in his chest that hashish which he had swallowed." Also, it seemed to him that his "eye-lashes were lengthened out indefinitely, and rolled like threads of gold around ivory balls." One of his experiences lasted fifteen minutes, but he thought that it had lasted for three hundred years.[56]

* * *

Although Americans could read about hashish use in foreign lands, their own accounts of pleasure-seeking drug use added to the public discussion in the 1850s. Poet and travel author Bayard Taylor decided to "make a trial of the celebrated *Hasheesh*" while visiting Damascus in the mid-1850s. He provided the earliest firsthand account of the drug's effects by an American. His narrative, first published in *Putnam's Monthly Magazine* in 1854, was reprinted the following year in his book *The Lands of the Saracen*. Taylor and his friends withdrew to his hotel room so as to conduct their experiment unobserved. His friends reclined on a sofa, and Taylor sat in the center of the room. The first dose produced no effect, so Taylor encouraged them to take more. After eating it in the form of a paste, he felt a "nervous thrill," and he had a burning sensation in his stomach. Then, his "sense of limitation" disappeared, and he perceived himself as existing "throughout a vast extent of space," as if he were omnipresent. He felt, however, that the "demon" drug "had entire possession of me."[57]

Taylor explained that he had taken hashish to satisfy his curiosity about it and that, although he hallucinated, he was not completely under the drug's influence. In one dream, Taylor envisioned moving through the desert aboard a ship "made of mother-of-pearl, and studded with jewels" over sand that was "grains of gold."

Yet he insisted that he retained a critical distance from the scene. "When I was most completely under" the influence of hashish, he insisted, "I knew myself to be seated in the tower of Antonio's hotel in Damascus, knew that I had taken hasheesh, and that the strange, gorgeous and ludicrous fancies which possessed me, were the effect of it." While he enjoyed the visions, "in some other chamber of my brain, Reason sat coolly watching."[58]

Taylor had, however, inadvertently consumed a dose of hashish large enough "for six men," and his initial visions gave way to painful perceptions, despair, and a long sleep. As the evening progressed, he imagined that he was "a mass of transparent jelly" that a confectioner was pouring into a mold, and he "writhed . . . to force my loose substance into the mould." He conceded that his contortions would appear "ludicrous" to observers but insisted that, to him, "they were painful and disagreeable." He later felt as if his blood were rushing through his system. It seemed as if his throat were "filled to the brim with blood," as if blood were pouring from his ears, and as if his heart were pounding so intensely that his ribs might break. In that state, he lay on his bed. After thirty hours of sleep, he awakened "prostrate and unstrung" and found it "painful" to engage in conversation. He suspected that those attending him understood his condition, as they gave him "a glass of very acid sherbet" that produced "instant relief."[59]

Taylor's travel accounts were popular with American audiences, and his enthusiasm for immersing himself in foreign cultures was key to his appeal.[60] In the mid-1850s, audiences thronged to see him on the lecture circuit, and many Americans bought copies of *A Morning in Damascus*, a portrait of Taylor that was mass-produced.[61] In the painting, Taylor is dressed as a member of the Ottoman elite, and he holds the mouthpiece of a hookah pipe. Historian James Todd Uhlman has suggested that Taylor presented a new version of masculinity that included "boundless raw energy fueled by primal passions," accompanied by a degree of "moral latitude" that earlier generations would have denounced, and that this combination was central to his appeal. This suggests that American audiences found hashish use to be enticing and daring. With that said, Uhlman also suggests that Eastern-inspired images of Taylor, which merchants used to sell cigars and steam baths, were also popular because audiences knew that he was white.[62]

In 1857, Fitz Hugh Ludlow would add to the literature on hashish use by producing "the first U.S. autobiography of drugged experience," as literary scholar Susan Zieger has noted. Ludlow based his work on experiences that began while he was a student at Union College.[63] He first used cannabis while in the shop of a friend who worked as a druggist. During his visits to "Anderson the apothecary," Ludlow had also tried opiates, chloroform, and ether out of curiosity. He believed his experiments were safe, as he assumed that only pleasure seekers risked developing drug habits. "Research and not indulgence was my

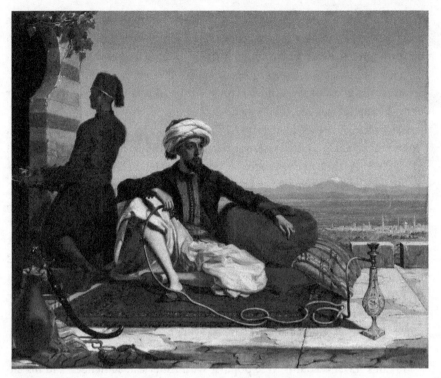

*Figure 3.1.* Thomas Hicks, "Morning in Damascus," 1855. Hicks depicts travel writer
Bayard Taylor in the garb of a member of the Ottoman elite. Taylor was one of the first
Americans to write about the effects of hashish, which he used while visiting the ancient
city. Many Americans likely approved of his use of the drug since he contributed to the
general knowledge regarding it. Courtesy of the National Portrait Gallery, Smithsonian
Institution.

object," he explained, adding that his ventures preceding his use of hashish had
never caused him to become "the victim of any habit." When he spied a vial
marked "Cannabis indica," Anderson warned him that it was a "deadly poison."[64]
Ludlow read up on the drug and learned that hashish's pleasant effects had
made it popular in Asia. In the volume he consulted, *The Chemistry of Common
Life* (1853), Scottish chemist James Johnston wrote that its physical effects
were "generally very agreeable," adding that people in India regarded it as "the
increaser of pleasure, the exciter of desire, the cementer of friendship, [and] the
laughter-mover."[65]

Ludlow tried hashish and found that it distorted his perceptions. On one
occasion, he asked a friend to let him know if he were talking "loudly or im-
moderately" and later criticized the friend for not intervening when Ludlow was
"shouting and singing." His friend replied that Ludlow "had not uttered an au-
dible word"—an assertion that the author, at the time, could not believe.[66] On

another occasion, Ludlow chatted with people who sat three feet away from him. As the hashish took effect, he discerned "great spaces surrounding me on every side."[67]

Fittingly, some of the Americans' hallucinations evoked impressions of the nation at the time. A friend of Taylor's thought he was a locomotive, and "for the space of two or three hours," he paced "to and fro with a measured stride." He correlated his speech with his motions, "turning his hands at his sides, as if they were the cranks of imaginary wheels." On one occasion, Taylor believed he saw the Great Pyramid of Giza first from its base, then from its peak, at which point he discovered that it was made of "huge square plugs of Cavendish tobacco!" The "ludicrous" scene, he recalled, put him in "an agony of laughter."[68] Ludlow once envisioned himself "in a large apartment, which resembled the Senate-chamber at Washington." On the walls were "grotesque frescoes" of animals and monsters that kept changing, "like the figures of the kaleidoscope." In Congress sat witches made of purple yarn, who were "knitting old women like themselves!" And on another occasion, a dose of hashish led Ludlow to believe he was in a Greek garden where a "horde of Indian braves burst whooping, in their war-dance; and writhing in savage postures, with brandished club and tomahawk." They called for Ludlow. He lay down to hide from them, and the scene changed.[69]

Ludlow believed that the drug's effects depended on the user's race, because he believed that some cultures were more open to enjoying hashish than were others. According to Ludlow, hashish shaped "the Eastern mind" and imparted an Asian quality on all users—it "makes both the Syrian and the Saxon Oriental," he wrote.[70] He believed, however, that only those with a rich imagination could truly enjoy it. As a consequence, it was better suited to "Eastern races" than to "the Anglo-Saxon race," he asserted, because Asians had a "warmth and activity of imagination" that was rare among the English. To him, this explained why many Europeans and Americans who used hashish experienced "insensibility" and then a "general and painful disturbance of the nervous system" rather than enjoying a "hasheesh fantasia." In 1858, he insisted that Americans were "in very little danger of becoming a nation of hasheesh-eaters."[71]

In *The Hasheesh Eater*, Ludlow celebrated nature's beauty and the potential of the human mind, following the Romantics, while criticizing the pursuit of profit. "In our minds," he wrote, "we possess a far greater wealth than we have ever conceived." He believed that this should make material things less important, and that people should "live well for the sake of a spirit which possesses fathomless capacities for happiness [and] knowledge." He criticized those who exploited nature to make money. Under their control, "the whole face of nature is staked off into building-lots or manufactory-sites," he lamented. The ideal man, meanwhile, prized "the roses leading from the door-step to the gate, the lake below him, [and] the mountains on the other side." For the ideal man, it was a sad day when a mill was built. Soon thereafter, "the waters began to run foul with dye and sawdust, gigantic band-wheels spun and hummed where birds had sung." The man could be forced to move to avoid what he saw as a desecration of nature; but others would think he should be glad to have modern conveniences, such as "bathing apparatus, with warm, cold, and shower cocks" and "shopping conveniences for your wife."[72]

Ludlow ultimately ended his use due to hashish's negative effects, but the world without the drug seemed mundane, and he defended his preference for hashish-enhanced visions. He quit because "shadows of as immeasurable pain" were eclipsing his hashish-inspired euphoria. He believed that, were he to continue, he would one day experience nothing but misery. Yet he could not forget the images that hashish had provided him, and he missed them. "I refused to worship earth," he stated, "when I had seen heaven." While sober, he felt as if he were in an "earthly prison." The world was "utterly distasteful, like a heavy tragedy seen for the fortieth time." To try to recapture a bit of his "hasheesh-sky," he blew soap bubbles. And because reality seemed so drab in comparison, he believed he should not be criticized for his drug use. From his perspective, he had aspired to something greater than the natural world offered. For some men, he concluded, the world, as it was, was not enough. He believed that such men should be supported rather than being told that their wish was "unnatural and sinful." Instead, they should be told, "Your wish is approved by Heaven, for from Heaven came the constitution which made you capable of such a wish." Ludlow believed that all people wanted to alter their consciousness and to experience the visions and understanding that were otherwise unavailable. He thought that humanity's "tendency toward stimulants" existed due to "the soul's capacity for ... deeper insight, [and] grander views of Beauty, Truth, and Good than she now gains through the chinks of her cell."[73]

The experience of American hashish users at the time was lonely, because they were few in number and there was little public discussion regarding how to end problematic usage. Ludlow's use had become habitual, and he felt isolated. "Within a circle of one hundred miles' radius," he explained, "there was not a living soul who knew or could warn me of my danger." For this reason, he was happy to discover the writings of Bayard Taylor. One fall morning in 1856, Ludlow took his "ordinary dose" of hashish and bought the latest issue of *Putnam's Monthly Magazine.* In it, he found Taylor's article "The Hasheesh Eater." Ludlow's "utter isolation" had ended. "I had supposed myself the only hasheesh-eater upon this side of the ocean," he admitted, and he initially suspected that it was an article about himself, penned by an acquaintance. He was amazed to read that the author *"had forever abandoned hasheesh."* Ludlow wrote to Taylor, asking for advice regarding "the best means of softening the pathway of my escape." Taylor obliged.[74] He recommended that Ludlow try writing when he craved hashish.[75] According to Ludlow, Taylor's article was his "prime motor to escape."[76]

Some people recommended a ban on works such as Ludlow's to reduce the number of hashish experimenters. Although memoirs such as *The Hasheesh Eater* contributed to knowledge, one reviewer believed that the damage they did outweighed their value. They had been produced "under the guise of scientific ardour," the reviewer acknowledged, but they inspired readers to engage in risky experiments. For this reason, he believed that such works should be "forbidden lore."[77] Regarding *The Lands of the Saracen*, a writer for a Unitarian journal chided Bayard Taylor for writing about drug use in a way that could inspire imitators. "The chapter upon Hasheesh had better not have been written," he wrote. He placed Taylor's behavior on a par with that of a man who, to satisfy his curiosity, "thrusts his head into the lion's mouth." And Taylor had made "the sensuality so dreamful that others may imitate it to their cost."[78]

\* \* \*

American women occasionally published accounts of their hashish use, and they tended to have concerns about potential negative effects. In 1868, New Yorker Adele Fielde enjoyed smoking hashish while working as a missionary in Bangkok. She had endured loneliness and clashed with the head of the mission, who objected to single women serving as missionaries. She observed the Siamese using hashish and decided to try it—secretly, to avoid criticism from colleagues.[79] Smoking "six thimblefuls" of the drug led her to feel "luxuriously quiet." She then became "conscious of dual being." While she remained aware of her circumstances, she believed she was in a hall where the walls and furniture were "encrusted with tinted gems." She felt "infinitely joyous" and thought she was in heaven. On another occasion, her hashish use gave her so many ideas that, if she had written them down, she would have "filled the world with new books." (When she awakened, however, she could no longer remember the ideas.) She only used hashish three times, because she had seen it lead to the "gradual destruction of mind and body" of habitual users in Siam.[80] Twenty years later, she published her account in a medical journal. Few readers realized that the author was a woman. She used the name "A. M. Fielde," and she did not mention the impetus for her use. When the staff of the journal *Science* summarized the article, they erroneously referred to her as a man, and other journals then republished the flawed article from *Science*.[81] Most accounts of drug use were penned by men, and this error appeared to exaggerate the already lopsided ratio.

Another woman who published an account of her hashish use considered the experience to have been an ordeal. In 1883, writer Mary C. Hungerford took an excessive dose to avert a headache and fainted, and her family summoned the doctor. As she later described, she experienced distortions of time while under the influence. When the doctor asked if she had taken a large dose of hashish, she nodded and believed that her nodding continued "for seven or eight hours." She perceived herself as dying and sinking "through the bed, the floors, the cellar, the earth," like "a fragment of glass dropping through the ocean." She feared that she would not be accepted into heaven. At one point, she heard a "great and terrible voice" say, "You denied the power of Christ in time" and that she would remain "in lonely agony forever." Forces seemed to hold her down, and she fought back as if she were in a "struggle against death." Then, she awakened.[82]

In the early 1860s, Frances Eells had a negative experience with the drug, which she admitted in a letter to her boyfriend. When eighteen-year-old New Yorker Ned Homans went off to fight in the Civil War in 1862, he sent Frances his "weed divine." A month earlier, he admitted, "I would have thought of renouncing my parents as soon as the use of it, but to that & to 'hash' a long farewell."[83] Eells tried it and had a bad experience, and Homans teased her when he heard about it. "So you have been experimenting with the weed!" he wrote. "'Tis a pity it did not hurt you twice as much. 'Twould have been but a deserving reward for your curiosity." He encouraged her not to use it again.[84] In January 1864, he was impatient for their wedding, which was three months away, and wrote that he would like to "take a big dose of hasheesh that I might dream of you & not wake up til April."[85]

In some fiction of the era, hashish facilitated romance among the well-to-do, which reinforces the notion that many in the upper class regarded its use as daring and intriguing. In Louisa May Alcott's story "Perilous Play," which appeared in *Frank Leslie's Pleasant Hours* in 1869, a group of wealthy, young white adults are bored one afternoon and eat "hashish bonbons" to entertain themselves. A doctor in the group tells them that those who take it will "be amused in a new, delicious, and wonderful manner." He promises to give them safe amounts of it and adds that physicians prescribe it because it is "very efficacious in nervous disorders." In the story, the drug brings about a happy ending. Two members of the group, Mark and Rose, are romantically interested in each other, but she is aloof, and he lacks the courage to tell her how he feels. After taking the hashish, however, Mark summons the courage to confess his love to Rose, and she becomes "soft and lovable." The story ends with Mark's comment, "Heaven bless hashish, if its dreams end like this!"[86]

Hashish was popular among elite women, who appeared to have little regard for society's opinion of them. According to writer Elizabeth Fries Ellet, some nouveau riche women in the 1860s used hashish. Upon moving to New York, they "create[d] a sensation" with their wealth and outrageous behavior. One, for example, was "building a splendid house near Central Park" and would "get herself up with hasheesh for dissipation." "Dissipation," of course, meant that she used it for amusement rather than for medical purposes. Ellet contrasted such behavior with the "old-fashioned articles" of "morality and good taste," which the city's "pure-blooded, pure-mannered aristocracy" still cared about.[87]

It appeared, however, that beyond the possible negative effects of the drug itself, there were few negative repercussions for well-to-do users of hashish. When *The Hasheesh-Eater* was published, for example, John Hay was a student at Brown University. According to one of his classmates, Hay wanted to try hashish to "see if it was such a marvelous stimulant to imagination" as Ludlow had asserted. Other students did likewise. The experiment ended late that night with a professor being awakened "to minister to the very sick boys who had participated in the adventure," according to biographer Tyler Dennett. Later secretary to President Lincoln and Theodore Roosevelt's secretary of state, Hay would refer to Brown as a place "where I used to eat Hasheesh and dream dreams."[88] In 1884, the *Baltimore Sun* ran a story about a "well-dressed young man" named Binns who had tried hashish, become disoriented, and gone to a hospital. He was unsure of "the locality of his face," the reporter explained, and believed it was "situated at least two feet from where it really was." Binns also "was dubious whether he had any legs or was simply walking on his chin," and he feared that someone might steal one of his limbs. Although the reporter characterized Binns's plea for help as "pitiful," he did not criticize the man's lack of productivity or sobriety or suggest that his usage had an ominous portent for the nation. He noted that Binns had not taken hashish due to medical need but because he had had "a strange desire for several days" to try it. And the reporter included a happy ending: "After medical treatment Binns felt better."[89] The *Sun*'s editor was not the only one who saw the story as amusing rather than concerning; the next day, the piece was reprinted in the *New York Times*.[90]

\* \* \*

In the late 1860s, drug habituation in America was only beginning to enter public discussion. Before the discourse ensued, Americans learned about dependency—including hashish use—from travelers' accounts of pleasure-seeking drug use in foreign lands, including parts of Africa, the Middle East, and Asia, where the practice was more visible and widespread, in part due to proscriptions on alcohol. From these accounts some Americans learned, for example, that hashish use was followed by lethargy. Some concluded that widespread use could devastate a society. In 1892, a writer for the *St. Louis Post-Dispatch* would state that hashish use had "played havoc with many of the Oriental peoples and has been a curse in Egypt." He expressed relief that

America had few hashish habitués. Otherwise, he explained, "we should have a race of dreamers and visionaries in place of a sturdy ambitious people."[91] Because reports from abroad—some of them accurate, others less so—shaped understanding of drug habituation, it is important to explore those travelers' accounts and what they reveal.

# PART II

# LEARNING FROM A WORLD OF USERS

# The Global Context, 1774–1862

Until the late 1860s, few publications aimed at a popular audience addressed habitual drug use in America, and those that did tended to focus on specific examples—a laudanum habitué, or a hashish habitué—rather than describing a widespread problem. As a result, the earliest public information in America about pleasure-seeking drug use and drug habituation came from Europeans' accounts of their travels in parts of Africa, Asia, and the Middle East. These early chroniclers did not necessarily condemn the drug use that they observed. Some acknowledged that it provided respite from cares and could enhance users' productivity by, for example, forestalling the need for sleep. Others described drug tolerance and other consequences of drug dependence.

By the nineteenth century, however, many Americans would associate certain populations with their drug of choice, and there was a growing tendency, when envisioning this geography of intoxicant use, to link a society's preferred psychoactive substance with its level of productivity. Dr. David Cheever, for example, regarded populations along a spectrum from "civilization" to "barbarism," and he believed that their place on that scale determined which psychoactive substances they would crave. He asserted that "perhaps, the majority of the most civilized people" were content with the "gentler stimulants," while those with "barbarous habits of thought, from tropical and sensuous imaginations," pursued "the dangerous use of the true narcotics." He added that they did this "almost insensibly," thus reinforcing the perception that non-Western populations exerted little self-control and did not consider their decisions.[1]

He pointed out that while populations had different drugs of choice, people who partook of a certain substance could use it in different forms and have different experiences. For example, although opium was eaten "in Turkey and Persia," it was drunk "among Christian nations; and smoked in China and the islands of the Indian Archipelago." The form of opium that was smoked—called "smoking opium"—differed from the form that was eaten. Smoking opium was processed extensively, and it contained less morphine. Meanwhile, people's

*Habit Forming.* Elizabeth Kelly Gray, Oxford University Press. © Oxford University Press 2023.
DOI: 10.1093/oso/9780190073121.003.0005

beliefs and the settings where they used the drugs also shaped the effects of their use. As Cheever warned readers, while taking opium could give them a wonderful experience, it could also produce "uncomfortable, and even devilish visions."[2] Psychiatrists support the notion that a drug user's expectations and the setting in which a drug is consumed can shape a person's experience with the substance.[3]

\* \* \*

In the early 1790s, Maryland native Hast Handy studied opium's impact on users while he was pursuing his medical degree at the College of Philadelphia (now the University of Pennsylvania). In the introduction to his dissertation, he explained that he depended on "facts only" in his research and avoided "mere speculative assertions." He based much of his work on the writings of respected physicians of the time, but he also included accounts of laypersons—elite men who had observed opium use in the non-Western world and then published accounts of their journeys. He devoted a page and a half of his work, for example, to a lengthy quote from Sir Jean Chardin's *Travels in Persia, 1673–1677*. Chardin had journeyed to Persia to buy jewels for his father's business and while there observed nonmedical drug use. Handy included Chardin's observations about opium's appeal: users experienced "pleasant visions, and a kind of rapture," he reported. He also shared Chardin's comments about the drug's drawbacks. After its initial, beneficial effects, the user would be "dull and indolent . . . till the dose is repeated." And a habitual user who stopped using it would experience "depression of spirits, and a languor and debility."[4]

Whether he anticipated it or not, Chardin contributed to Western medicine by providing information on a topic—pleasure-seeking drug use and its effects—about which Westerners had known little. Portions of Chardin's work first appeared in English in the early eighteenth century, and Handy was not the only medico to find it useful.[5] Scottish physician John Leigh had quoted Chardin in his own study of opium in 1786.[6] In 1803, Dr. Franklin Scott used Chardin's work as evidence that vinegar was not an antidote to opium.[7] For *Medical Inquiries and Observations* (1805), Dr. Benjamin Rush also turned to Chardin. When Rush recommended using opium to treat ailments associated with the elderly, he added that "Chardin informs us, that this medicine is frequently used in the eastern countries to abate the pains and weaknesses of old age, by those people who are debarred the use of wine by the religion of Mahomet."[8] Information from *Travels in Persia* would also appear in the *Boston Medical and Surgical Journal* in 1837 and the *New-York Mirror* and the *New York Evangelist* in 1840.[9] By this point, Chardin's writings were more than a hundred fifty years old, but they were still valuable to the medical community and of interest to the American public.

Chardin's work was just one of many travel accounts of the East that informed Western understanding of nonmedical drug use. Publication of these accounts had begun in the sixteenth century, following the 1497 discovery of the route to the East Indies around the Cape of Good Hope. That discovery had initiated a new kind of travel and a great interest in Europe for travel literature.[10] Many of these writers described pleasure-seeking drug use. The impact of their writings on Western doctors' knowledge of the non-Western world, including drug use there, was profound. John Leigh's *Experimental Inquiry into the Properties of Opium*, for example, was a valuable source for nineteenth-century American doctors. In writing it, Leigh drew on the writings of Chardin as well as the works of several doctors who had traveled to the non-Western world: Garcia da Orta of Portugal, who in 1563 wrote on medicine in India; German physician Engelbert Kaempfer, who traveled in Persia, Siam, and Japan in the 1680s and 1690s; and Italian doctor Prospero Alpini, who spent three years in Egypt in the 1580s. Leigh also incorporated the writings of other European travelers: Charles Marie de la Condamine, a Frenchman who explored Latin America in the 1730s and 1740s; Pierre Belon, a French naturalist who visited Asia Minor and Egypt in the 1540s; Johan Albrecht de Mandelslo, a German who visited Persia and India in the seventeenth century; and Jean-Baptiste Tavernier, a Frenchman and the author of *Travels in India*, which was published in the 1670s.[11] In 1871, American physician Alonzo Calkins estimated that more than one hundred fifty "non-professional explorers . . . have made opium-eating a subject of individual examination." They included "Travellers in the Far East, Missionaries, English and American, Chinese officials, Civilians in British India and Malacca, and at Chinese ports, experts not a few of them."[12] Before reading such accounts, Westerners likely knew little about using opium or cannabis for pleasure-seeking reasons, and except for those who stumbled upon it themselves, few might have conceived of the possibility.

While many of these travelers shared their observations in a non-judgmental manner, their writings collectively produced the impression that habituation was an Eastern phenomenon—"something that existed only with the Indians, Chinese, Persians, or Turks," as sociologist Albert Hess has pointed out.[13] In contrast with the West, such usage was both widespread and visible. In his *Inquiry into the Nature and Properties of Opium* (1793), Dr. Samuel Crumpe explained that "in the eastern countries, where Opium is taken in very large quantities, its enlivening and exhilarating effects are universally known and acknowledged."[14] Although some of these accounts appeared as early as the sixteenth century, many were still being cited and quoted well into the nineteenth century, before

Americans dwelled on drug dependency—other than alcohol consumption—
as a domestic problem.

European travelers provided useful information about nonmedical drug use,
but some of their information was inaccurate even though it would become
widely accepted. It was true, as they reported, that some people used psychoactive substances for restorative purposes, a practice akin to Westerners' use
of alcohol, and that the drugs could enhance users' endurance or suppress
their appetites. They also shared important information about intractable dependency and the consequences that would become known as tolerance and
withdrawal. Some, however, perpetuated the erroneous assertion that ongoing
habituation derived from a lack of self-control. Also, some wrongly suggested
that habitual users were destined to die young, and others asserted that habitués
could be identified on sight by their weakened condition.

Although the appeal of the non-medical use of drugs, including alcohol, was
practically universal, many excerpts that appeared in American publications
criticized such use in non-Western societies, which bolstered an apparent distinction between a productive West and a lethargic East. Some impoverished
non-Western users told European observers that drugs provided a respite from
their cares, and some Europeans described an almost ubiquitous tendency to
seek solace in an intoxicant. They also pointed out that the drugs were helpful
as appetite suppressants and that they could boost users' productivity. More
visible were accounts implying that Eastern users consumed their drugs un-
thinkingly. The assumption that all populations should aspire to productivity as
defined by the West reinforced a growing notion that drug use created laggard
societies. Some writers also exaggerated the extent of problematic use in the East
and suggested that there was no endemic concern with habitual use when, in
reality, Eastern doctors and political leaders addressed it much as their Western
counterparts later would. The misrepresentations, however, provided a pretext
for colonization.

* * *

The medical and pleasure-seeking uses of opium and cannabis began in ancient
times, and patterns of use often spread along routes of trade or conquest. In
part of what is now Iraq, Mesopotamians cultivated opium around 3400 B.C.E.
Sumerians would refer to it as the "joy plant." Its use had reached Egypt by
1300 B.C.E., and the Minoans, on the island of Crete, introduced it into Greece.
Hippocrates recognized its medical value, and it was also a valued medicine in
Rome and among Arab physicians. In 330 B.C.E., Alexander the Great brought
opium to Persia and India, and Arab traders introduced it in China around the
seventh century C.E.[15] As noted in Chapter 3, cannabis use originated in Central

Asia, and around 2000 B.C.E., it spread to other parts of Asia, including India, as well as to parts of Eastern Europe and the Middle East. It became popular throughout the Islamic world. Cannabis had reached Egypt by the mid-twelfth century C.E., and Arab merchants had introduced it in eastern Africa by the thirteenth century. Its use spread thereafter down Africa's east coast and into the central and southern parts of the continent.[16] Government leaders' concerns with its use increased as the practice became more widespread. In the mid-thirteenth century, for example, the founder of Egypt's Mamluk Sultanate sought unsuccessfully to ban hashish consumption. There were, however, no similar government attempts after the fourteenth century.[17]

The spread of these drugs was hastened by their effects, but religious beliefs and transportation obstacles also affected the pace at which they were adopted. Plants that "provide human pleasure" tend to be dispersed "more quickly and freely than staple foods," as David Courtwright has noted.[18] Religious strictures also informed the patterns. While the Qur'an proscribed Muslims' use of alcohol, for example, neither opium nor hashish was explicitly banned, and use of them was consequently adopted.[19] Europeans learned about coca and its uses as early as 1505, when explorer Amerigo Vespucci wrote on the topic, but use of the coca leaf did not spread beyond its native South America until the nineteenth century.[20] Part of the reason for the delay was that when coca leaves were shipped, they often lost much of the cocaine alkaloid by the time they reached their destination. In 1860, a German doctoral candidate became the first person to isolate cocaine.[21]

\* \* \*

Some European travel writers chronicled the benefits of nonmedical drug use, such as noting that the intoxicants provided pleasure to those who used them. In his *Geographical Historie of Africa*, for example, Leo Africanus asserted that hashish delightfully disoriented those who ate it. Africanus, born Al-Hasan al-Wezaz al-Fasi, was a Spanish-born Berber who traveled through much of Africa in the early sixteenth century; the first English-language edition of his work was published in London in 1600. He had learned about the Tunisian use of hashish, which he called "Lhasis," and explained that "whosoeuer eateth but one ounce falleth a laughing, disporting, and dallying, as if he were halfe drunken; and is by the said confection maruellously prouoked unto lust."[22] Nicolas Monardes, a physician in sixteenth-century Seville, described the benefits of the cannabis-based drink called bhang. He wrote that in the "Oriental Indies," there was "an Hearbe, which is called Bague." Consisting of "hashish, cloves, mace, nutmeg, and camphor," it was used to make "a confection of excellente smell and taste." Upon eating it, Indians would "see visions that doeth give them pleasure." Monardes's books were widely reprinted and translated.[23]

European travelers often reported that non-Western men used drugs for restorative purposes—to banish their cares. In the 1570s, German doctor Leonhart Rauwolf wrote that in Aleppo, "Turks, Moors, Persians," and others took opium habitually, some in order "to take away troubles and deliriums, or at least to alleviate them."[24] By 1614, when Englishman Samuel Purchas published *Purchas His Pilgrimage*, he could report that "slaues and souldiers" used Bangue and that it "made them drunke-merrie, and so to forget their labour."[25] Purchas based much of the work on travel writings that were available in England.[26] And in 1578, Portuguese physician Cristóbal Acosta wrote that some Hindus consumed bhang "to forget their worries and sleep without thoughts."[27]

Some suggested that those who derived the most enjoyment from these drugs were members of the lower class, who had a greater wish than others to seek respite from daily life. According to Egyptian historian Al-Maqrizi, impoverished people in fifteenth-century Cairo explained that they ate hashish to help them "escape their miserable condition." More than a century later, Egyptian peasants consumed hashish for the same reason as well as "to mimic the alcohol consumption of wealthier classes," according to historian David Guba Jr.[28] In the accounts of Dr. Alexander Russell and François Baron de Tott, a Frenchman who lived in Constantinople for many years, "opium-eaters imagine themselves to be more prosperous than in reality," as noted by historian Richard Davenport-Hines. This suggested a class dimension.[29] And when German explorer Carsten Niebuhr visited Arabia in the 1760s, he specified that "the lower people are fond of raising their spirits to a state of intoxication." To reach this state, they would "smoke *Haschisch*, which is the dried leaves of a sort of hemp."[30]

Some Western writers presented recreational opium use as merely the East's alternative to smoking tobacco or drinking alcohol. Such a characterization addressed the differences among cultures while also underscoring the universal desire to have something to cope with life's challenges. Using "*Turkish* Histories," English physician John Awsiter pointed out that opium was first used "to dissipate Anxieties, Pains, and Perturbations of the Mind." In his *Essay on the Effects of Opium* (1767), Awsiter concluded that such use was "not unlike the Use of intoxicating Drinks, so much requested in *Europe*." Everyone endured significant "Labours of Mind and Body," he pointed out. As a consequence, "a temporary Relief becomes indispensably necessary." Englishmen drank, for example, and with tobacco, "the Soldier can perform his March, and the Sailor his Service, through the rudest Storm, in a Nightwatch upon Deck."[31] In 1803 Franklin Scott, a medical student at the University of Pennsylvania, stated that people in "eastern nations" were said to "use Opium as we do tobacco."[32]

Meanwhile, some writers maintained that these drugs enhanced productivity by allaying the user's thirst and hunger. In the late 1490s, Amerigo Vespucci observed coca chewing in South America and believed that Indigenous people used it to avert thirst.[33] José de Acosta, a Spanish Jesuit who traveled to South America in the 1570s, wrote that coca fortified "the Indians . . . so as to go some days without meat, but only a handful of Coca, and other like effects."[34] According to Samuel Purchas, in "*Cafraria*"—South Africa—the people cultivated "*Bangue*." They would dry its leaves, crush them to powder, "eate a handful" of it "and then drinke water, and so sustaine themselues many dayes."[35] And in *The Botanic Garden*, English physician Erasmus Darwin noted that a messenger in India could "travel above a hundred miles without rest or food, except an appropriated bit of opium for himself, and a larger one for his horse." An American edition of the work was published in 1807.[36]

As Darwin indicated, opium could also enhance the user's endurance. It prevented weariness, and this was why "the *Turks*, and other *Eastern People*, do, by the Help of *Opium*, perform prodigious *Journeys* without being tired," as Dr. John Jones explained in *The Mysteries of Opium Reveal'd* (1701).[37] In a medical study in the 1830s, German doctor F. W. Oppenheim noted that opium enabled "Tartar couriers" to conduct their work with "astonishing celerity," an observation that was reprinted in American publications.[38] In 1862 Dr. David Cheever, drawing on Oppenheim's writings, agreed that narcotics enabled users to endure "long and exhausting physical labor."[39]

Some stated that employers approved of their employees' use of these drugs, or at least accepted it, which suggested that such usage could be part of a well-functioning society. In *The Present State of the Cape of Good-Hope* (1719), astronomer Peter Kolb wrote that the Khoikhoi received "*Dacha*"—that is, cannabis—from the Dutch as "Part of their Wages."[40] Some reports suggest that the arrangement became standard. Cannabis use in southern Africa had waxed and waned before the arrival of the Dutch, and they revived its use, likely inadvertently. When the Dutch arrived, they encouraged the Khoikhoi to smoke tobacco, and this made it valuable in trade. They also planted hemp, perhaps to make rope. By the early eighteenth century, many Khoikhoi were smoking cannabis. A number of Dutch settlers grew it in part "to ensure their [workers'] continued presence," according to Martin Booth.[41]

Others maintained that the extent of a population's drug use was determined by their climate, another approach that presented such use in the East in a manner that was, for the most part, non-judgmental. In an article that appeared in Philadelphia's *Literary Magazine* in 1804, a writer asserted that the warmer the climate, the greater the population's eagerness "for heating liquors and intoxicating drugs." This was said to affect not only the people native to a region but also to those who moved there. The "incessant heats" in the "torrid zone," the writer explained, would diminish the energy of all who lived there and would change "the constitution of the Europeans transplanted thither." All inhabitants would need "the hottest spices and the most inflammatory liquors" in order to "keep their stomach and the other organs of digestion in order." He added that this craving was also determined by "the higher or lower dignity, and the higher or lower refinement of nations": the craving, he suggested, was greater among less "refined" people.[42] Others agreed that the climate had a significant effect on drug use. Eleventh-century Iranian scholar Al-Bīrūnī, for example, noted that many people who lived in hot climates took a daily dose of opium to soothe themselves, to help them sleep, and "to relieve the body from the effects of scorching heat," according to David Courtwright.[43] Some observers would mistakenly attribute the Ottomans' apparent ability to consume much larger amounts of opium than Europeans could consume directly to their climate rather than to tolerance built up over years of use. Dr. Charles Caldwell, for example, wrongly suggested that Ottomans could do so because they were "long accustomed to a vitiated atmosphere."[44]

\* \* \*

Other European travelers described problems that could result from pleasure-seeking drug use, such as tolerance. Habitués need to take larger and larger doses of a drug to continue to feel its effects. As Jean-Baptiste Tavernier put it in 1677, Turkish *"takers of Opium"* might begin with a dose "no more . . . than the head of a pin" and eventually consume an amount "the quantity of half a wall-nut."[45] In his 1702 study of poisons, Richard Mead, who served as physician to King George II, wrote that *"Turks* and *Persians"* began "with small Doses" of opium but, over time, needed "more and more to raise themselves to the same *Pitch."*[46] He learned this in part from the writings of Pierre Belon.[47]

European travelers to the non-Western world also described withdrawal—the negative feelings that result when habitués go too long without their drug. According to Tavernier, if Turkish opium eaters "omit to take [opium] for a day . . . they are as cold and stupid [in a stupor] as before, which obliges 'em to take it again."[48] Sir Jean Chardin, a contemporary of Tavernier's, also noted that anyone who "accustoms himself to those Poppy Pills . . . must constantly use them," and that failure to do so would put him into "a languishing State."[49] In 1855 the *National Magazine,* a New York publication of the Methodist Church, ran an account of a doctor who had worked in China in the 1840s. Dr. G. H. Smith had reported that if a Chinese habitué was deprived of his drug, "Coldness is felt over the whole body, with aching pains in all parts; diarrhoea occurs; the most horrid feelings come on; and if the poison be withheld, death terminates the victim's existence."[50]

It was not necessarily true that a habitué would die prematurely, whether he stopped using the drug or not, although that notion became widespread. In *Natural History of Aleppo* (1756), Alexander Russell wrote that those who were "addicted" to opium "seldom live to a good old age."[51] In 1830, Irish physician Richard Robert Madden agreed that it was "very rare" to see an opium eater live past the age of thirty, "if he commence the practice early," because the habit had a terrible effect, "both moral and physical," on the user.[52] Ending opium use, however, was said to be deadly, too. Chardin stated—in a piece that was published in Philadelphia in 1804—that an opium habitué who only missed taking a dose by a few hours "will certainly pay for the neglect with his life." He went on to state that a Persian prince had met this sad fate.[53] In 1846, New York's *Water-Cure Journal* published the account of a "writer in India" that an opium eater, after two years of the practice, "must expect to die, and a death most terrible, and which makes one tremble to think of."[54]

Some habitués stated that being deprived of the drug would end their lives, though they had an incentive to say this. In 1578, for example, Cristóbal Acosta asserted that habitual users could not "give up their pleasure and addiction without great risk to their lives," unless they drank wine. He learned this from an opium habitué—a "discreet and wise Turk"—while aboard a ship in the Indian Ocean. The man and other habitués with him lacked an opium supply. As Acosta recalled, the man told him that he "could not live two days if I did not give him Opium," but Acosta had none to provide. The man then told Acosta that his own life and those of the others could be saved only if, each morning, Acosta would give them "a drink of pure wine, increasing the amount during the day." The doctor did so and added that "none of them died, and after a month they refused the wine, and did not suffer any harm for lack of Opium."[55] One wonders whether the notion that habitual users would die without their drug became widespread, in part because suffering habitués found this assertion to be persuasive as they pled for more. Using Acosta as a source, Samuel Purchas wrote that opium was "vsed much in Asia and Africa" and "must daily be continued on paine of death" unless wine was provided.[56] In *The Mysteries of Opium Reveal'd*, John Jones wrote that the consequence of ending opium use "after a long, and lavish Use thereof" was "commonly . . . a most miserable *Death*, attended with *strange Agonies*, unless Men return to the *Use of Opium*."[57]

Western travelers also described the health problems that resulted from compulsive use. The visible effects of habitual use—such as significant weight loss and tremors—suggested that a person could always recognize an opium habitué on sight. Thinking back to his visit to Constantinople in 1792, barrister William Hunter described "debauchees." "Their limbs are emaciated," he recalled, "their features are cadaverous and distorted." He could see in their faces, he added, that they were "slaves of bestial appetite and sensuality."[58] When Franklin Scott was studying opium as a medical student in Philadelphia, he drew on travelers' accounts. "In those countries where it is used as an article of luxury," he wrote of opium, "those who take it to excess are affected with tremors, paralytic affections of the lower extremities, which travellers have compared to the rickets."[59] This could explain why, later on, some Americans would incorrectly aver that there were no opium eaters in their midst because nobody around them fit these descriptions.

Some drug use took place in public, with spectators observing habitués' erratic behavior. A few described what they saw, and their accounts were published and republished, further making known the possible results of habitual drug use. In 1784, for example, François Baron de Tott observed Turkish opium users. In the early evening, he explained, men would gather in "the market of opium eaters," sit on sofas, and eat opium pills, some of them "larger than olives." The men's unhealthy appearances would "inspire only compassion" from onlookers, Tott admitted, if the distortions of their bodies were not so bizarre. Their "stretched necks, their heads twisted to the right or left, their backbones crooked, one shoulder up to their ears . . . present the most ludicrous and the most laughable picture," he wrote. The spectacle was not over. About an hour after they took the opium, the baron explained, it took effect and "the scene becomes most interesting." Apparently the men did not object to having an audience, if only because the drug brought them joy and made them oblivious to mockery. They would "gesticulate in a hundred different manners," Tott recalled, "but they are always very extraordinary and very gay." Opium gave them a happiness that they were otherwise denied. And they were "Deaf to the hootings" of people who were "making them talk nonsense."[60]

Several editors published this account, likely believing readers would find it interesting, informative, or both. The New-Haven Gazette and the Pennsylvania Packet published excerpts in 1788.[61] English physician Samuel Crumpe included Tott's description in his 1793 work An Inquiry into the Nature and Properties of Opium, as did Philadelphia scientist George W. Carpenter in his 1828 study of the drug.[62] In 1848, the editor of the American Phrenological Journal chose to reprint the sixty-four-year-old narrative.[63] In 1803, Daniel Wilson published his medical school dissertation about opium's "Morbid Effects," and he quoted the same passage. Wilson did, however, distance himself from Tott's "reasoning on the propriety or impropriety of conferring our pity on these poor wretches."[64] The extensive use of this account shows its medical influence as well as the scope of popular interest. Meanwhile, it reinforced Americans' association of pleasure-seeking opium use with the non-Western world since its nonmedical consumption in America was hidden.

Travel accounts could perpetuate misinformation about nonmedical drug use, such as when writers mixed up the drugs. Dutch explorer Jan Huyghen van Linschoten, for example, borrowed a great deal of information from the writings of Garcia Da Orta when he published his *Itinerario* in 1596. The work was a bestseller that was translated into other languages, including English.[65] Van Linschoten, however, distorted Da Orta's words and, as Martin Booth notes, he "gave the impression that hashish and opium produced similar hallucinogenic effects, a misconception that was to linger in the literature of drugs for a long time." In 1698, John Fryer, who worked as a doctor for the British East India Company, indicated in his own writings that opium was "a mixture of *bhang* and belladonna," another inaccuracy.[66] Belladonna is a plant that apothecaries were studying for its medical value. Its alkaloids would later be included in a variety of medicines, including sedatives and painkillers.[67]

\*\*\*

Many travelers suggested that non-Western opium habitués lacked qualities that Westerners generally believed men should have: fortitude, stoicism, courage, and self-control. Readers could conclude that if drug use became widespread, the consequences would be disastrous, because there would be a dearth of "manly" men to do the work that a society needed to thrive and progress.

In the late eighteenth century, some Western observers likened Eastern opium-using men to stereotypical women, due to their apparent inability to endure pain and their emotional response to adversity. In *Dissertation on the Gout* (1771), British physician William Cadogan suggested that "Asiatics" kept themselves in an "effeminate state free from pain."[68] In 1792, Dr. James Mease asserted that Turks' "immoderate use of opium" made them excessively sensitive—in Mease's mind, akin to emotional women. For these men, he explained, "the slightest noise, such as the sudden shutting of a door" would cause "involuntary startings and tremors, similar to what we observe in women who are highly hysterical."[69]

Many Europeans who traveled in Eastern countries reported that some men took opium to give them courage, an insinuation that they were naturally timid. In 1546, Pierre Belon wrote that Ottomans ate opium "because they think they will thus become more courageous and have less fear of the dangers of war. At the time of war, such large quantities are purchased it is difficult to find any left."[70] In *The Mysteries of Opium Reveal'd*, John Jones wrote that opium could inspire "*Courage,* [and] *Contempt of Danger*" in users. The "*Turks, &c.* use *Opium* before *Engagements,* desperate *Attacks, &c.* (as is most notorious,) to make them Courageous," he wrote.[71] In 1788, an edition of *Father's Instructions*—English physician Thomas Percival's collection of moral lessons—was published in Philadelphia. In the work, Percival stated that "Pusillanimity"—that is, timidity—was a characteristic of "the inhabitants of the East Indies." He had heard that

East Indians "take opium before any arduous and dangerous enterprise, to give them vigour and courage."[72] Such observations also appeared in American medical texts. When studying opium at the University of Pennsylvania, Valentine Seaman consulted Guillaume Raynal's *Philosophical and Political History of the Two Indies* to describe the behavior associated with opium "drunkenness." Some chose to "intoxicate themselves" if they wanted to commit "some desperate action," he wrote, quoting Raynal. In that state, they would then take on "the first object that presents itself, upon strangers as well as upon most inveterate enemies."[73] Such reports were not so much indictments of the drugs themselves as of the men who took them.

Although some characterized opium as an aphrodisiac, the drug in fact led to impotence. In 1563, Garcia da Orta referred to the use of hashish and opium as aphrodisiacs in India.[74] It appeared, though, that opium worked this way only with moderate users. With habitual users, da Orta observed, it had the opposite effect.[75] John Jones recorded that a large dose of opium could lead to "*Venery, Erections, &c.*" and stated that this was a major reason it was used by "the *Infidels of Turky,* and the *Eastern Nations* (especially where *Poligamy* is allow'd)."[76] Cristóbal Acosta wrote that while opium use led to impotence, users imagined that it worked as an aphrodisiac and thus "commonly employ it to increase their lacivious [*sic*] carnal pleasures."[77] Extensive opium use, therefore, could affect population growth. Some concluded that opium use had slowed the population increase in both China and the Indian province of Assam. In China, Alonzo Calkins wrote, the rate of natural increase had been reduced by two-thirds, and in Assam "impaired fecundity" had slowed population growth to a degree that could be easily observed.[78]

Others asserted that those who used the drug habitually became fickle and physically weak. In 1591, Prospero Alpini, an Italian physician who had lived in Egypt, wrote that people resisted doing business with opium eaters because they were inconstant—"first affirming, then denying a thing," as historian Glenn Sonnedecker put it—and were therefore untrustworthy.[79] In the 1790s, William Hunter acknowledged that Constantinople's "opium-eaters" experienced "luxurious dreams of ideal happiness." These positive effects, however, did not last, and the drug drained their energy. They would experience "the lassitude and languor of life," he explained, and this would "unhinge the whole system."[80] In 1804, Benjamin Waterhouse, one of the first professors at Harvard Medical School, noted in a public lecture that "travellers inform us, that the visage and general appearance of the opium-eaters in Turkey are the most disgusting imaginable; even worse than our most abandoned rum-drinkers."[81] Dr. David Cheever quoted the Reverend Walter Medhurst's account of Chinese opium smokers as being "haggard, dejected, with a lack-lustre eye, and a slovenly and feeble gait."[82]

German physician F. W. Oppenheim's description of Ottoman opium eaters underscored their miserable condition and was widely quoted:

> The habitual opium-eater is instantly recognized by his appearance. A total attenuation of body, a withered, yellow countenance, a lame gait, a bending of the spine, frequently to such a degree as to assume a circular form, and glossy, deep sunken eyes, betray him at the first glance. . . . The sufferer eats scarcely anything, and has hardly one evacuation in a week! his mental and bodily powers are destroyed. . . . These people seldom attain the age of forty, if they have begun to use opium at an early age.[83]

This reinforced the association of destructive opium eating with Turks. Also, it likely suggested to American readers that they would be able to identify opium eaters by a decrepit appearance.

If a habitual opium user were married, his wife would likely have to work excessively hard, observers reported, to compensate for her husband's inaction. In 1796, for example, the *Massachusetts Magazine* published an account by Edward Moor, a soldier for the British East India Company. According to Moor, men with an opium habit—such as Canary Islanders, off the coast of Morocco— were unproductive and thus burdened their wives. "If they live on the produce of a garden," Moor explained, "the labor of cultivation falls to her share." Her husband would stay at home "stupefied with opium" and would offer no kind word to his wife when she returned home. "On a journey," he continued, "he mounts a bullock; she, with a child in her arms, pants after him to drive it." Such information reinforced the notion that pleasure-seeking opium use was inconsistent with Western notions of masculinity and suggested a society in disarray.[84]

The man Moor described did not take care of his family, but others told of situations in which drug users abandoned their families or even became murderers. Charles Alexander Bruce, a Scotsman who was in charge of tea production in Assam in the 1830s, wanted to eliminate Assam's opium supply because of its effects on Indian men. A male user, Bruce wrote, would "sell his property, his children, the mother of his children, and finally, even commit murder for it." Bruce believed that they had no qualities that a man should have. According to Bruce, the Assamese could not do the work that needed to be done: to "fell our forests, to clear the land from jungle and wild beasts, and to plant and cultivate the luxury of the world"—that is, tea. The "enfeebled Opium consumers of Assam" were, Bruce concluded, "more effeminate than women." In 1850, American physician Nathan Allen quoted Bruce in his influential *Essay on the Opium Trade*.[85] According to Alonzo Calkins, Assamese men had been "vigorous and thriving," but opiate use had rendered them "the most demoralized and degenerate of all the tribes of India." Calkins repeated the assertion that an Assamese man would trade his wife and children for the drug, which indicated the man's lack of both morals and shame. Due to opium use, Calkins concluded, Assamese men did not match the West's masculine ideal. Instead, they were barely getting by, "eking out existence in a miserable effeminacy."[86]

Some European observers suggested that pleasure-seeking opium use was responsible for some countries' troubles. In 1788, when the Ottoman Empire was at war with the Habsburg Monarchy and the Russian Empire, a writer for the *New-Haven Gazette* provided context for the Turkish role in the conflict. The writer suggested that the Turks had grown weak—he referred to their "decay"—and then gave reasons why this had happened. One cause, he insisted, was "the excessive use of opium." Nothing else, he stated, could "more enervate the body and mind." He concluded that as a result, the Ottomans were indifferent to their lack of freedom, rather than fighting for it. He said that opium "divert[ed] their minds from their melancholy reflections on the ill conditions of their fortunes and lives, which depend on the caprice of their grand signiors and vizirs."[87] In 1807, a writer for Philadelphia's *Port-Folio* asserted that the Turks were "more indolent and inactive" than the Chinese and Indians. The writer mused that one reason for this could be their "continual use of opium."[88] And when the Chinese were fighting the First Opium War with Great Britain in 1840, the *New-York Mirror* summarized an English lecture that stated that at least four thousand Chinese men in Guangzhou were unable to serve their nation in its time of need because they had been "rendered utterly unfit for service by the use of opium."[89] These accounts suggested another dimension of what could happen if opium use became widespread: the population would be unable to fight against tyranny or outside aggression.

* * *

Some Europeans criticized non-Western populations' use of drugs in order to bolster the case for colonial control, while those who were colonized sometimes used drugs to help them to endure colonial oppression. Many Europeans in seventeenth- and eighteenth-century South Africa, for example, disdained the Khoikhoi's contentment with subsistence. They refused "to work for material reward," as scholar Mary Louise Pratt has noted, and European commentators derided them as guilty of "idleness and sloth."[90] Drug use shaped perceptions of productivity or a lack thereof. By 1800, Europeans regarded cannabis smoking as signifying a user's "exotic, non-European character," as geographer Chris Duvall has noted. The pleasure-seeking use of cannabis, he adds, evoked a "dreamy, sensuous hedonism" that was "an inversion of idealized Western pragmatism and industriousness."[91] In reality, cannabis use and industry could coexist. Some

Khoikhoi, for example, were compelled to work excessively for farmers, as they plowed fields all day and were then required to guard cattle at night. Some drank alcohol or smoked cannabis to cope with the conditions, as one laborer stated in 1769.[92]

Some commentators at the time provided evidence of non-Westerners' diligence to combat suggestions that drug use had enervated their societies. In 1762, Philadelphian Anthony Benezet quoted Europeans who, around the turn of the century, had attested to Africans' industry. Frenchman André Brue had observed the extensive agriculture south of the Gambia River. He found the land to be "well cultivated . . . scarce a Spot lay unimproved, the low Ground divided by small Canals, were all sowed with Rice; the higher Ground planted with *Indian* Corn and Millet, and Pease of different Sorts." Merchant Willem Bosman had described a productive society on the Dutch Gold Coast, which is now part of Ghana. It "abounded with fine well-built and populous Towns, enriched with vast Fields of Corn, Cattle, Palm Wine and Oil." The people would be "sowing Corn, pressing Oil, and drawing Wine from Palm Trees" while others fished. Referring to Africans, Benezet wrote that these observations were "sufficient to shew them to be entirely different from the stupified and malicious People some would have them thought to be."[93] Historian Jayeeta Sharma has noted that some of the stereotype of laziness could have derived from the people's unwillingness to work for colonizers more than parttime because they needed to work in their fields. Some Englishmen in mid-nineteenth-century India admitted that "most peasants did not find wage labour attractive" because there was so much available land. Other Britons, however, attributed the refusal to do such work as demonstrating "innate indolence" and maintained that the people's easy access to opium also "induces great laziness."[94]

Some scholars assert that in many cases, European travelers' tendency to identify and criticize idleness derived from a wish to justify colonialism and that criticism of drug use arose for the same reason. According to sociologist Syed Hussein Alatas, Europeans used "the idea of the lazy native" throughout the colonization era to justify conquest. The implication was that colonial leaders would modernize and "civilize" the people.[95] Novelist J. M. Coetzee describes this pattern in South Africa. Few travelers who visited before 1652, when the Dutch East India Company arrived, described the Khoikhoi as idle. The characterization appeared later on and was connected to "the desire of the colonists to impress them as labourers."[96] Hans Derks, meanwhile, asserts that the "production, consumption and distribution of opium and its derivatives" did not constitute an "opium *problem*" until colonial powers became involved in Asia, beginning in 1660, when the Dutch established a trade empire on India's west coast.[97] Sharma has noted that opium was "a commercial crop under peasant control" in India's Assam state in the nineteenth century, and some doctors acknowledged opium's medical usefulness, due to the prevalence of malaria. But colonial officials, rather than recognizing the people's productivity and control, responded with "the usual colonial reaction," Sharma adds, which was to dismiss opium cultivation as a "needless luxury" and to accuse the people of "sloth and indulgence."[98] Scholars of imperialism emphasize that writings denigrating non-Western populations abetted the colonization process. Such writings reinforced these tropes for "at least two centuries in thousands of books and reports written by administrators, scholars, travellers and journalists," according to Alatas.[99] Their writings could include descriptions of the bodies of colonized people, especially when they suggested the people's "degradation," as David Spurr points out in his study *The Rhetoric of Empire*.[100]

Some asserted that habitual opium use caused users to lose self-control and thus put others in danger, and the accounts—without the context of colonial exploitation—became medical dogma. Before the colonial era, for example, "amok" had a heroic connotation in Batavia—now Jakarta, Indonesia. It referred to "war or self-sacrificial behaviour for one's lord," as researchers at Kyoto University have noted. Dutch colonial leaders, however, sought to extinguish this concept. They redefined "amok" as connoting violent, manic behavior that was typically caused by opium use, and they punished such conduct. The measure obscured heroic behavior and suggested that those who were colonized were inclined to be irrational and violent, while it advanced colonial domination.[101] John Hawkesworth traveled to Batavia with Captain James Cook in the early 1770s, and Hawkesworth's memoir of the journey was published in New York in 1774. In it, he explained that running amok meant to "get intoxicated with opium, and then rush into the street with a drawn weapon and kill whoever comes in the way," until the person—typically someone enslaved, but sometimes a freeman—was killed or captured. Such events, he added, occurred in Batavia on an almost weekly basis.[102] The information appeared in American medical accounts. In *Medical Inquiries and Observations* (1812), Dr. Benjamin Rush wrote that "the intemperate use of opium" led to "madness of a furious kind" in Java. The response would depend on the person's status. If he were poor, Rush wrote, he would be "put to death," whereas the wealthy could afford care and "generally recover."[103]

* * *

In the mid-nineteenth century, some American writers reinforced the association of non-Western drug use and a lack of dynamism by connecting populations that were relaxed but appeared to be unproductive with the population's opium use. In 1857, the Boston literary journal *Flag of Our Union* ran an illustration depicting a "Café and Divan" in Algiers and explained that

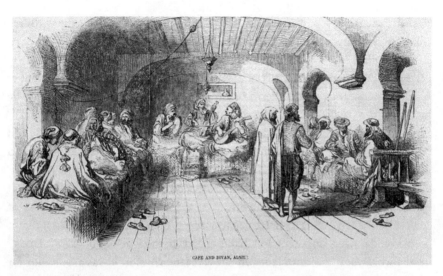

CAFE AND DIVAN, ALGIER

*Figure 4.1.* "Café and Divan, Algiers," *Flag of Our Union*, April 11, 1857. This image captured "the dreamy indolence of the East," according to the accompanying article. It shows Algerine men not at work but at a café where they would smoke opium and listen to music. Some commentators contrasted such characterizations with presentations of Westerners as productive. Drug habituation in America received little attention at the time. Author's copy.

this image best conveyed "the dreamy indolence of the East." Although few of the patrons drank alcohol, the writer explained, the "fearful drug *opium* is smoked to a fatal excess by all those who resort thither."[104] The next year, a writer for *Scientific American* presented a similar portrait by referring to the "drowsy appearance and indolent character of Eastern nations." The writer attributed it to the nations' climate, their natural abundance—which "in a great measure render[ed] labor unnecessary"—and "the use of powerful narcotic drugs."[105]

Many early American writers characterized Ottomans as inactive and as lacking intellectual curiosity, and they often linked these reported qualities with the Turks' opium use. In *American Universal Geography* (1805), Jedidiah Morse stated that Turks focused only on their immediate existence and that opium alone attracted their attention. Opium, he stated, gave users "sensations resembling those of intoxication." Otherwise, the people's thoughts were "simple and confined, seldom reaching without the walls of their own houses." They showed "little curiosity," he added, "to be informed of the state of their own or any other country."[106] In another geographical dictionary in 1806, Richard Brookes wrote, "Learning is at a very low ebb among the Turks."[107] John Aiken similarly depicted a sedentary and incurious people. "The pleasures of the Turks are almost all of the indolent and sedentary kind," he wrote, adding that they

lacked "science, art, or liberal curiosity." Instead, they spent their time with "tri-
fling amusements or sensual indulgences" and enjoyed the "stupefying exhilaration of opium."[108]

Many Ottoman men used opium, but some writers exaggerated the extent of
use. In 1546, for example, Pierre Belon misrepresented the situation when he
asserted, "There is no Turk who would not buy opium with his last penny."[109]
Opium use was an official concern, as authorities issued edicts against its use and
warnings regarding the consequences of use.[110] A contrary account appeared in a
manuscript that dates to around 1700, in which an anonymous Ottoman writer,
likely living in Constantinople, acknowledged opium's widespread use but
insisted that it served most frequently as a medicine or an appetite suppressant
rather than as an indulgence. He acknowledged the criticisms of opium: that it
could render users impotent and that it added "to the woe of the Islamic lands,"
in the words of historians Hatice Aynur and Jan Schmidt. It was a "stimulus for
the spirit" and the "companion of all men, common or privileged," but the author insisted that it was favored by "the weak and frail, those on a diet, and by the
elderly," as Aynur and Schmidt note.[111]

By the mid-eighteenth century, the practice appeared to have diminished.
In *Natural History of Aleppo, and Parts Adjacent* (1756), Dr. Alexander Russell
wrote that he could not "find the taking it [opium] so general a practice in *Turky*
as is commonly apprehended, being chiefly practiced only by debauchees."[112]
Dr. Samuel Crumpe reprinted Russell's observation in his 1793 work, *An Inquiry
into the Nature and Properties of Opium*. Crumpe then suggested that opium
played the same role in "eastern countries" that alcohol did in Europe; both,
he stated, were used by the unfortunate. These substances were, he wrote, "the
support of the coward, the solace of the wretched, and the daily source of intoxication to the debauchee."[113] In 1824, Pennsylvania's *Susquehanna Democrat*
and the Boston publication *Spirit of the English Magazines* also acknowledged
that "the practice of eating opium does not appear to be so general with the
Turks as is commonly believed."[114] And in 1829, the *Long-Island Star* quoted an
American missionary who insisted that "the Turkish character . . . is viewed by
most persons in too unfavorable a light." He added that "opium eating does not
exist to any considerable extent"—that he had "seen tens of thousands of Turks,
and never observed one making use of that drug."[115] The stereotype, however,
endured.

Also, non-Western doctors recognized the problem of drug habituation. In the
sixteenth century, Cristóbal Acosta noted that "Arabic, Persian, Turkish, Indian,
Malay, Chinese and Malabar doctors" opposed the widespread use of opium due
to the risk of developing dependency on it, as Martin Booth has noted.[116]

Some non-Western leaders believed that widespread drug use was causing
problems and tried to restrict usage, with punishments often including the

death penalty, but they had only partial success. In 1360, for example, several decades after Chinese merchants had begun bringing opium to what is now Thailand, King Ramathibodi I banned its trade and use. The prohibition remained in place for almost five hundred years. And in 1665, King Canh Tri III prohibited opium in Vietnam, a policy that remained in place until 1858, when French colonization began.[117] (Although colonizing powers highlighted nonmedical drug use to justify the imposition of colonial rule, France and Great Britain spread opium use in Indochina and Burma as "a way to finance empire," according to historian Ronald D. Renard.)[118] Some travelers reported on non-Western efforts to restrict drug access and the limited effectiveness of those measures. According to Sir Jean Chardin, Persian rulers had tried to diminish the use of opium, due to its "fatal Effects," but without success. The government tried "several times to prevent the Use of that Drug," he wrote, but usage remained widespread. It was "so general a Disease," he wrote, "that out of ten Persons, you shall not find one clear from that ill Habit."[119] In his 1804 account *Travels in China*, Sir John Barrow wrote that although the Chinese government banned the importation of opium, it remained popular with elites. A great deal of it was smuggled into the country, because some customs officers accepted bribes.[120]

There was also official opposition to opium usage in Constantinople; as a consequence, the practice became less visible. This somewhat modified Westerners' perceptions of Turkish use, though some still sought it out. American writer Nathaniel Parker Willis was interested in seeing opium eaters when he visited Constantinople, but he explained in *Pencillings by the Way* (1835) that this was not possible. While there, his traveling companion asked a coffee shop proprietor "whether there was any place at which a confirmed opium-eater could be seen under its influence," and the man replied that an "old Turk" who patronized his shop might arrive in an hour or two, "in the highest state of intoxication." They did not, however, have time to wait.[121] When Stephen Olin recalled his time in Constantinople, he saw coffee houses that had been "the great resort of the opium eaters." The former president of Wesleyan University had hoped to see "some remains of this race" but was disappointed. In response to inquiries, he was told by residents and "intelligent Franks" that "no such persons at present exist." Some attributed it to the increase of alcohol use there. They also insisted that the popular perceptions of opium use, "if not wholly fabulous, are grossly exaggerated."[122]

Some difference in usage over time derived from changing preferences rather than from new policies. By 1910 in Java, opium smoking had become "a mark of being old fashioned, if not uncivilized," as historian James Rush has observed. These views had begun with the elite and then spread to the general population.[123]

* * *

Westerners sometimes tried the drugs themselves, but in their accounts they presented such episodes as scientific experiments or one-time trials to satisfy their curiosity and thus escaped the ignominy of those who immersed themselves in such use. In 1829, Irish physician Richard Robert Madden wrote about opium use in Constantinople. Earlier, an "opium eater" had told him that his favorite reverie involved nymphs in a Muslim heaven: that he was "shampooed by the dark eyed *houris* of Paradise." As Madden did not trust others' accounts, he decided to try opium under the guise of medical research. As he put it, he had "heard so many contradictory reports of the sensations produced by this drug, that I resolved to know the truth." By explaining his reasoning, Madden distinguished himself from the "half a dozen *Theriakis*"—a derisive term for opium habitués—among whom he sat, who were "completely under the influence of the opium." His description of them suggests that they were almost incapable of presenting their perspectives or of accomplishing anything. While in their drug-induced state, he wrote, "Their gestures were frightful." They "talked incoherently, their features were flushed, their eyes had an unnatural brilliancy, and the general expression of their countenances was horribly wild." And while not under it, "they are miserable till the hour arrives for taking their daily dose." He also presented them as lacking self-control. Despite the drug's horrible physical toll, he added, "they cannot abandon the custom."[124]

Although Madden experienced the drug's delights, he emphasized his enduring self-control. He took small doses and heard "'the faint exquisite music of a dream' in a waking moment," he recalled. Yet he was mindful of how he appeared to others. The Turkish users "address[ed] the bystanders in the most eloquent discourses, imagining themselves emperors," he wrote, but when Madden began to feel opium's effects, he headed to his lodgings "as fast as possible, dreading, at every step, that I should commit some extravagance." Therefore, he suggested, he had a self-consciousness that others lacked. Also, he paid for the attempt, as the next day he endured a headache and loss of energy.[125] Several American editors published excerpts of Madden's narrative of his sojourn with the Turkish habitués.[126] The impact of such accounts was significant. In 1837, writers for the *Boston Medical and Surgical Journal* maintained that having read the accounts of Madden, the Baron de Tott, and other travelers, they believed they were "almost as well acquainted with the habits, the appearance, and the follies of the opium-eaters of Constantinople" as if they had been there themselves.[127]

Europeans appeared willing to be candid regarding their own drug use, even if they partook just to satisfy their curiosity. Captain Thomas Bowrey, along with fellow merchant seamen in the Bay of Bengal, tried cannabis in the 1670s. He and the others saw "the local people amusing themselves" with it in the form of bhang and therefore wanted to try it, as Davenport-Hines notes. Bowrey recalled the episode in *A Geographical Account of Countries Round the Bay of Bengal* (1680). The effects were not uniformly pleasant. One man "wept bitterly all the Afternoone," he recalled, and another "fought with one of the wooden Pillars of the Porch," losing much of the skin from his knuckles in the process. Others, however, were "Complimentinge each Other in high termes, each man fancyinge himselfe noe less than an Emperour." Davenport-Hines deemed the experiment "a pioneering episode in Western use of medicinal substances to satisfy curiosity and the desire for oblivious joy."[128]

\* \* \*

Descriptions of drug use in the non-Western world provided information about habituation that many Americans found interesting and that medicos deemed especially valuable. As these reports came from remote locales, they affected populations with whom few Americans identified. Although initial accounts were nonjudgmental, many that appeared later—especially with the onset of colonization—criticized the society for the drug use and accentuated an apparent divide between East and West. In the 1820s, consequently, many white Americans would be shocked to read about drug dependency among well-educated Englishmen including Thomas De Quincey. In his *Confessions of an English Opium-Eater*, De Quincey described the "pleasures" that opium gave him and insisted that ending drug use was agonizing, once the habit had formed. His work prompted curious American readers to experiment with the drug, and his captivating account would long remain one of the most influential sources in the field.

# Habitual Opiate Use in Great Britain, 1821–1877

Reports of habitual or pleasure-seeking drug use in parts of Asia, Africa, and the Middle East had expanded American knowledge regarding the effects of such use. The accounts also led many white, middle-class Americans to associate these practices with people of color and to identify them with societies that did not appear to be progressing—that were not "civilized," in the parlance of the day. The theory had a corollary, if a tacit one: that white, well-educated Westerners could avoid habitual drug use. This assumption enhanced the impact of Thomas De Quincey's *Confessions of an English Opium-Eater* (1821). In it, De Quincey provided the habitué's perspective. He described "pleasures" that opiates gave him, his intense dependency, and the extent of use in England. His story demonstrated that there was no immunity to compulsive use along lines of race or class.

In his study, "Narcotics," Dr. David Cheever reviewed *Confessions*, which was more than forty years old by that point. It had remained valuable to doctors and laypersons alike because De Quincey had provided rare first-person insights into drug dependency. Cheever trusted the accuracy of De Quincey's account, quoting him at length. For example, he shared the Englishman's assertions that opium use was not necessarily followed by "a proportionate depression" and that opium consumption did not lead to "torpor and stagnation," so long as the person received the correct dose. Cheever found it noteworthy that, according to De Quincey, in England there was "a pretty large amount of opium-eating," a conclusion based on the habituation of people he knew as well as his conversations with druggists.[1]

Cheever also emphasized the intractability of habituation. He described the drug use of English poet Samuel Taylor Coleridge, who "struggled desperately to break the habit." Coleridge paid people to keep him from the drug, but when he craved it, he insisted that, as his employees, they should let him have it. He also

*Habit Forming*. Elizabeth Kelly Gray, Oxford University Press. © Oxford University Press 2023.
DOI: 10.1093/oso/9780190073121.003.0006

put himself under a doctor's care in order to end his use but was "all the while buying laudanum secretly," while his friends assumed that he was being cured.[2]

\* \* \*

An American who purchased a copy of *Saturday Magazine* in 1822 had the opportunity to read the first work in a new genre: the confessional memoir of a person addicted to drugs.[3] The Philadelphia publication printed in serial form *Confessions of an English Opium-Eater*, which had debuted in *London Magazine* the previous year.[4] In this cautionary tale, Thomas De Quincey, who initially published the work anonymously, chronicled his descent into opium dependency and his partial emergence from it. He had discovered the drug's delights at age nineteen, when he bought it as a painkiller and unexpectedly experienced "divine enjoyment." "Happiness might now be bought for a penny, and carried in the waist-coat pocket," he marveled in *Confessions*. De Quincey was not the only Englishman who discovered this and had become habituated. After considering how many dependent users he knew personally and discussing the subject with druggists, he had concluded that British opium habitués were "very numerous indeed." Druggists had told him that the number of people "to whom habit had rendered opium necessary" was "immense," and it was especially popular with workers who bought opium because they could not afford alcohol.[5]

In the preface to his work, De Quincey explained that he was sharing his story to save others from his fate, but *Confessions* had the effect of encouraging use. He took the drug sporadically for several years because it inspired pleasant dreams and heightened his enjoyment of the opera. In his late twenties, however, he became a daily user, terrified by nightmares and unable to accomplish basic tasks. Therefore, although his dependency ultimately made De Quincey feel "agitated, writhing, throbbing, palpitating, [and] shattered," he acknowledged that, early on, the drug had given him several years of "exquisite pleasure."[6] Because he described "The Pleasures of Opium" before describing its "Pains," the memoir might have inspired more drug experimentation than it prevented, and this risk is perhaps inherent to the genre. Richard Davenport-Hines has pointed out that the memoirs of people addicted to drugs have dual appeal, as they uphold society's moral strictures while at the same time violating them. *Confessions* "set the pattern," he observed, for "individuals who wanted to transgress, shock or rebel without abandoning utterly the moral rules of their time."[7]

*Confessions of an English Opium-Eater* was flawed, but it provided Americans with a detailed account of habitual drug use, and many American doctors used it as a resource. De Quincey exaggerated some aspects of his tale to appeal to readers and unwittingly misrepresented others, such as the amount of time that people who ended their use would endure withdrawal. *Confessions*, nonetheless, had an extensive impact on Western understanding of drug dependency. Its unique content and high-quality prose attracted readers. De Quincey showed that susceptibility to drug dependency was universal—that neither race, nor nationality, nor level of education conferred immunity. Also, he emphasized the intensity of habituation. According to a recovering habitué who later reflected on the memoir's impact, *Confessions* helped physicians to understand "how easily the habit of using it could be acquired, and with what difficulty when acquired it could be left off."[8] Doctors would treat it as a trustworthy account even fifty years after its publication, in part because they trusted him but also because so few sources on the topic existed.[9]

Many Americans who read *Confessions* tried opium, because De Quincey touted the drug's "pleasures" and because he suggested that intellectual people like himself—he contrasted himself with "any Turk"—would derive the most from its use. In this respect, De Quincey supported an ongoing belief that drug use by white Westerners was merited in a way that use by others was not. Many members of America's white middle-class concluded that they would benefit from such use or at least wanted to see what the results would be. The theory that opium provided inspiration to poet Samuel Taylor Coleridge popularized the notion of opium as a kind of psychoactive muse.

The accounts of De Quincey and Coleridge, however, revealed some negative consequences of opium dependency. De Quincey asserted that opium's effects were preferable to those of alcohol since it produced clarity of thought while the latter led to intoxication. Others concluded that habitués were self-absorbed. While people drank alcohol in social settings with friends, opium users preferred solitude and focused on themselves. Also, following Coleridge's death, acquaintances of his recalled his persistent pleas for money, which he spent on laudanum while he was neglecting his family. This sparked discussions about the intensity of habituation but also lowered the poet's reputation in many readers' estimations.

\* \* \*

Thomas De Quincey first took opium as a painkiller in 1804, when he was nineteen years old, and that dose changed his life. He had suffered from "excruciating rheumatic pains of the head and face" for three weeks when he ran into a college friend who recommended it. He bought some from a druggist in London's Oxford Street. Expecting only pain relief, he marveled at the drug's impact. "The abyss of divine enjoyment [was] suddenly revealed," he recalled. He took the drug "occasionally" for almost ten years thereafter and experienced "those trances, or profoundest reveries, which are the crown and consummation of what opium can do for human nature." In *Confessions*, he dismissed negative perceptions about opium and thus further heightened the drug's appeal. For example, he denied that the "elevation of spirits" that opium produced would be followed by "a proportionate depression." The day after he used opium, he insisted, "was always a day of unusually good spirits." Despite his apparent advocacy for the drug, he insisted that he was not making light of the subject, for "nobody will laugh long who deals much with opium."[10]

De Quincey had difficulty accomplishing things as his usage continued, and he began to experience nightmares in 1813, when he became a daily user. He stressed, however, that he wanted to remain productive. "The opium-eater," he explained, "loses none of his moral sensibilities or aspirations"—he still wants to accomplish things and believes that he should, but he had difficulty doing so. Those inclinations were overwhelmed by "intellectual apprehension" regarding what he could do or even try to do. In this "state of imbecility," he could not read "with any pleasure" and was barely able to reply to correspondence. He was fascinated by David Ricardo's *On the Principles of Political Economy, and Taxation* (1817) and wrote a response to it, for example, but he lacked the energy to complete it, so his reply remained unpublished. Intellectual "torpor" by day was succeeded by nightmares that he insisted were "incommunicable by words," though he tried to describe them. In them, he seemed "literally to descend, into chasms and sunless abysses" and saw no chance that he "could ever reascend." He dreamed that he was "buried, for a thousand years, in stone coffins." Yet even while chronicling opium's worst aspects, he mentioned its positive impact on his memory and creativity, aspects that could have intrigued readers. His dreams included the "minutest incidents of childhood," which led him to conclude that humans retain all their experiences—that "there is no such thing as *forgetting* possible to the mind." And the terrible visions were so striking that "horror seemed absorbed, for a while, in sheer astonishment." But the drug no longer brought him pleasure. He kept using it to avoid the "tortures" that he would otherwise experience when he tried to end his dependence. Although he was able to greatly reduce his use, at the end of the work he admitted that "my sleep is still tumultuous."[11]

Although De Quincey stated that he wrote *Confessions* to save others from his fate, he also did so to make money. To appeal to a middle-class audience, he made "the waste of money, by himself and others, into a recurrent lament of his memoirs" and "advocat[ed] productivity," as Richard Davenport-Hines has noted.[12] Literary scholar Colin Dickey has pointed out that "for all its shocking revelation," the work was "bound by moral conventions of the time: it follows an arc of rise, fall and redemption." The redemption section implied— erroneously—that De Quincey was no longer using opium.[13] In 1841, a writer for the *Southern Literary Messenger* was impressed by the work's "melancholy details, the moral lessons, [and] the episodes of eloquent reflection"—the qualities that would define the genre.[14] This narrative structure, in which a person of promise tries a drug, enjoys it greatly, but then suffers terribly, has endured in depictions of drug use. It summarizes T. S. Arthur's bestselling 1854 temperance novel *Ten Nights in a Barroom*, the 1936 film *Reefer Madness*, and numerous celebrity memoirs.[15]

The work also interested readers because it suggested that habitual opium use was a problem that could persist without being noticed. From the perspective of a writer for the *Southern Literary Messenger* who reflected on the memoir's impact in 1850, it was "as if some one had discovered, for the first time, some horrible malady that had been scourging society in secret for a very long period." *Confessions*, he added, led readers to wonder "if their neighbours whom they met daily, really concealed beneath their stolid countenances, the horrible agony inflicted by this fearful Nemesis." There was additional concern that habitual users accepted their dependency. As he wrote, men discussed "if it were true that so large a number of their fellow-citizens were enduring the pangs of this fatal infatuation without an effort to disenchant themselves."[16] Drug habituation was thus a concern because people either suffered silently or accepted a condition in which they lacked both independence and sobriety.

*Confessions* shaped popular American perceptions of addiction, but in several respects, it was inaccurate. For example, De Quincey wrote that abstaining from opium caused him four months of agony, but opium withdrawal does not last nearly so long. De Quincey biographer Robert Morrison concludes that the Englishman either exaggerated his misery for literary effect or he did not realize that he was habituated to both opium and alcohol, and this aggravated his efforts to end his use. He took laudanum—which consisted of opium and sherry "flavored with cinnamon, cloves, and saffron," according to David Musto—and he took it in huge quantities.[17] Therefore, he likely suffered from a poly-addiction—to opium and alcohol—and tried to give up both at once, an incredibly challenging undertaking.[18]

Some writers ignored the most nettlesome aspect of De Quincey's dependency: that medical use, which was socially sanctioned, could lead to habitual use, which was not. Willard Phillips, a lawyer and author, reviewed *Confessions* for the *North American Review*.[19] In his article, he presented De Quincey's opium use as having always been pleasure-seeking in nature, and this allowed him to ignore the more complex reality. Phillips glossed over De Quincey's explanation that he first took the drug as a painkiller and was unaware of its euphoria- and habit-inducing potential. He stated only that De Quincey's first use "put him into an ecstacy" and that later he would occasionally decide to "commit an excess in opium." Presenting De Quincey as aware of opium's effects and as using it solely for hedonistic purposes, Phillips deemed it "incredible" that someone "would cooly, and with deliberate purpose" ingest something that would cause "pain, weakness, melancholy, and early decrepitude." Phillips did not envision a future of American opium eating, perhaps because he paid scant attention to the origins of De Quincey's dependency. He wrote that Americans should read *Confessions* "more as an object of taste and literary curiosity" than as a warning, because "very few persons, if any, in this country, abandon themselves to the use of opium as a luxury."[20] In reality, the search for pain relief sometimes led to decades-long dependency.

Not all the initial reviews in American publications were condemnatory. Some journals reprinted British reviews of the work, and these reviewers tended to note the appeal of nonmedical opium use and to downplay its risks. A reviewer in the *United States Literary Gazette*, for example, accepted De Quincey's defenses of the drug, namely, that it "never did and never can intoxicate," that one would experience "uncommon happiness" the day after using it, and that it "clarifies the intellect." He stated that use of the drug could be fatal but then pointed out De Quincey's assertion that he had almost completely stopped using it. The reviewer insisted that the book bore "the impress of genius" and did not seem bothered that it could lead some readers to try opium.[21] The review of *Confessions* that appeared in the *American Medical Recorder* was written by former British opium eaters. They believed that De Quincey had overstated the difference between alcohol and opium. Like De Quincey, they had "suffered the horrors of vivid dreaming" due to their use. They also, however, "well recollect . . . the inexpressible delight produced by opium." They insisted that it was a valuable medicine and acknowledged that it could produce "beatific visions" and "dreams of ideal happiness" that words could not express.[22] None of these early reviews suggest that the authors or editors regarded addiction as a problem that Americans would face. They appear to have assumed that this was a peculiar and interesting practice in a foreign land that they might not hear of again.

\* \* \*

Despite De Quincey's chronicling of opium's "pains," his work long inspired nonmedical opium use among readers who were intrigued by his assertions that opium could enhance a user's creativity and abilities. A US Navy chaplain tried it when he visited Constantinople in the 1830s. "My imagination was once so kindled," he explained, "by the perusal of a little book called the 'Opium-Eater.' " He experienced the drug's pleasures but also its pains and concluded, "Let no one test, like me, the dreaming ecstacies and terrors of opium."[23] In 1851, a Yale student lamented that *Confessions* gave readers a sense of "fascination" with the drug. He believed that younger readers might follow De Quincey's "fascinating though ruinous course."[24] In the late 1870s, Jane Addams sought "to understand De Quincey's marvelous 'Dreams' " during a school break from Illinois's

Rockford Seminary. The future Nobel Peace Prize laureate and some friends "drugg[ed] ourselves with opium," she later recalled, but she was sorry to say that she did not experience a "mental reorientation."[25] And in the 1880s, a doctor in St. Louis agreed that *Confessions*, with its "overdrawn picture of the pleasures of opium," was "largely responsible for the spread of this insidious curse and disease."[26] De Quincey denied that he was to blame for readers' usage, as he believed that those who did not hear about opium's pleasures would find out on their own when they took it medicinally, as he had. Yet he revised his memoir in 1856 to give greater emphasis to the "pains" the drug caused.[27]

In this respect, De Quincey's memoir undid the efforts of some eighteenth-century English doctors and druggists who had hidden information about opium from the public to prevent improper use. Greenwich apothecary John Awsiter knew that writing about opium could encourage use and lead to habitual use. He noted that earlier in the century Dr. Richard Mead had written about opium's effects on dogs but had not addressed its effects on humans.[28] Awsiter suggested that Mead did that because, had he included opium's effects on people, his readers would lose their "Fear and Caution" regarding the drug and would then "indiscriminately use it." Awsiter applauded Mead's decision. There were "many Properties" of opium, he explained, that "if universally known," would "make it more in Request with us than the *Turks* themselves, the Result of which Knowledge must prove a general Misfortune."[29]

Others, however, believed that it was better to let the public know. In 1753, Dr. George Young defended his decision to publish *A Treatise on Opium*. He admitted that the work could contribute to "fatal blunders," as charlatans could use its information to pass themselves off as skilled doctors. But Young also believed that he could help readers by warning them, for example, that small doses of laudanum administered improperly could be lethal. Without this information, well-intentioned people could commit "this fatal error," and because the cause of death would be unclear, there would be no warning for potential users. Furthermore, Young believed that laypersons would use opiates regardless. Doctors must "either assist the unskilful by our experience," he had concluded, "or they will proceed boldly without us."[30]

Several American imitations followed the publication of *Confessions*, a sign of its popularity and influence. In 1833, poet John Greenleaf Whittier wrote a story called "The Opium Eater" that began with a quote from *Confessions*.[31] In 1842, New York's *Knickerbocker* magazine published "An Opium-Eater in America." Author William Blair, an English immigrant, described his descent into habituation in the account, which he modeled on *Confessions*.[32] American poet and habitué John Lofland penned his own "Confessions of an Opium Eater" in the late 1840s.[33] In 1857, New Yorker Fitz Hugh Ludlow acknowledged his debt to De Quincey in the preface of his work *The Hasheesh Eater*. And almost a century after that, William S. Burroughs gave his memoir *Junky* the subtitle *Confessions of an Unredeemed Drug Addict*.[34] Some maintained, however, that none of the nineteenth-century works equaled the original. In reviewing *The Hasheesh Eater*, a writer for the *Knickerbocker* likened the men who sought to emulate De Quincey to those who had imitated Lord Byron's dress and style. They could resemble Byron in some respects, he explained, but they lacked his "features, mind, knowledge, GENIUS." Similarly, he explained, those who had tried to write à la De Quincey were "weak-minded aspirants," most of whom could not turn their experiences into a full-length work, as De Quincey had.[35]

Many criticized *Confessions* and subsequent works on the topic for inspiring risky drug use. Reflecting on the work's influence, a writer for the Boston Methodist publication *Zion's Herald* insisted that "De Quincey and his imitators have done a world of mischief by seducing weak-minded persons, who yearned for a new sensation, into tasting the delights of opium."[36] And in his account of his own dependency much later in the century, William Rosser Cobbe asserted that "the evils of the fascinating 'Confessions of an English Opium-Eater' have been beyond estimate and are daily luring innocents to eternal ruin."[37] Some were critical of the book but hesitated to criticize it publicly. A writer for the Unitarian *Christian Examiner* asserted that *Confessions'* influence was primarily "injurious." He could not, however, explain why "without doing the same mischief as the book."[38]

\* \* \*

De Quincey's dependency surprised readers because many had assumed that an intelligent Englishman would have the wherewithal to avoid habituation. Earlier reports of habitual use had focused almost solely on people of color in the non-Western world, and the people who wrote about them provided no information regarding the habitués' lives, beliefs, levels of intelligence, or motivations for use. Many readers perhaps concluded that these users made no effort to avoid dependency but that a European would—and could. Before *Confessions*, many believed that "the Asian was more susceptible to absolute moral enslavement than the British addict, who retained the ability to act autonomously," as literary scholar Peter Melville Logan has observed.[39] Readers, accustomed to accounts of emaciated Turks ingesting the drug in public settings, were shocked to learn that "English opium eating was possible," as historian Virginia Berridge and psychiatrist Griffith Edwards have noted.[40] De Quincey had emphasized his intelligence. He began his use while a student at Oxford University, and he characterized himself as "a Scholar." In the 1870s, when American concern with domestic habituation was growing rapidly, a writer in Chicago mentioned that *Confessions* revealed the drug's "absorbing power," given the fact that De Quincey's "strong intellect was scarcely proof against its tenacious clutch."[41]

And as De Quincey had mentioned, opiate use was extensive in Great Britain. Some Americans had assumed that white Westerners would consider the risks of nonmedical opiate use and that, in contrast, other populations partook of them without a thought. Reports that educated Englishmen regularly resorted to opiates, therefore, seemed to suggest that anyone might do so. As American writer Henry Tuckerman mused, when even British ministers and writers resorted to laudanum and alcohol use,

> we can scarcely wonder that the unfurnished mind of a Japanese should yield to the feverish charm of his rice-distillation; the limited understanding of a Chinaman dwindle to imbecility amid the sedative vapor of opium; the American Indian forget his woes in fire-water; and the idler in the gardens of Damascus fall an unresisting victim to the enchantments of Hasheesh.

Tuckerman characterized these people as "imprisoned in blind instinct, unsustained by faith, wisdom, or love" and was unsurprised that, bereft of these, they sought solace in something to help them to forget their problems.[42]

Some Americans wondered whether opium enhanced natural talents or if it could bestow insights and eloquence upon those who were not naturally gifted. De Quincey insisted that opium's effects correlated with the user's natural abilities and lived experiences. The author, who called himself "a philosopher" and boasted that he had been a prodigy in Greek, had fascinating dreams. Yet the opium-inspired visions of those who lacked exceptional skill and training, he maintained, would be uninteresting and, one could infer, not worth the effort. "If a man 'whose talk is of oxen,' should become an opium-eater," he wrote, "the probability is, that (if he is not too dull to dream at all) he will dream about oxen."[43] Writers for American publications tended to accept this explanation. In 1858, the Reverend J. Townley Crane wrote that "a man of scanty ideas and no fancy" could experience opium's highs and lows, "but his fantasia would be narrow and common-place."[44] In 1860, a writer for the *Dial* agreed that opium could not make "an unimaginative man imaginative."[45] The discussion continued, in many cases because individuals appeared to wonder what opium could do for them. In 1877, a writer for the *Saturday Evening Post* doubted that the drug "did anything more than intensify [De Quincey's] splendid faculties."[46] This made some want to try it—to see what would happen if, in the words of writer Martin Booth, they "embellished what already existed."[47]

There was evidence that opium could spark intellectual inspiration, the best-known example of which was Samuel Taylor Coleridge's poem "Kubla Khan."

According to the poet, he was inspired to write it one day in 1797 after reading about Kublai Khan, the leader of the Mongol Empire, in Samuel Purchas's *Purchas, His Pilgrimage*. Coleridge took a painkiller, fell asleep, and dreamed a poem of almost three hundred lines. Upon awakening, he began to write it down but was then interrupted and forgot most of it. The result was the fifty-four-line poem "Kubla Khan, or a Vision in a Dream. A Fragment." It begins:

> In Xanadu did Kubla Khan
> A stately pleasure-dome decree:
> Where Alph, the sacred river, ran
> Through caverns measureless to man
> Down to a sunless sea.

In an unpublished note on an early draft of the poem, Coleridge acknowledged opium's role in the composition: "This fragment with a good deal more, not recoverable, [was] composed in a sort of Rêverie brought on by two grains of Opium," he wrote.[48] Scholars have long debated opium's importance in the composing of the poem, and most have accepted that its role was significant.[49]

Opium's alleged ability to inspire led some, such as American poet Julia Ward Howe, to regard writers' use of it as tantamount to cheating. In the 1850s, the future author of "The Battle Hymn of the Republic" accused British poet Elizabeth Barrett Browning, an opium user, of writing her work under the influence.[50] In the poem "One Word More with E.B.B.," Howe wrote that she herself could only write about "pictures of the things I see," but that others used a "nameless draught" to reach "unearthly things." She would not adopt the practice, however, because of its dangers: "If a drug could lift so high, I would not trust its treacherous wings," she explained.[51] It is unclear to what extent Howe objected to the practice and to what extent she was smarting from the lack of attention that Browning and her husband, Robert, had given to her work.[52] Other Americans, meanwhile, were eager to see what opium could do for them. In 1860, a writer for the *Dial* stated that many opium and hashish users had "cultivated and highly susceptible minds" and used the drugs to attain "insight into the profound mysteries of the human soul, which they alone can give."[53]

De Quincey suggested that a user's ethnicity shaped how he or she would experience drug use, with Westerners faring best, and others also believed that race and ethnicity were determinative. In *Confessions*, De Quincey expressed doubt that "any Turk" using opium could "have had half the pleasure I had" and went on to state that "I honor the barbarians too much by supposing them capable of any pleasures approaching to the intellectual ones of an Englishman."[54] Others reinforced the idea that Westerners would derive the most enjoyment from the intoxicants. In 1855, the *Ladies' Repository*, a Methodist Episcopal magazine based in Cincinnati, republished a British article that explored the impact of various substances on human beings. The writer contrasted "the miserable Theriaki who haunts the coffee-houses of Constantinople, with his withered visage, his bent spine, his shattered frame" with "those two gifted men of our own country"—De Quincey and Coleridge—"whose genius shaped its fumes into gorgeous dreams." The writer went on to state that opium's effects varied, based on the user's "temperament and race." When taken by "excitable people, like the Javanese, the Negro, the Malay," he wrote, "it exerts a terrible power" and could make users "frantic" and possibly homicidal.[55] In 1862, Dr. David Cheever stated that De Quincey "surpassed all other opium-eaters . . . in talent and in highly intellectual visions," whereas "Turks and Hindoos manifest the pernicious effects of opium consumption in indolence, ignorance, and degeneracy."[56]

Different populations' experiences with drugs could vary, but these differences derived from the form of the drug they consumed and its role in their society—not on the user's ethnicity or race.[57] As psychiatrist Norman Zinberg has noted, people's experiences with drugs are shaped by their expectations regarding the use, by the settings in which they consume them, and of course, by the drugs themselves.[58] Commentators, however, often treated different drugs as if they were identical. De Quincey's decanter of ruby-colored laudanum was not the olive-sized ball of opium that some Turkish habitués ate at dusk, nor was it the viscous "smoking opium" that the proprietor of an opium den in China heated and then gave to a habitué to inhale through a pipe.[59] Yet many believed that race and ethnicity were the determinative aspects, a belief that De Quincey shared.

* * *

Many maintained that a habitué would, as a result of his dependency, accomplish little, and they held up De Quincey and Coleridge as examples. Writers for the *Yale Literary Magazine* wondered in 1851, while De Quincey was still alive, "what heights his genius might have borne him, had it been untrammeled" by his opium habit.[60] Two years later, regarding Coleridge, a writer for the *Universalist Quarterly* asked, "What might" he have done, "had it not been for opium?"[61] According to a writer for *Harper's Magazine*, Coleridge wrote little after he placed himself in the residential care of a physician to try to end his usage.[62] Several other writers echoed the notion that De Quincey and Coleridge could have accomplished much more had it not been for their habituation.[63] Others suggested that opium negatively affected not only the quantity of their output, but also the quality. "It seems to me that what is best in a man will be developed more perfectly in a state of health than in a state of disease," writer Ellen M. Mitchell mused in her article about De Quincey for *Arthur's Home Illustrated Magazine*.[64]

One can wonder, could they have done much more? As English professor Paul Youngquist has observed, despite being addicted for more than half his life, Coleridge kept publishing "at a pace that would make any Dean of Humanities proud." With the poet's collected works filling fourteen volumes, Youngquist quipped, "If Coleridge failed as a writer, he failed prolifically."[65] The same is true of De Quincey, regarding both the quantity and quality of his work. It is true that he could not finish the response to David Ricardo's book. A writer for the *Southern Literary Messenger*, however, noted that, after publishing *Confessions*, De Quincey continued to write "wonderfully metaphysical, yet passionate, and eloquent prose poems."[66] A writer for the *Saturday Evening Post* called De Quincey "the chief and most artistic prose writer of the nineteenth century."[67] And a writer for the *National Era*, in reviewing De Quincey's *Essays on the Poets and Other English Writers*, insisted,

> In harmoniousness of mental organization, in extent and variety of culture, in profundity and directness of thought, in force of expression and purity in style, probably no living English writer surpasses Thomas De Quincey.

In fact, he gave partial credit to opium for the high quality of De Quincey's prose, stating that "that terrible vice" had been "providential" for him, "so far as intellectual and psychological development are concerned." He added that, in De Quincey's writings, "Every word he uses is exactly the right one."[68] The *Southern Literary Messenger* writer agreed, suggesting that opium use contributed to "the peculiar originality of his views."[69] Its impact on a user's work was not always detrimental.

Conventional wisdom also suggested that opium use shortened the user's life, but the examples of Coleridge and De Quincey call this into question. Both writers were born in eighteenth-century Great Britain, and people in their cohort, on average, lived for 49.4 years, with members of the royal family living about ten years longer.[70] Both Coleridge and De Quincey exceeded even the royals' average life span, reaching sixty-one and seventy-four years old, respectively.[71] It is true that they were born later in the century—Coleridge in 1772, De Quincey in 1785—at a time when life spans would have been increasing. And perhaps they would have lived longer had they never consumed an opiate. The lengths of their lives, however, call into question the notion that opium eaters were destined to die young.

An 1832, Scottish court case further called into question the notion that opium habitués could not reach old age. The case pertained to the death of John Thomas Erskine, the Earl of Mar. He had been a habitual laudanum user for decades but had not informed the Edinburgh Life Assurance Company of his dependency when he took out a policy on his life in 1826. He died two years later of jaundice and dropsy, but the company refused to pay on the grounds that his dependency, of which they had been unaware, had caused his death. When the policy had been issued, he had declared he was in good health and suffered from nothing that tended "to shorten life." The company maintained that the earl was guilty of "misrepresentation and Concealment of material facts" and that the contract was therefore void.[72]

Some witnesses challenged the theory that an early death was a habitué's inevitable fate. Several physicians did testify in the trial that habitual opium use was "very injurious." Yet the case also revealed "that a fair proportion of opium-eaters reach an advanced age," as the *American Journal of the Medical Sciences* reported. Dr. Robert Christison, whose comments were widely reprinted, acknowledged that opium dependency could damage "the digestive organs and . . . the nervous system," that it was at least as "destructive" as "the vice of drinking spirits," and that opium dependency had likely foreshortened the lives of "many" habitual users. He warned, however, against concluding that this was the norm—that "the practice of using opium in excess tends to shorten life." One woman, for example, had ingested laudanum "daily for nearly forty years" and had "enjoyed tolerable health" until her death at the age of eighty. A seventy-year-old woman who had used laudanum daily for almost forty years was still alive, Christison relayed. She "enjoys tolerable health," he asserted, and "every year travels great distances to visit her friends." He traced popular misperceptions regarding opium users' fates to early Westerners' accounts of habitual users in Asia and the Ottoman Empire. He stated that "eastern travellers" had probably "given an exaggerated view of the facts" and that laypersons and even many doctors had trusted these unreliable sources. Christison's evidence was eye-opening, but the verdict was anticlimactic. The judge ruled against the insurance company not because he accepted that someone could indulge in opium safely, but because he concluded that the company had not done due diligence when they issued the policy.[73] As British physician R. H. Semple explained, the company "did not make sufficient inquiries into his lordship's health and his habits."[74]

* * *

De Quincey suggested that opium use was safer and more gratifying than that of alcohol, an intoxicant that English society had long embraced, but many Americans were not persuaded. By comparing its nonmedical use with that of alcohol, he made such use seem more familiar than it otherwise would have appeared. De Quincey had used opium every few weeks from 1804 to 1812, and he surmised that it had not harmed him any more than eight years' use of port or Madeira would hurt his readers. And where alcohol made users less focused, he added, opium made them more so. Wine "disorders the mental faculties," De Quincey explained, but opium, if taken properly, "introduces . . . the most exquisite order, legislation, and harmony." He was so certain of opium's superiority that he believed English workers who bought opium instead of alcohol to save money would not switch back if their wages increased, given opium's "divine luxuries."[75]

Alcohol would remain the more socially acceptable drug, not because opium made some users ill, but because, for centuries, alcohol had been a part of Western sociability—a role that opium could not play. Alcohol brought people together, while an opium user focused on his own mind and well-being: with the exception of opium smoking, it was not a drug that users enjoyed communally. Wine could lead men to "shake hands, swear eternal friendship, and shed tears," De Quincey acknowledged. Meanwhile, opium's value was experienced inwardly—helping the user to "compose what had been agitated" and to remove "deep-seated irritation," he explained.[76] Opium users preferred to explore their minds rather than to engage with others. De Quincey asserted that it was for this reason that intellectuals could experience the drug best. These perceptions help to explain why opium users came to be perceived as selfish and elitist.[77] American physicians also saw this dichotomy. In 1830, a writer for Philadelphia's *Journal of Health* noted that people who drank did so while enjoying the company of other people—they "jovially quaffed from the glass and the bowl amid songs, and joyous shouts," he explained. The laudanum devotee, meanwhile, "carefully meted out" his dose at home, alone.[78] In 1871, Dr. Alonzo Calkins wrote that the "*alcohol family* lean towards festive association," but the "opium-eater" opposed such "fraternization" and was instead "withdrawn to the seclusion of his solitary hauteur."[79]

\* \* \*

Public understanding of an ailment increases when a person of renown struggles with it openly, and Coleridge's battle with drug dependency advanced conversation about habituation. The poet first took laudanum for medicinal purposes in his schooldays, then used it later in life to ameliorate both "physical pain and mental worry," including relief from "rheumatic affections and knee-swellings" that had rendered him practically bedridden.[80] His pains remained with him into adulthood.[81] He also used the drug for its sedative effects. In 1796, for example, he took it when he was "tottering on the edge of madness," as he described it, when his pregnant wife was seriously ill. His usage became habitual. He hid his use from most of his friends, but his dependence became known, and he openly acknowledged it in 1816.[82] He then made trips to the druggist "in full daylight . . . without disguise or false pretence" according to Seymour Porter, who had worked as the druggist's apprentice. Porter recalled neighbors treating Coleridge with "pity rather than . . . reproach."[83]

There is evidence that Coleridge wanted to end his use, despite his failure to do so. Repeatedly, he took measures to distance himself from the drug, only to give in. At one point, he hired men to prevent him from buying laudanum. When his craving became intense, however, he told them, as their employer, to disregard his earlier instructions, and they obliged.[84] In 1816, he became "the first celebrity to enter rehab," as Paul Youngquist has observed.[85] Coleridge moved in with Dr. James Gillman, who was supposed to keep the poet away from laudanum. Coleridge lived with the Gillmans for the last eighteen years of his life. Although he still consumed laudanum, he decreased his doses.[86] Coleridge wanted his story to serve as a cautionary tale for others. In an 1814 letter to a friend, he expressed his wish that, after his death, "a full and unqualified narration of my wretchedness, and of its guilty cause, may be made public, that at least some little good may be effected by the direful example!" He rued the negative consequences of his opium use. "In the one CRIME of OPIUM, what crime have I not made myself guilty of!" he exclaimed. "Ingratitude to my Maker! and to my benefactors—injustice! *And unnatural cruelty to my poor children!*"[87]

After Coleridge's death in 1834, some people who had known him published their recollections of him, and they described a man who had cared only about his drug habit and who treated his friends and family poorly. Their criticism is understandable, not only because they were directly affected but also because few at the time grasped how intractable drug habituation could be. Joseph Cottle, a Bristol bookseller and former friend of the poet's, characterized Coleridge as having been dishonest, self-indulgent, and neglectful of his children. Cottle had tried to persuade him to end his opium use "and to return to that family whom for years he has utterly abandoned," as a reviewer noted in *Harper's Magazine*.[88] At one point, Cottle had suggested to Robert Southey, Coleridge's brother-in-law, that they raise money for him, but Southey objected, saying that Coleridge would just spend it on drugs. The *North American Review* quoted Southey's reply to Cottle: "*He promises, and does nothing.* Nothing is wanting [needed] to make him easy in circumstances, and happy in himself, but to leave off opium."[89] In 1847, a reviewer for *Graham's Magazine* predicted that Cottle's memoir would bring "deep pain" to the poet's fans. He emphasized that Coleridge was as

> given over to sloth and self-indulgence, as careless of his word, as indifferent to the happiness and comfort of his wife and children, as a deceitful and unsafe friend, as a kind of sublime charlatan and vagabond.

This behavior included asking friends for money for necessities and then spending it "gratifying his debasing habit." And Coleridge paid a great deal for opium "at the very time his family were suffering, and he himself was living on the charity of a friend."[90]

Although Coleridge likely experienced genuine remorse, it appears that he often expressed contrition to spur his correspondents to loan him money. He dwelled on his failures in an 1815 letter to Cottle. After lamenting his shortcomings, Coleridge asked Cottle to "advance him thirty or forty pounds" against his upcoming writings. Cottle sent him only five pounds. He knew how Coleridge would spend the money, since he "uses from two to three quarts of laudanum weekly," as a writer for *Harper's* explained in relaying the episode. Cottle received another letter from Coleridge three days later, in which he "still more piteously" asked for money. It was the last letter that Coleridge would send him.[91]

Some Americans hoped that such stories would prevent youth from trying the drug. A writer for the Presbyterian *Princeton Review*, for example, was glad that Cottle had revealed the "revolting truth" about the drug's effects and hoped the information would reach "all who may be venturing on this species of sensual indulgence." Writing in 1848, he reported that it was "fashionable" among "youth in some literary institutions, and doubtless elsewhere," to use "Turkish and other tobacco prepared with an infusion of opium." He also drew attention to the fact that Coleridge's dependency negatively affected his family: "His wife and three fine children were wholly neglected by him," he wrote. "He did not even write to them or open their letters to him."[92]

There were disagreements regarding the degree to which Coleridge deserved blame or sympathy. The year after the poet's death, Gillman learned that Cottle planned to allege that Coleridge's poor health "had been solely due to self-indulgent opium habits." The doctor contacted Cottle and tried to convince him that it traced back to a different ailment.[93] And Dr. James Davenport Whelpley, in the Whig publication *American Review*, acknowledged that Coleridge's life "became one of almost entire depend[e]nce." Yet he forgave him for lying to his friends. He likened the behavior to that of a "convalescent, who will venture upon harmless lies to obtain a larger quantity of food." He maintained that Coleridge's falsehoods derived not from "depravity of heart," but "solely out of physical weakness and a desire to escape the surv[ei]llance of friends."[94]

Similarly, the publication of *Confessions* had inspired a debate regarding the habitué's culpability for his condition. De Quincey denied that he was to blame for his state on the grounds that he began using opium for medical purposes. He asserted that "infirmity and misery do not, of necessity, imply guilt," and he refuted the idea that he "brought upon myself all the sufferings which I shall have to record." He also explained that he began to use opium daily "not for the purpose of creating pleasure, but of mitigating pain in the severest degree." The distinction addresses an important and enduring aspect of perceptions of addiction: then as now, there was greater sympathy for habitués who began using a drug after being prescribed it for an ailment rather than for pleasure-seeking reasons. That is, there is greater sympathy for those who take a drug in order to remain productive than those whose use will cause them to abnegate their responsibilities. From his writing, it is clear that De Quincey had faced many critics. They would ask him, how could a "reasonable being knowingly ... fetter himself with such a seven-foot chain?"[95] The focus was on the intention regarding the first use. Many treated him, in the words of Tobias Smollett, as "the author of his misfortune."[96] This helps to explain the defensive tone of De Quincey's work.

De Quincey was somewhat vulnerable on this count, as he acknowledged in *Confessions* that although he began to use the drug for medicinal purposes, he would have "a debauch of opium" once every three weeks or so for several years, to enhance his enjoyment of the opera.[97] Richard Davenport-Hines has pointed out that "these musical opium evenings established De Quincey as among the first Europeans consciously to take a drug to enhance aesthetic pleasure rather than to desensitize pain."[98] Of these years, De Quincey would insist that he had been "ignorant and unsuspicious of the avenging terrors which opium has in store for those who abuse its lenity." Therefore, he argued, he should not be blamed, because he had no way of knowing that he was playing with fire. Furthermore, he only became a "confirmed opium-eater" in 1813, due to personal challenges—a "very melancholy event" in 1812 and a subsequent "appalling irritation of the stomach."[99] He came to rely on the drug not for enjoyment but to try to restore a sense of well-being. As Virginia Berridge and Griffith Edwards have noted, however, both Coleridge and De Quincey demonstrate an "intertwining of 'social' and 'medical' usage so much a feature of opiate use at the time," as "self-medication could easily shade into recreational use."[100] This reality helps to explain why people could reach different conclusions and judgments about such usage.

Part of the criticism derived from the assumption that willpower should be sufficient to end problematic use. Consequently, many regarded active users as either weak-willed or selfish. A writer for the *Universalist Quarterly* referred to Samuel Taylor Coleridge's "record of his indulgence and weakness of will."[101] A writer whose article appeared in *Harper's New Monthly Magazine* stated that De Quincey had "the most potent of brains, and the weakest of wills, of almost all men who ever lived."[102] De Quincey, however, tried to impress upon readers that stopping use of a drug, once dependency had developed, was more difficult than they could imagine. When he began to use opium on a daily basis in 1813, he insisted, "I could not have done otherwise." And when he tried to diminish his usage, the people around him insisted that he end the endeavor, due to his suffering: "Those who witnessed the agonies of those attempts, and not myself, were the first to beg me to desist," he recalled. He spoke critically of "inhuman moralist[s]" he encountered, and he believed that people should "show some conscience in the penances they inflict," especially when dealing with someone in "the infirm condition of an opium-eater." He insisted that although a user could diminish the amount that he took, he could not reduce it past a certain level without "intense suffering," distress that non-users could not comprehend.[103] To try to appeal to his audience or to resolve his tale, he stated that he had almost completely weaned himself from the drug—a feat that few had accomplished.[104]

An American doctor who saw drug dependency up close corroborated De Quincey's views. In 1834, the physician chronicled his own efforts to help a patient who was trying to end his opium use. After working with the patient, the doctor "fell in with a book, which treats of the very subject," as he recalled. It was *Confessions*. He noted that De Quincey's conclusions coincided with his own regarding "the nature and operation of the medicine" and confirmed his beliefs regarding "the difficulties attending a relinquishment of the habitual use of it."[105] Not everybody, however, shared this recognition.

\* \* \*

One story of addiction could be illuminating, but it cannot be regarded as typical or as capturing all the dimensions of such a complex experience. *Confessions* did not mirror the American experience of drug habituation at the time. De Quincey referred only to male habitués—although many Englishwomen were also habituated—and he focused on opium's ability to bestow clarity and new insights to its users.[106] Most Americans dependent on the drug at the time were women who began using it under a doctor's care and who continued using it to avoid withdrawal. Evidence exists that it served as a kind of Valium, to allay boredom, unhappiness, or loneliness, and some experienced opium's pleasures.[107] Women's reasons for continuing to use the drug after the immediate medical need had passed, therefore, appear far different from De Quincey's efforts to increase his enjoyment of the opera or to explore his dreams. Also, while De Quincey dwelled on the negative impact of opium use on himself, he did not address the hardship that his use created for his family. As Keith Humphreys has observed, De Quincey, "like many heavy drug users," focused on himself when addressing "the costs of his behaviour." His "long absences from and poor treatment of his wife and children are never mentioned."[108]

*Confessions* would, however, remain in the American consciousness when concerns with domestic drug use grew. Writers still referred to it in the 1880s, when American drug addiction was receiving extensive public attention. By that point, the initial, casual interest in overseas drug use had been replaced with grave concern for American youth. Over time, Americans who read *Confessions* had derived different lessons from it, as domestic sentiment regarding drug dependency changed. At first, De Quincey's account was intriguing but not relevant. It inspired readers to consider how far the drug might expand the limits of their own minds. At midcentury, some suggested that opium could curtail the productivity of those who used it, while others insisted that it could enhance users' intellectual potential. In the atmosphere of anxiety in the 1880s, it would be read as the cautionary tale that Thomas De Quincey had intended it to be.

\* \* \*

Some Americans who wrote about De Quincey were surprised that he could not avoid habituation, as they had assumed that well-educated white people could summon the fortitude required to prevent drug dependency. The following decade, many Americans would be dismayed to learn that Great Britain supplied China with opium for nonmedical use despite its illegality and its demoralizing effects on the Chinese population. News from China would also demonstrate to Americans the national consequences of widespread habituation, and the First Opium War between Great Britain and China would indicate how determined some countries were to ensure that the trade would continue.

# The Drug Trade and Habitual Use in China, 1804–1881

Reports of opiate dependency in England had established that Westerners were among the habitués, and Thomas De Quincey's memoir had provided insights about the effects of opiates from the user's perspective. Even so, most Americans continued to believe that dependency was much more common in the East, a belief that was strengthened by information coming from China. Descriptions of opium smoking in that country and reports of the first Anglo-Chinese Opium War, in the early 1840s, demonstrated the possible implications of widespread dependency. To many Americans, China was the quintessential example of how extensive drug abuse could ravage a nation. In his study of "Narcotics," Dr. David Cheever addressed the devastating effects of opium habituation in China. He included the oft-quoted comments of American missionary Dyer Ball who stated that habitual drug use in China produced "walking skeletons," people who had lost their homes, and families "wretched and beggared by drugged fathers and husbands."[1]

Cheever blamed the Chinese to some extent for their situation but saved most of his ire for Great Britain. There was, he admitted, extensive opium cultivation in China itself. There were "valleys upon valleys of fine, rich land covered with poppies" beyond the mountains that surrounded the Ningbo plain. Still, he blamed "English avarice" for much of China's "misery," as Great Britain grew wealthy from the cultivation of opium in India and its sale in China. Great Britain had promoted a habit that had become so widespread that laws in China against opium's importation and use were "practically a dead letter."[2] Like Cheever, many Americans were aghast at Great Britain's determination to sustain the opium trade in China, and the first Anglo-Chinese Opium War educated them on important aspects of the trade.

\* \* \*

*Habit Forming.* Elizabeth Kelly Gray, Oxford University Press. © Oxford University Press 2023.
DOI: 10.1093/oso/9780190073121.003.0007

Around 1840, American missionary Henrietta Hall Shuck visited a Chinese opium den, an establishment that catered to opium smokers. Opium smoking had begun in Southeast Asia soon after the introduction of tobacco, and the practice had proliferated in China in the eighteenth century.[3] In the dens, smokers could find pipes and the rest of the smoking "layout," assistance in preparing the pipes for smoking, and perhaps a sense of community.[4] The den that Shuck entered was not one of the "*respectable* opium shops," she later explained, yet many less respectable ones existed throughout China. The room was filled with "old couches," and the floor was the "damp ground." The proprietor stood in the middle of the room, eyeing her suspiciously. A customer, an "old man, of haggard countenance," was lying down, resting his head on a wooden block. He heated a ball of opium, then applied it to his pipe and took "several quick whiffs." He repeated the process and entered a state of "silly stupefaction." Shuck surmised that another customer, a young man of about twenty, would rather "go supperless" than forgo his pipe. Opium smoking had become a national problem. Although the practice had long existed, Shuck explained that it had been "only within the last fifty years that its consumption has been so enormous." And users were failing to meet their obligations. Customers were "inhaling the stupefying poison, while their families are starving at home," she lamented. She considered the trade "one of the most enormous national sins known upon earth." Yet many participants justified their roles in it. For example, the shop's proprietor told Shuck that " 'if *he* dont supply the poison, some one else will.' "[5]

Many Americans back home read about opium smoking in China and were shocked at the toll it seemed to be taking on the nation. Most opium-related news pertained to the First Opium War, in which China, in 1839, challenged Great Britain in an effort to end that nation's importation of the drug. Drug abuse had grievously affected the country, despite its long and proud history and extensive resources. Francis Wharton, a Yale graduate who was beginning his career in the law, noted in 1843 that China's story "goes back centuries behind the Christian era." Its "population exceeds three hundred and fifty millions," he added, and its "agricultural resources are richer than those of all Europe together." Yet, due to opium, the nation was "tottering on its foundations."[6]

Reports about the First Opium War educated Americans about the international drug trade, including the moral issues that it raised and the parties involved. These included Indian cultivators who were compelled by the British East India Company to grow poppies, British merchants who pursued enormous profits, and huge numbers of besotted Chinese customers. Updates about the conflict revealed how lucrative the trade was and, consequently, how determined merchants were to preserve it. Earlier accounts of global drug use had not focused on those who sold the drugs without the pretense of medical need. Some merchants in China rationalized their participation by suggesting that smoking opium was no worse than drinking alcohol, while others pointed to users' complicity or to Chinese officials who facilitated the trade. Some American merchants were involved in the trade but, at the time, few of their countrymen back home suspected their participation.

American publications included descriptions of smokers who seemed unable to speak for themselves, but Chinese efforts to end the importation of opium provided a clear Chinese voice rejecting the trade. The fact that the British government, which was Christian and Western, defended the trade shocked many Americans, as did the realization that the non-Christian Chinese were behaving in the more principled manner as they sought to end it. American merchants who were involved in the trade justified their role, much as their British counterparts did. News of the war sparked a discussion about whether a society had the right to ban a drug that had a detrimental effect, and many Americans agreed that it did.

\* \* \*

The type of opium that is smoked differs significantly from that used as a medicine. In China, crude opium from India was refined into opium for smoking.[7] The process involves repeatedly soaking crude opium in water and letting the water evaporate until it becomes "a treacle-like mass," as ethnographer Stewart Culin has explained.[8] The process takes several months. Someone who smoked medical opium would feel no effects from the practice.[9] Because it was onerous to convert medical opium to smoking opium, the two can be regarded as distinct substances.[10]

The effect of opium smoking was different from that of other opiates, and many nineteenth-century doctors regarded it as less harmful than opium eating and morphine habituation.[11] It was not without negative effects; it could cause constipation, lethargy, and pulmonary disease, and many users would become addicted. But the opium-smoking habit took longer to form than did addiction to other opiates, and it was typically easier to break. Its impact on users helps to explain its appeal and the reduced level of risk associated with it. When someone smokes opium, the morphine vapor is "absorbed across the lining of the lungs into the bloodstream, and reaches the brain within seconds," according to pharmacologist Harold Kalant. Its impact is more rapid than that of eating or drinking an opiate, thus enhancing the attraction of smoking. But its effects are less enduring, and the amounts that are absorbed are smaller—"a little at a time, from each separate puff," Kalant points out.[12] Because of its rapid effects, users can adjust their consumption more easily than those who consume opium in other forms. The likelihood of an overdose is also diminished since users are likely to "pass out, fall asleep or otherwise lose consciousness" after smoking, as historian Carl Trocki observes.[13]

The perception that opium smoking led to "social and physical ruin" has been overstated, according to historian Richard Newman, whose research focused on the 1870s. For only "a small proportion" of smokers did the practice become ruinous, and some of them could have been self-medicating to treat a chronic illness. Even many habitual users were able to remain productive.[14] For many Chinese, in fact, opium smoking enhanced their productivity. The practice could relieve fatigue and suppress hunger, helpful effects for those who worked hard for long hours, including police officers, rickshaw drivers, waiters, and waitresses.[15]

Chronic opium smoking, however, can be ruinous. In addition to enduring constipation and pulmonary disease, habitual users can experience loss of memory, reduced fertility, and weight loss, which results from the appetite suppression. They also become unproductive. As Kalant notes, these opium smokers are often deemed lazy because, as a result of their "tiredness and lethargy . . . they sleep late and work only sporadically." This leads to loss of income and neglect of their families.[16]

By the time the First Opium War began, the Chinese government had been trying, unsuccessfully, to end the opium trade for more than a hundred years. The Portuguese had begun selling opium in China in the early seventeenth century, and the Chinese used it as a medicine. Pleasure-seeking opium use became widespread among the Chinese over the course of the century.[17] In 1729, China's emperor forbade the sale and distribution of the form of opium that is smoked. Penalties were harsh: possession could lead to a ten-year prison sentence or a hundred lashes, while opium merchants and den operators risked execution. Nonetheless, consumption continued to increase.[18] In 1773, the British East India Company secured a monopoly on the opium in Bengal, and Company officials worked with smugglers who delivered the drug to China.[19] In 1780, China limited opium importation to what was needed for medical use, and in 1799, the nation banned its importation altogether. Subsequent Chinese emperors also inveighed against the traffic. These actions, however, were ineffective.[20]

For Great Britain, opium profits reversed a negative balance of trade, but the arrangement was precarious. By 1800, the British were drinking twenty million pounds of Chinese tea annually, which they paid for with silver. Extensive British demand for Chinese silk and porcelain added to the trade imbalance. To address the situation, the British had sought a product that would be popular in China, and they found it in opium. By the 1830s, opium sales were bringing in about £1 million annually to Great Britain and thus shifted the balance of trade in its favor.[21] The trade was, of course, morally problematic at best, but those who tried to end it or diminish it were unsuccessful. The Company forced the Bengalese to cultivate poppies, and Governor-General Charles Cornwallis wanted to end the monopoly in order to end the oppression, but Prime Minister William Pitt overruled him, because the Company depended so heavily on the commerce.[22] In the 1790s, Warren Hastings, the governor of Bengal, spoke out against the increasing use of opium in India. He deemed the drug "a pernicious article of luxury" that should be allowed "for the purposes of foreign commerce only."[23] Great Britain, however, would fight to preserve that trade.

China's government was concerned with the opium traffic's effects on its economy and its population. In the early nineteenth century, opium was *"probably the largest commerce of the time in any single commodity,"* according to economic historian Michael Greenberg.[24] In China in the early 1830s, the growing trade was leading to both the "increasing demoralization of the people, and the swelling drain of sycee silver in payment," according to a writer for New York's *Merchants' Magazine.* The silver payments increased China's deficit and prompted higher taxes. By 1837, opium constituted about 57 percent of China's imports. When China tried to suppress the trade, they saw how determined Great Britain was to sustain it. Other efforts to combat the trade, such as destroying opium poppies and seizing opium in transit, failed to diminish consumption.[25]

Great Britain's economic dependence on the opium trade helps to explain the nation's determination to preserve it. In the 1830s, opium "constituted about two-thirds of the value of all British imports into China," according to Greenberg.[26] Despite bans on the commerce, opium importation increased from the 1820s throughout the century.[27] The outcome of the Opium War would have huge implications, regardless of the result. Either Great Britain would lose a major portion of its revenue, as Seeley and Glover law clerk E. W. Stoughton opined, or China would "fall an easy unresisting prey to a rapacious and powerful adversary."[28]

In assessing the situation, it is important to recognize China's role in creating its opium problem. The Chinese demand for opium predated Great Britain's role in selling it, and the Chinese cultivated poppies, with some selecting such lucrative work instead of growing much-needed grains.[29] In addition, the timing of the Chinese crackdown on opium smuggling could have resulted from politics between the Han Chinese and Manchu people rather than being shaped by British actions. In the 1830s, Han scholars believed that advocating opium prohibition could help them to challenge Manchu aristocrats and thereby enhance their own power, and the emperor supported prohibition.[30] Moreover, Chinese smokers made the decision to smoke opium. All this said, Great Britain still deserves censure for promoting the trade. As Dr. H. H. Kane wrote in 1881, "The Chinese *smokers* themselves are not free from blame, but every honest observer *must* believe that if China had been allowed to have her own way the vice, to-day, would be nearly dead."[31]

\* \* \*

Some American merchants imported opium into China. Americans had entered the China trade in 1784, when the *Empress of China* sailed from New York to Macao.[32] Many of these merchants were scions of respected families in Boston, Philadelphia, and elsewhere who traveled to China to make fortunes. They began bringing opium from Smyrna—now Izmir, Turkey—to China around 1804.[33] By 1818, American merchants were supplying China with between one-fifth and one-third of its opium supply.[34] Their work violated Chinese law. Because they were so far from home, however, they were able to conduct this business for decades while Americans back home were none the wiser. Many American merchants who were involved in the trade obscured the source of their wealth, and those who did not were publicly criticized.[35]

American merchants knew the importation of opium into China was illegal, but many participated nonetheless, and for a long time, the trade proceeded largely unimpeded. In his memoir, Samuel Shaw, who served as America's first consul to China, acknowledged that opium in China was "absolutely contraband, and cannot legally be admitted into their ports." He added, however, that the trade could turn a "handsome profit" and that a merchant could smuggle it in at Guangzhou (Canton) "with the utmost security."[36] In an 1806 letter, Stephen Girard admitted knowing that opium was "prohibited at Canton." He also knew that there was "no difficulty in shipping" if one exercised care.[37] And in 1819, even though a member of the American firm Perkins and Co. wrote from Guangzhou that the opium trade was "considered a very *disreputable* business," the company became involved in it because "the benefit is great."[38]

American merchants who dealt in opium rarely saw the merchandise. As historian Jacques Downs has explained, the "Lintin system" was arranged in such a way that they kept it out of sight. With this system, Western ships would drop off their opium at Nei Lingding Island (Lintin), near Guangdong. Chinese smugglers would then buy "opium chits" in Guangzhou and present them at Nei Lingding Island, along with a bribe, to get their opium. As Downs notes, the Chinese dealers handled the "dangerous and unpleasant part of the business—bribing officials, delivering the narcotic ashore, and retailing to addicts." He adds that Americans' technological superiority served them well: their opium schooners were faster than any Chinese craft.[39] John Latimer of Wilmington, Delaware, who oversaw opium sales, believed the system of selling the illegal drug was "perfect," because "we never see it."[40] As historian Peter Fay observed, "One might almost suppose that to diffuse and dilute responsibility had been the whole intent of the arrangement."[41]

American merchants were aloof from aspects of the trade, but they were aware of opium's negative effects on its users. There were two opium dens not far from their "factories," the term for establishments where overseas merchants conducted business. And in 1844, Edward Delano visited several dens in Singapore. In one, he recalled, he found a man who was "prostrate under its effects—pale, cadaverous, death-like." When Delano took the man's pipe from him, "he offered no resistance, though his eyes tried to follow me."[42] When writing to his wife from Guangzhou in 1839, Robert Bennet Forbes admitted that the opium trade in China was "demoralizing the minds, destroying the bodies, & draining the country of money."[43] Part of what made the trade possible, Downs has suggested, was that American merchants regarded the Chinese people as so different from themselves that they had no reservations about selling them a dangerous drug. It appeared that the "rules of proper behavior somehow do not apply" when selling to "strange foreigners," Downs observed. Because the merchants defined the Chinese as "alien and somehow bad," he added, they believed they could treat them in an unprincipled manner. This made the opium trade "psychologically possible."[44]

\* \* \*

In 1839, the Chinese government sought to end the commerce due to the negative social consequences of widespread opium use and the growing unfavorable balance of trade.[45] According to Downs, the trade was an "unmixed evil" for China. It was "corrupting its officialdom, demoralizing its people, . . . draining its specie, raising the cost of living and generally undermining its authority, [and] its finances."[46] Lin Zexu, governor of the Huguang province, feared that soldiers would become habituated, thus leaving the country unable to defend itself. The emperor put Lin in charge of the crackdown on the trade. In 1839, Commissioner Lin compelled foreign merchants to surrender their opium. He confined the merchants in their factories for several weeks and confiscated more than twenty thousand chests of the drug, which were then destroyed.[47] The amount that was confiscated demonstrates how determined Great Britain was to pursue the trade, as historian Steffen Rimner has noted. Each chest weighed about 140 pounds. It took five hundred men more than three weeks to empty the opium "to the bottom of the sea."[48]

For the British, the crackdown posed a significant economic threat. Their opium was produced in India, and as long as India and China cooperated in the commerce, the British East India Company realized huge profits. Loss of China's opium market would upend that lucrative arrangement. There was also a wish to avenge the Chinese treatment of British merchants, which the government regarded as humiliating.[49] Commissioner Lin had anticipated that Great Britain, distant and comparatively small, would find the prospect of war with China daunting and would not want to risk losing the rest of the nation's trade.[50]

The British government, however, emphasizing their concern with the Chinese government's conduct, sent warships to China. After two and a half years of skirmishing, the Chinese government capitulated. In the 1842 Treaty of Nanjing (Nanking), the British gained access to five ports. Two years later, in the Treaty of Wangxia, the United States received the same rights.[51] Following another Opium War in 1858, China allowed for the legal importation of opium, making it subject to a tariff.[52]

*　*　*

The Opium War introduced American observers back home to the moral and economic complexities of the pleasure-seeking drug trade, in which both sellers and buyers bore responsibility. The trade could not have thrived without the involvement of the Chinese who participated in the commerce as well as the Chinese habitués. Some depicted Chinese smokers as if they played no conscious role in their dependency. In 1842, for example, missionary William B. Diver wrote of Chinese opium smokers that "the deluded inhabitants have been seduced into a destructive habit."[53] To focus solely on Great Britain's role ignores Chinese agency: the degree to which the Chinese people participated in the commerce voluntarily, either by buying the drug or by helping to make it available. Such a perspective also reinforces the notion, as seen with earlier travelers' accounts of the non-Western world, that Eastern populations indulged in intoxicants thoughtlessly, and the concomitant belief that Western habitués' inclination to think about their situation distinguished Eastern from Western users. British and American merchants asserted that their trade was possible only with Chinese customers and cooperative Chinese officials, and they were not wrong.

Opium merchants, however, blamed the Chinese for the trade and tried to diminish their own culpability in three main ways. They suggested that it was not truly illegal, since some corrupt Chinese officials participated. They suggested that the emperor was mainly concerned with the trade's financial consequences, rather than with opium's effects on its users, to try to downplay the seriousness of those effects. Finally, they suggested that if they were to abandon the trade, new sellers would take their place; therefore, their exodus would do no good. Pierre Caquet notes that all three arguments had "partial validity," yet he points out that these arguments constituted their entire defense. Advocates for the opium trade did not defend it "on its own terms."[54]

American opium merchants tended to justify the trade, publicly or privately, in part by suggesting that selling opium was akin to selling liquor. In his 1876 memoir, Robert Bennet Forbes acknowledged that opium was "demoralizing to a certain extent" but suggested that it had no worse effect on users than "the use of ardent spirits."[55] In a letter to his family Warren Delano agreed, stating that importing opium into China should be no more objectionable than importing "wines, Brandies & spirits into the U. States, England, &c."[56] And in his recollections of his time in China in the early 1850s, where he worked for a merchant company, Henry Blaney made the habit sound harmless. Many members of China's upper class smoked opium secretly, he explained, "just as many an old lady at home takes a quiet Cordial" and then blames her red nose on the sun.[57] A missionary in Batavia in 1834 agreed with the analogy, but he saw both situations as worrisome. He acknowledged that the scene in an opium den resembled what someone might have seen in a Massachusetts "country grog-shop" at sunrise. He maintained that both were awful, and the only difference was a matter of scale. Americans familiar with intemperance had seen "the living putrid carcass of a drunkard," he wrote. "But where rum has slain its thousands," he added, "opium has slain its tens of thousands" in Southeast Asia.[58]

Some American opium merchants suggested that were they to leave, others would simply take their place in the trade, so they might as well continue with it. John Jacob Astor, for example, sold opium because "inasmuch as 'everyone else does it,' he saw no reason why he should not profit from the illicit business," according to historian John Upton Terrell. Astor was not alone. By 1830, Boston merchant Thomas Handasyd Perkins had personal wealth valued at more than $700,000, most of it earned through selling opium. And when American merchants asked Congress for protection during the Opium War, they acknowledged their involvement in the "extensive opium trade." Meanwhile, some opium dealers had characterized merchants who abstained from the trade not as law-abiding, but as "squeamish," thereby suggesting that the abstainers' behavior—not their own—was out of step.[59] The New York firm Olyphant and Co. was unusual in that it steered clear of the opium commerce. Although the trade's illegality made it risky, it appears that D. W. C. Olyphant, the firm's head in Guangzhou, made his decision based on religious considerations. His piety had originated during America's Second Great Awakening, and a missionary friend explained that Olyphant "conscientiously declines dealing in the pernicious drug." Other merchants might have found it unnerving that a merchant could succeed with an approach that was legal and morally sound. They called the company "Zion's Corner," a nickname that they intended to be derisive.[60]

Time and again, the British pointed to the involvement of Chinese officials in the trade to justify their continuation of it, suggesting that official Chinese opposition was insincere; but Americans back home questioned this argument. The British maintained that some Chinese officials "who issued prohibitory edicts with one hand extended the other to receive bribes from illegal traders," as sociologist Richard Harvey Brown has explained.[61] Owners of opium clippers sometimes received advance word if their boats were going to be searched.[62]

Some tried to assert that the trade was, therefore, legitimate. George Davidson, the author of *Trade and Travel in the East* (1846), insisted that no more than 1 percent of the opium brought into China was smuggled in. On almost all of it, he wrote, merchants paid "a heavy duty (miscalled a bribe)," much of which went to the Chinese government. He added that residents of Beijing's "imperial palace" consumed "large quantities" of the drug. As a result, he dismissed criticisms of the trade. The staff of *Hunt's Merchants' Magazine*, which carried his comments, stated in the preface that the "morality of his remarks . . . [is] rather questionable."[63]

Some Americans, however, appeared to support the notion that British opium merchants, because they were esteemed men of high station, should not be regarded as criminals. In 1848, the *American Journal of Pharmacy* reprinted, without comment, observations of Robert Fortune, a Scottish botanist who had spent three years in China. Fortune insisted that the entire "civilized world" regarded British opium sellers as "merchants of the first class." Society, he added, should condone their behavior despite its illegality. He admitted that opium was "contraband" but believed the merchants' work was "so unlike what is generally called smuggling" that the term, in this instance, was misleading.[64]

Also, some well-to-do Americans insisted that the opium commerce could not be eliminated and that China should therefore legalize it, despite its destructive effects. In 1857, for example, businessman George Francis Train averred that keeping opium out of China would be as difficult as "keep[ing] back the waves of the sea." He believed that East India Company officials should ignore criticism of the practice. As long as they "continue to derive $18,000,000 revenue per annum," he wrote, "what do they care for newspaper squibs and Buncom [pretentious and insincere] editorials?"[65] In 1853, Dr. William Ruschenberger in the *Southern Literary Messenger* recommended legalizing the trade, which the Chinese "do not approve but cannot prevent." In the same paragraph, he urged legalization of the international slave trade, "another contraband trade which all deprecate but cannot prevent."[66] In the 1850s, it was not unusual for the domestic slavery debate to influence Americans' opinions of news from abroad.[67]

American missionaries in China wanted the nation to be more open to the world, and some interpreted the Opium War as providential, since the conflict helped to open China to Christianity. From their perspective, something evil was being used for good purposes. Dr. Peter Parker, a medical missionary in Guangdong, regarded the war "not so much as an opium or an English affair, as a great design of Providence to make the wickedness of man subserve his purposes of mercy towards China," with the goal of "bringing the empire into more immediate contact with Western and Christian nations."[68] Henrietta Shuck shared this interpretation. She acknowledged that the war had caused "much devastation, and many deaths" but pointed out that it had "been the means of opening the closed doors to the heralds of the cross."[69] In 1840, a writer for the *United States Magazine and Democratic Review* agreed that "Providence" had brought about the war. The Chinese, he explained, were "bigoted, intolerant, incommunicative, and selfish," and their aloofness from the world had blocked the spread of Christianity in their land. Since other efforts to open China had failed, he maintained, it was likely "destined" that this would be accomplished through the "force of foreign arms."[70]

\* \* \*

Many Americans, however, sided with China, seeing Great Britain's actions as illegal and immoral. A writer for the *New York Herald* wrote, "What cause of grievance the British originally had, does not so clearly appear. They smuggled opium contrary to law, and the Chinese destroyed it."[71] In the midst of the war, New York lawyer Edwin Stoughton wondered what would have happened if American merchants had been "smuggling goods into the Liverpool market, in open defiance of English laws." He doubted that they would have been let off simply by turning over the goods and agreeing to "go and sin no more." He regarded the British system as immoral. For the British to see the effects of their policies, Stoughton suggested that British statesmen "look upon the dark face of their vast Indian empire, and there mark the gloomy bondage of millions and tens of millions, chained to the cultivation of a drug."[72]

Many Americans were shocked and disappointed that "Christian" Great Britain would fight to preserve a trade that they knew the Chinese were right to oppose. A writer for the Congregationalist *Boston Recorder* expressed dismay: "When has a Christian and civilized nation been engaged in a more disgraceful enterprise!"[73] A writer for the *Christian Examiner* also saw the profound inconsistency. The nation that was "foremost in the great duty of christianizing the world," he wrote, should not "[poison] a whole people" "for purposes of national aggrandizement."[74]

And just as many Americans were appalled by the British determination to preserve the trade, so were they heartened by the Chinese priorities, as they destroyed the confiscated opium. In his 1877 travel memoir, the Reverend Henry Martyn Field wrote that the Chinese had destroyed the opium, "throwing it overboard, as our fathers destroyed the tea in Boston harbor."[75] A writer for the *Christian Register and Boston Observer* deemed it "truly sublime" that the "sovereign of a great nation" had used its power "for the destruction of its chief social evil."[76] Nathan Allen agreed. In his 1850 study of the opium trade, he marveled that the Chinese government could have made millions of dollars by selling the confiscated opium, but they destroyed it rather than profit from "the ruin of their own people."[77]

Some who criticized the opium trade were disturbed that men who had every advantage had chosen an immoral career, pointing out that because of their high class standing, they avoided criticism. In 1855, a missionary, writing about the trade for New York's *National Magazine*, asserted that one of its "most painful features" was the merchants' high level of refinement. "They are not low, vulgar, degraded outlaws," he wrote, nor were they unsuccessful businessmen whose destitution could explain their participation. Instead, they were "gentlemen of intelligence and fortune." He was dismayed that these men—wealthy, well educated, and "accomplished in all the arts and elegancies of social life"—had chosen such an "unworthy trade." He added that they would have gotten "the contempt and hatred of the world" had they been "low, ignorant, and impoverished retailers of the fatal poison."[78] It was, he asserted, a "great moral evil" to manufacture opium for the purpose of "creating and gratifying an unnatural and morbid appetite for its momentary exhilaration," and it would lead to "physical, intellectual, and moral consequences of the most deplorable character." When defenders of the trade pointed to the profits, he responded, "For three millions sterling, must China and India be sacrificed?"[79]

Some Americans asserted that the opium trade was more exploitative than slavery, perhaps to attract readers' attention at a time of intense focus on slavery's future. In *Travels in South-Eastern Asia* (1839), the Reverend Howard Malcom, a Philadelphia native, had asserted that "the horrors of the opium trade" were "worse to its victims than any outward slavery." Nathan Allen reprinted these comments in his *Essay on the Opium Trade* (1850).[80] When Allen's essay was published, Congress was debating the compromise that would address, among other things, whether slavery would extend into the Mexican Cession. In 1853, a writer for the *New-York Observer* similarly maintained that when compared with the opium trade, "the slave trade in its worst forms, loses all its horrors." He maintained that there were more "*slaves of opium*" than enslaved African Americans and that the number of smokers who died annually from their habit exceeded the number of enslaved people who were, in a given year, separated from their families through sale. For many reasons, such comparisons were inapt. Smokers, for example, bore some responsibility for their circumstances. The writer, who opposed slavery, drew the comparison to challenge the notion that England was superior to the United States. He criticized "English travellers and writers" who denounced American slavery and who pointed out that Parliament had abolished slavery in the British Empire. He suggested that, while Great Britain had abolished slavery, it still permitted grave forms of exploitation that should be condemned.[81]

Unsurprisingly, some who declared the opium trade worse than slavery were proslavery themselves. In 1840, South Carolina Senator John C. Calhoun suggested that the opium trade was more damaging than the slave trade. In doing so, he derided slavery's critics. He stated that had China not challenged the opium commerce the previous year, Great Britain would be providing enough opium for "thirteen or fourteen millions of opium-smokers." That would have meant "a greater destruction of life annually" from opium, he asserted, than there were black people in the British West Indies, "whose condition has been the cause of so much morbid sympathy."[82] As historian Alastair Su has observed, slaveholders saw the opium trade as "a potent cudgel to defend chattel slavery" and to accuse the British of hypocrisy.[83]

\*\*\*

Reports from China suggested that widespread nonmedical opium use would not just affect the lives of its users, but it could have devastating effects for the nation as a whole. Several writers presented widespread opium smoking as having brought China's centuries of progress to a halt. Many Americans had known of China's achievements. In 1787, the *New Haven Gazette* had presented China as "a ravishing idea of the happiness the world might enjoy, were the laws of this empire the model of those of other countries," given its apparent ability to feed such a large population.[84] A writer for the *United States Magazine and Democratic Review* pointed out that when Europe was still "in barbarism," China could "boast of education, of printing, of civilization, of arts, and the conveniences and many of the luxuries of life."[85] In 1829, however, Benjamin Ellis wrote that the Chinese, after advancing a great deal as a civilization, had "suddenly stopped short in the career of improvement" and were unusual in that they were "stationary in the arts and sciences." The "consumption of drugs in that country is said to be immense," he added.[86] During the war, a writer for the *Advocate of Peace* stated, erroneously, that "this pernicious drug" had caused the country's rate of population growth to drop from 3 percent to 1 percent. There was a drop, but scholars have concluded that it was less pronounced and that it resulted primarily from natural disasters, including famines.[87] In 1841, a writer for the *Christian Examiner* warned that unless opium smoking were limited in China, "it will bring in a short time to the lowest pitch of degradation, an empire the most ancient and populous in the world."[88]

Others focused on the degree to which opium smokers became dependent on public support, a problem throughout much of Asia. In 1842, a doctor in Pulo Penang, an island in Malaysia, reported that "the hospitals and poor-houses are chiefly filled with opium-smokers." A Boston publication shared the observation.[89] In 1850, the *American Journal of the Medical Sciences* reported that thirty-five of the forty Chinese prisoners in the Singapore House of Corrections were opium smokers.[90]

Some writers suggested that opium smoking had diminished Chinese men's "manly" resolve, thus disrupting their households and weakening the nation. One suggested that even healthy Chinese men were not assertive, and they could not afford opium's debilitating effects. In 1862, a writer for *The Evangelist*, based in New York, asserted that "John Chinaman is not a giant at best" and that "the free use of opium destroys the little manhood that he has left."[91] Others criticized the fact that opium use shifted the burden of work to women. In 1871, a female missionary reported that a Chinese woman's husband might lounge "at home smoking tobacco, or, worse still, opium, while he sends her forth to plough, dig, or carry burdens for him."[92] Others focused on the national implications of widespread opium use. In 1853, a writer for *Gleason's Pictorial* stated that at least three million Chinese were "excessively addicted" to opium use, and the drug's influence was "debasing and brutalizing to the lowest degree. No wonder the nation is so weak and effeminate!"[93] In 1862, Dr. David Cheever wrote that men who became habitual opium smokers "lost their manliness." As a result, they "were unable either to resist their invaders or to live without them, since they supplied them with opium."[94]

*  *  *

The 1878 account of Zhang Changjia, a Chinese opium smoker, suggests that Chinese smokers' perspectives and the family dynamics that resulted from their drug use resembled those of their Western counterparts. His account was not available to American audiences at the time. Little is known about Zhang, whose text appeared in a collection of writings edited in Shanghai in the late nineteenth century. In it, he provided a rare first-person perspective of a Chinese opium smoker, as well as the perspectives of other habitués. According to Zhang, those who began to smoke opium knew the practice could lead to habituation, but they assumed they were "intelligent enough" to avoid it. Some young men, he asserted, planned to " 'wait until I'm on the verge [of addiction] and then I'll stop.' " As their use became compulsive, they maintained that they could control it, and they were later shocked to learn that they could not.[95]

Zhang stated that other Chinese criticized compulsive opium smokers and that opium use frayed smokers' relationships with friends and family. His assertion that opium use ruined "countless reputations" indicates that many Chinese neither smoked opium nor approved of it. Many smokers cut off ties with non-smokers, he wrote, reaching out to old acquaintances only to try to borrow money. Opium smoking also led to quarrels among friends and family members: "Fathers and brothers exhort the addict to quit," he wrote, "brothers fight and split up because of it, husbands and wives clash, friends cut you off."[96]

Zhang's brother disapproved of his opium smoking and once, pointing to his opium layout, angrily asked him, "'What do you get from it that makes you so transfixed?'" He encouraged Zhang to focus on "flowers and beautiful women" instead. Zhang maintained that men who smoked opium and had families to support "should be ashamed" of themselves, since their decisions could have the consequence of "starving their wives and families," while they spent time and money on opium. He insisted that parents should forbid their sons from smoking opium. "Whoever tells him to smoke at home and be 'a little more sparing,'" he wrote, "is already at the stage of absolute hopelessness."[97]

Zhang included poems written by other habitués, who identified the drug's origin as Western but who also enjoyed its effects, while others criticized them. One habitué stated that "In famine," he would "willingly put it [opium] before food." In another poem, titled "Singing of the Western Drug," a user described opium smoking as making him feel "sweet and free." A friend of Zhang's contrasted the notion of opium as a curse with the positive feelings that it could impart:

> Foreign ships from afar deliver their tribute of mud.
> From such earthly flames we turn into immortals.

Zhang also, however, quoted a friend who hated opium and who pointed out that smokers would fail to attain their potential. His poem read, in part:

> I know, sire, you have abandoned lofty ambition,
> happily taking up the company of your opium clouds.

Zhang wrote that reading this was like "being clubbed on the head and berated."[98]

While Zhang acknowledged that Chinese users bore responsibility for disregarding opium's risks, he also noted that ending use was more difficult than many non-smokers realized. He stated that opium smoking replaced gloominess with feeling "free and uninhibited" and left his eyes "sparkling with fresh energy." He acknowledged that England brought the opium but emphasized users' responsibility, especially as they knew of the risks of their use. "Once the Western lamp is lit," he wrote, "those whose eyes it meets come like moths flying into a flame." He emphasized the severity of addiction. At best, he had discovered that he could avoid the need for ever-increasing doses by avoiding smoking "until the urge to smoke is at its extreme." He considered his own habituation "irreversible," however, and stated that he had "entered a bitter sea and left the shore too far behind."[99]

\* \* \*

The First Opium War caused some Americans to consider whether a community had the right to ban a product that it deemed damaging, and many believed
that it did. Francis Wharton believed that the heart of the conflict was "whether
China shall be allowed the right of . . . rejecting such [articles] as she may think
injurious."[100] Edwin W. Stoughton, in the *Merchants' Magazine*, deemed Chinese
law forbidding opium to be "clear, absolute, and unlimited."[101] In 1853, New
Jersey senator Jacob Welsh Miller agreed, as he believed it was crucial that a
nation conduct its foreign commerce in a moral manner. Otherwise, it could
"require centuries to eradicate the evil." As examples, he pointed to African involvement in the slave trade as well as "the opium trade of the east, . . . the early
slave-trade of Spanish America, and . . . our whiskey dealings with the northern
tribes of Indians."[102]

Writing in 1850, Nathan Allen acknowledged that China still had laws against
the opium trade. Even so, the laws were "a dead letter," he lamented, as the
Chinese had made almost no effort to enforce them since the war.[103] Soon thereafter, Dr. Albert Welles Ely wrote in *De Bow's Review* that although importing
opium into China was still officially a capital offense, the law was disregarded.
"The smuggling of it is reduced to a regular system," he wrote, "and carried on
to a very great extent."[104] Throughout the nineteenth century, China had "one
of the highest rates of opiate addiction of any nation in the world," according to
David Courtwright.[105]

From the Western perspective, the connection between the Chinese and
opium smoking would persist. The opium pipe "became as much a symbol of
Chinese culture as the queue or the tea cup," as social scientist Stuart Creighton
Miller has observed, and publications after the First Opium War gave readers
the impression that "Chinese adults of all classes" were compulsive drug users. It
was not just American travelers or even adults who had this perception. In 1850,
students in three New York City public schools were asked to write down what
they knew about China. Among the students whose comments departed from
aspects such as population and commercial products, half cited habitual opium
use.[106] The association would endure. At the Louisiana Purchase Exposition in
St. Louis in 1903, the exhibit about Chinese culture would include a manne-
quin of an opium habitué and a display of opium pipes. Chinese visitors were
furious.[107]

* * *

By following news of the First Opium War, Americans saw some of the ways in
which widespread opium use could affect a society, and they saw the international trade networks that made such extensive use possible. News from China
and other foreign lands had provided Americans with information about many

aspects of drug habituation at a time when domestic dependency received little attention. Many Chinese men would soon emigrate to the United States, disheartened by the domestic turmoil caused by the Opium Wars and enticed by employment opportunities and the lure of gold. Some brought the practice of opium smoking with them. When American reporters and others would write about domestic, habitual drug use in the 1870s, many would focus on Chinese immigrants' opium smoking. A major reason for this attention was availability: while much domestic consumption was hidden, opium smokers gathered in public dens. Also, many native-born Americans regarded the Chinese as culturally different and unwelcome, partly in objection to the job competition they presented. Xenophobia would bolster support for some of the nation's first antidrug laws, which focused on opium smoking.

# PART III

# AN OPEN PROBLEM

# American Opium Dens, 1850–1910

Many Americans criticized Great Britain's determination to sustain the opium trade in China, but their identification of the Chinese and Chinese Americans with opium smoking would become more ingrained, as some Chinese men who immigrated to the American West brought the practice with them. Americans tended to regard pleasure-seeking drug use as a foreign practice because, for so long, cases of habituation among native-born Americans received little attention. Dr. David Cheever, however, noted that some people in "Christian nations" used laudanum as a "narcotic indulgence," and he correctly predicted that white Americans would increasingly avail themselves of opiates. Meanwhile, he pointed out, the United States's increased trade with Asia was leading some Americans to pursue "the imitation of Oriental habits."[1]

At the time that Cheever wrote, opium smoking in America was practiced only by some Chinese immigrants in the West.[2] Soon thereafter, members of the "white underworld" would pick up the practice, and it would move eastward. It then extended to members of "the so-called respectable class of men and women," at which point the first laws in the nation restricting access to drugs other than alcohol were passed.[3]

\* \* \*

One evening in 1875, writer Samuel Williams visited one of San Francisco's opium dens in the company of a police escort. Many white Americans were intrigued by the communities of Chinese immigrants, and entrepreneurs advertised tours of the neighborhoods, including their dens.[4] On their way to the establishment, Williams and the others had to "grope our way through a dismal court" and "squeeze through a narrow entry," he explained in *The City of the Golden Gate*. Once inside the den, he sensed the "fumes of the deadly drug" and saw the smokers, who were lying down. Although some were cheerful, he wrote, others "are sullen and scowl viciously at us." Others appeared to be

*Habit Forming*. Elizabeth Kelly Gray, Oxford University Press. © Oxford University Press 2023.
DOI: 10.1093/oso/9780190073121.003.0008

dreaming. One man, with an expression of "hopeless imbecility," disregarded the policeman's warning that the habit could kill him. Many of these men practically lived in the dens, Williams added, while others had jobs but spent all their money on opium.[5] Descriptions of the dens were popular with readers. Excerpts of Williams's book were reprinted in *Scribner's Monthly* magazine and elsewhere, and many similar accounts were published.[6]

With the exceptions of alcohol and tobacco use, opium smoking was the most visible form of habitual drug use in late nineteenth-century America. Users smoked it in public spaces, and many reporters wrote about it, because the topic interested the public. It was less harmful than other habit-forming drugs and was problematic for only a fraction of its users. It would, however, be the first drug banned in America, primarily due to its association with the marginalized Chinese American community and its lack of medical application. Anti-Chinese sentiment was widespread in this era, because some native-born Americans competed with Chinese immigrants for jobs and because many Americans were suspicious of a culture that seemed so different from their own. Some advocates of the 1882 Chinese Exclusion Act, which barred the immigration of Chinese laborers, pointed to opium use to suggest that Chinese immigrants were a menace.

The criticism intensified with reports that white Americans were smoking opium. Some members of the "white underworld" took up the habit, and later some members of the middle class did, including middle-class youth. The most ardent anti-Chinese comments focused on opium use by young white girls. Some white Americans accused Chinese den proprietors of luring them to the dens, but many of these allegations would be exposed as lies.

\* \* \*

A large number of young men left China in the mid-nineteenth century to escape difficult conditions at home and to pursue enticing opportunities abroad. The Opium Wars of the early 1840s and mid-1850s were devastating, and the subsequent famine and disease caused more than twenty million deaths.[7] By opening China more to the West, those wars had also made possible the large-scale recruitment of Chinese men to work abroad.[8] News of California's gold had reached China, and Californian entrepreneurs needed workers in mining and railroad construction. Between 1850 and 1880, America's Chinese population grew from 7,520 to 105,465.[9] Few Chinese women immigrated at this time for a variety of reasons. There was a Chinese cultural belief that married women should attend to their parents-in-law rather than travel with their husbands, and most of the men who came to America intended to return to China. Also, America's Chinese community endured "intense anti-Chinese hostility," as political scientist Sucheng Chan has pointed out, and the 1882 Chinese Exclusion Act severely restricted immigration. For a combination of reasons, as late as 1920, less than 13 percent of America's Chinese population was female.[10]

Many American railroad titans favored Chinese workers over Americans because they regarded the Chinese as especially industrious, dependable, and willing to work for low pay.[11] Also, Chester Crocker, superintendent of the Central Pacific Railroad, had had difficulty finding enough native-born workers to meet his labor needs.[12] He considered Chinese immigrants "nearly equal to white men in the amount of labor they perform" and "much more reliable" than their white counterparts. Leland Stanford, the railroad's president, deemed Chinese workers "quiet, peaceable, industrious, and economical"—"economical" likely referring to the fact that labor costs with a Chinese workforce were about three-fourths that of white employees.[13] By 1867, Chinese immigrants constituted 90 percent of the railroad's workforce.[14] Some Americans envisioned them as possessing additional useful skills. Industrialist Aaron H. Palmer predicted that once railroad construction was complete, they could work in agriculture. "No people in all the East," he wrote in 1839, "are so well adapted for clearing wild lands and raising every species of agricultural product . . . as the Chinese."[15]

Chinese immigrants endured opposition from native-born workers with whom they competed for jobs, and anti-Chinese sentiment was exacerbated by the era's economic depressions.[16] Some believed that Chinese industry and frugality would be devastating to white workers. In 1876, Thomas J. Vivian, who wrote for the *San Francisco Chronicle*, criticized their willingness to work for low wages. In so doing, he maintained, they were "degrading white labor to a bestial scale." If immigration continued as it had, he insisted, the state would either end up "bereft of white labor" or there would be racial conflict deriving from their competition for jobs. "Either way," he insisted, "lies a calamity."[17] Some suggested that because white men could not find work, Chinese immigrants were indirectly compelling white women to become prostitutes in order to provide their families with an income.[18] In addition to racist sentiments, some Anglo-Americans feared that the Chinese planned to conquer the United States financially. In the 1879 play "The Chinese Must Go!," the character Ah Coy predicts "the Chinese takeover of American economy." Many labor organizations, including the Workingmen's Party of California, pressed for legislation barring the immigration of low-wage Chinese laborers.[19]

Some Chinese immigrants brought to America the practice of opium smoking, which was typically done communally, in dens. The process involved cooking a small amount of opium at the end of a steel needle over an open flame to the right consistency, then inserting the opium into a small bowl attached to the pipe—"not unlike a small low coffee cup," a writer for the *Christian Recorder* explained. The smoker, who was lying down, would inhale.[20] A person learning how to "cook" the opium could take "months to become proficient," Thomas Byrnes, a longtime New York policeman, explained in 1886.[21] Den owners, meanwhile, provided the paraphernalia—the "lay-out"—and the know-how. Smoking in dens also provided a sense of community. Many Chinese immigrants were "bachelors, de facto or otherwise," as historian David Courtwright has pointed out, and they smoked in dens to address loneliness and also, perhaps, because there were no family members nearby to dissuade them.[22] Also, opium smoking would have "suppressed sexual desire in predominantly male immigrant work environments," as Martin Booth has noted.[23]

By the 1870s, some native-born whites complained that Chinese immigrants were excessively industrious. "You find him at work when you get up in the morning, and when you retire at night," journalist Samuel Williams wrote of them. "And this tireless industry," he admitted, "is what fills the souls of his enemies with despair. If he would only be shiftless and lazy," he explained, "he might be endured."[24] Journalist George H. Fitch derided the immigrants' "abnormal capacity for work."[25] It appeared that even opium smoking did not prevent a Chinese immigrant from being productive. In 1875, the *Saturday Evening Post* quoted a British vice-consul in China, who had assumed that opium smoking was physically devastating to users. When he was aboard a ship with many of them, however, he saw them doing demanding work and eating heartily, which indicated that "their constitution was robust."[26] And at the Warrendale Cannery in Oregon, Chinese employees worked at least ten hours a day, six days a week. Many smoked opium frequently and yet, as archaeologist John L. Fagan has noted, "their work was never reported to suffer from the effects."[27]

Immigrants endured violence as a consequence of job competition. The anti-Chinese speeches of labor leader Dennis Kearney, for example, motivated some men to commit acts including "burning Chinese laundries, [and] stoning the Chinese to death at times. Boys of all classes caught the impulse to throw stones at them," according to Mrs. E. V. Robbins, who was active in the early twentieth century in an organization that assisted Chinese women who worked as prostitutes.[28]

Anti-Chinese sentiment was inscribed in state laws that limited Chinese and Chinese American economic opportunities. In 1859, for example, when the Comstock Lode was discovered in present-day Nevada, the Gold Hill Mine Workers' Union, whose members were white, passed a law that barred Asians from holding claims in that district.[29] As restrictive laws blocked Chinese immigrants from one field of enterprise they sought others but were repeatedly countered. Some opened businesses in service industries such as restaurants and laundries.[30] In 1880, however, Nevada senator-elect James Fair stated that white women had difficulty earning an "honest living" due to this competition.[31] California imposed several taxes on Chinese residents, including a "miner's tax," a hospital tax, and a school tax, despite denying them the privileges of citizenship.[32] Chinese immigrants tended to congregate in Chinatowns, which insulated them from prejudicial treatment, since whites visited these districts only for specific reasons—sometimes to buy food, to gamble, or to hire a prostitute.[33]

Smoking opium had restorative value, as it helped many Chinese endure homesickness and prejudice. The practice would bring about "a fine languor, a complete mental rest," writer Stephen Crane explained. "The problems of life no longer appear" and, under its influence, "wrong departs, injustice vanishes."[34] Historian Sharon Lowe has deemed the dens an "insulated sanctuary" for men who were "distant from their home and culture."[35] Opium smoking also likely comforted immigrants who realized that they might never return to China.[36] Writers at the time recognized the role of the drug. A Chinese immigrant smoked opium "in order to forget for a little time his sorrows and wrongs," reformer Sara Jane Lippincott—writing as Grace Greenwood—explained in an 1873 issue of *Youth's Companion*. These sorrows included homesickness and cruel treatment by other laborers.[37] Writer Miriam Leslie added that opium smokers were seeking "respite from toil and privation and home-sickness."[38] As noted in Chapter 6, although opium smoking is not safe, it is safer than other forms of opiate use. It could cause lethargy and pulmonary disease, and the practice could lead to addiction; but because of its rapid impact, users could adjust their consumption comparatively easily. And there was little likelihood of overdosing on the drug.[39]

Public dens were typically low-ceilinged, subterranean spaces that were open almost around the clock. In one such establishment, light came from a small window near the ceiling and from the lamps that were used to cook the opium. Two tiers of wooden bunks, with matting and headrests, lined the walls. A smoker would arrive, remove his "coat, collar, and shoes," then lie down on a bunk and ask for a pipe and twenty-five cents' worth of opium, as Dr. H. H. Kane explained. The proprietor would prepare the drug. After several puffs, a smoker "falls into a heavy sleep and indulges in those blissful dreams which render the practice so enthralling," a reporter explained in 1886.[40]

Some writers who visited the dens contrasted the professed pleasures of smoking opium with the establishments' remote, dark, and dirty character. The entrance to one den was at the end of a fifty-foot-long corridor.[41] Once inside, many commented on the gloom. When Mark Twain and a fellow reporter visited a den in Virginia City, Nevada, one night in the early 1870s, Twain saw "vagabonds" smoking "on a sort of short truckle-bed." He could see them only by the light of a "sickly, guttering tallow candle."[42] The setting could have some appeal. Writers for the *Saturday Evening Post* found the pervasive smoke in one den to be "stimulating" and "not unpleasing." Otherwise, however, their "senses rebelled at the situation," in particular with regard to the filth. "The beds, one above another," they wrote, "were dirty beyond description," and their fellow inhabitants were "nearly as dirty as the beds they occupied."[43] The Reverend Frederick J. Masters was overwhelmed by a California den's "opium fumes and foul gases."[44] As the culture of opium smoking moved eastward, reporters would describe the dens in those communities as similarly squalid. In 1880, for example, a midwestern journalist reported that smokers in a Chicago den were found "sprawling on a filthy floor," while "others had rolled into dirty bunks." White-run newspapers and some in the black press reprinted the article, a sign of the gulf that some Americans perceived between Chinese culture and their own.[45]

Many opium smokers anticipated the relaxation or joy that the pipes would bring, though they could later experience weakness or nausea. First-person accounts tended to come from white doctors or reporters who smoked to learn about the practice, or from white smokers they knew, rather than from Chinese or Chinese American users. Some den visitors did not notice the unpleasant surroundings. In the early 1880s, a smoker named Frank rejected the criticisms of his friend, reporter Allen Williams, who had accompanied him to the den. Instead, as Frank watched the attendant prepare the opium, he "purred" about the substance, "Is not that a beautiful golden brown?" According to Williams, their cook smiled, much as "the *chef* of the Hotel Brunswick might smile over a successful dish to which he had given his personal superintendence."[46] Some experienced the drug's enchantment but also its enervating potential. In the early 1880s, a Montana reporter wrote that opium smoking produced "a pleasant effect of dreamy insensibility, and a feeling as if there was no care in this world, nor fear of it." He felt "perfect calmness and restfulness" while under its influence. When he left the den, however, he found it difficult to walk, and he felt weary later on.[47] A thirty-five-year-old man named Frederick, who had begun smoking in 1881, found the practice "exhilarating," and it made him talkative. In a conversation with a physician, he admitted that too many pipes left him itching and nauseated. After several hours' sleep, he would feel like a person would "after a week's drunk."[48]

* * *

Although the earliest dens in America were in the West, Chinese immigrants—and, later, white Americans—established them farther and farther east, reaching the East Coast in the mid-1870s. In the 1850s and 1860s, almost all opium smokers in America were Chinese, largely due to the isolation of the Chinese immigrant community.[49] Historian Huping Ling attributes Chinese immigrants' movement eastward in the 1870s to the prejudice they endured on the West Coast; the decade's economic depression, which soured job opportunities in the West; and the 1869 completion of the Transcontinental Railroad.[50] By the mid-1870s, there were dens in Chicago, St. Louis, and New Orleans, and they were beginning to appear in New York City.[51] Outside of New Orleans, there was little opium smoking in the South, likely because Chinese laborers in the South tended to arrive not from China but from Latin America. They were less inclined to smoke opium, they were more likely to marry, and, therefore, they were less likely to seek out the company that the dens provided.[52]

Some presented smoking opium as a less damaging practice than drinking whiskey. In 1873, some Chinese Americans in New York admitted that opium could have "ruinous" effects but pointed out that some Americans "drink whisky until they are drunk." Therefore they wondered, as the reporter stated, why it was wrong for Chinese immigrants "to become senseless with opium."[53] Several years later, Chinese American journalist Wong Chin Foo also drew this connection. He averred that so-called opium fiends drowned their sorrows in opium much as "Christians" turned to whiskey but then added that alcoholism was much more common than the opium habit.[54] Some white Americans agreed. The Reverend Otis Gibson saw both practices as serious problems for users and their societies, but he admitted that opium users committed fewer crimes than did drinkers.[55] In 1893, journalist Allan Forman presented opium smoking as a way to relax—akin to the role of beer "among our German fellow-citizens." He added that he would rather deal with "an opium drunkard" than "a whiskey drunkard." "A Chinaman on an opium spree breaks no windows, beats no women, murders no companions," he wrote. He could not say the same of "Caucasians, on whiskey sprees."[56] And Helen F. Clark, who worked as a missionary in New York's Chinatown, stated in 1896 that she could invite opium smokers to her mission "with perfect freedom" but could not "go into an American saloon with the same safety."[57]

The analogy between opium smoking and alcohol consumption also suggested that the Chinese were not so different from Americans. In the context of intense anti-Chinese sentiment, there is something poignant about a cartoon that the New York humor magazine *Puck* published in 1885, three years after the Exclusion Act went into effect. In crafting the illustration, Michael Angelo Woolf, rather than characterizing a Chinese man's opium smoking as strange or objectionable, presented it in a humorous and recognizable context: as a substance providing solace to a henpecked husband. In "The Silver Lining to an Opium Cloud," a Chinese man sits at home, smoking opium while his wife complains. Although she is berating him, he ignores her and puffs away at his pipe, his eyes closed. According to the caption, opium enabled the man to experience "Mild Serenity" under "Very Trying Circumstances." Woolf implies that Chinese men smoked opium for reasons with which other men could perhaps identify. A sign on the wall reading "There's No Place Like Home," in a Chinese-inspired typeface, reinforces the notion that a Chinese household, though not identical to a Western household, was substantively the same.[58]

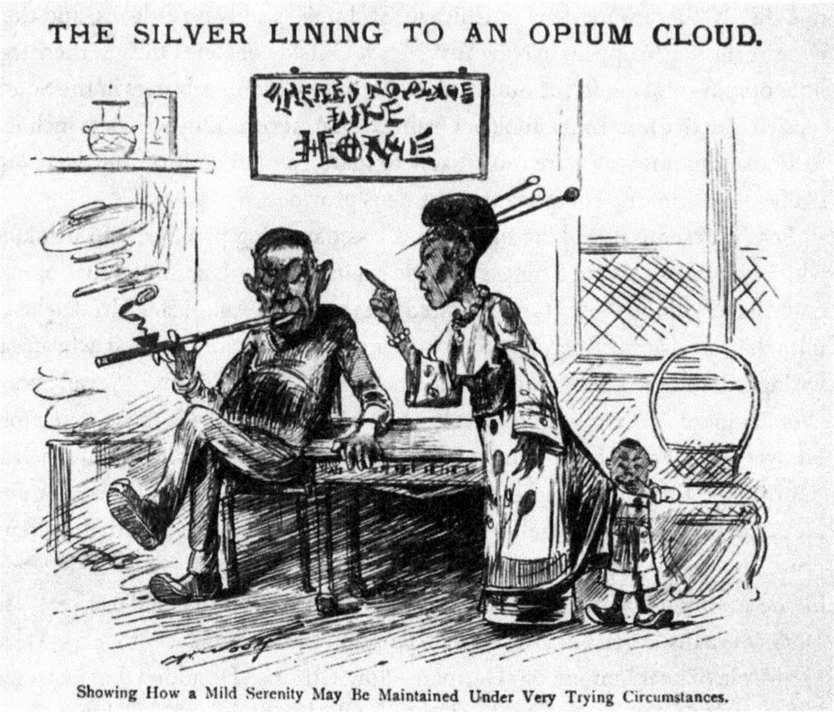

# THE SILVER LINING TO AN OPIUM CLOUD.

Showing How a Mild Serenity May Be Maintained Under Very Trying Circumstances.

*Figure 7.1.* Michael Angelo Woolf, "The Silver Lining to an Opium Cloud," *Puck*, August 12, 1885. Many native-born Americans criticized Chinese immigrants' opium use, but Woolf used humor to make this Chinese opium smoker relatable. In the image, the man's opium smoking helps him to endure his wife's critical comments. Courtesy of the Library of Congress, LC-USZC2-1211.

Some other Americans saw no reason to ban opium smoking. In 1879, the editor of Memphis's *Public Ledger* noted that many people were debating why one could not "smoke opium, eat hashish, or chew hen manure if they desire." He asserted that the practice was no more objectionable than others that were legal. "Tobacco chewers, cigar smokers—especially in the street car—and bibulous people," he maintained—the last referring to heavy drinkers—"have no more right to satisfy their appetites than opium smokers."[59]

Some anti-Chinese writers perpetuated the falsehood that usage was universal among Chinese immigrants.[60] In 1876, Thomas J. Vivian, in writing about San Francisco, erroneously reported that "every Chinaman uses the drug."[61] Several years later, on the East Coast, Augustine E. Costello stated of New York's Chinese population that "there is not one of them but 'hits the pipe' regularly every day."[62] In reality, some Chinese immigrants smoked only occasionally, many others not at all. In 1888, Wong Chin Foo stated that "most" Chinese men in New York smoked opium every now and then. For them, the pipe served as "an occasional mild sedative." A smaller group smoked frequently.[63] In 1901, New York physician Charles Brown agreed. Although he characterized Chinese immigrants who smoked opium as "the lowest type of Mongolian," he maintained that most Chinese Americans were "limited smokers and are absolutely unharmed by their practice." They were "hard-working" and smoked occasionally, "much as the holiday drinker of alcohol."[64] Many concluded that between a third and half of Chinese immigrants smoked opium, and about 10 or 15 percent were "sots," as the Reverend Frederick J. Masters put it.[65] The smokers themselves distinguished between heavy and occasional users. To those in the opium-smoking underworld, the former were "hop fiends," the latter "pleasure smokers."[66] Within the opium smoking community, Chinese immigrants were more likely than white users to smoke occasionally rather than habitually.[67]

\* \* \*

Many observers, however, regarded opium smoking as a greater concern than the more widespread domestic medicinal use of laudanum, due to the users' intent. While most laudanum habitués began using the drug for medical purposes—to restore health and, therefore, productivity—opium smokers had no such justification. A few doctors insisted that opium smoking could treat ailments such as coughs, hay fever, asthma, and migraine headaches.[68] Medical opium smoking, however, never caught on. Almost all those who smoked it took up the practice for enjoyment's sake or for its restorative quality—to experience tranquility at the end of a challenging day. As a consequence, very different profiles of smokers and laudanum users developed. Even other drug habitués could be unsympathetic. In 1895, Henry Cole, himself a recovering morphine habitué, deemed opium smoking "the worst type and apparently most degrading form of the opium curse."[69] That same year, William Rosser Cobbe chronicled his own addiction in *Doctor Judas*. Yet he stated that he divided "the vice of opium smoking from the disease of opium, because the two bear no relation to each other in morals." While the "disease of opium" derived from "physical infirmity," he contended, opium smoking was "instigated by moral depravity."[70] Distinguishing habitués based on their degree of "moral responsibility" was "one of the most common features in the discourse of addiction," as historian Timothy Hickman has noted.[71] Stephen Crane also saw the pattern. "Habit smokers have a contempt for the 'sensation smoker,'" he explained in 1896. He defined a "sensation smoker" as someone who was "won by the false glamor which surrounds the vice" and pretends to have "a ravenous hunger for the pipe. There are more 'sensation smokers,'" he added, "than one would imagine."[72]

Many regarded opium smoking, especially its habitual use, as "unmanly" because of its enervating effects on users. Opium smoking inspired behavior that was quiet and passive—not stereotypically masculine. As historian Diana Ahmad has noted, doctors "considered smoking opium feminine because it resulted in introspection, indifference, defeatism, and silence."[73] Also, many white Americans regarded Chinese men as effeminate. They kept their hair in a long queue, wore tunics, and tended to have a "slim body structure." These, combined with the fact that they worked in jobs "normally reserved for women," led white Westerners to regard them as unmanly.[74] There was also the notion that a habitual opium smoker was beholden to the drug and prized it more than self-respect. In 1881, a writer for the *New York Times* asserted that opium smoking "knocks all the manhood out of a man, physically, mentally, and morally; the victim loses all pride and conscience, and lives only for opium."[75] This concern made it difficult for den owners. In the late 1870s, for example, authorities in Deadwood, South Dakota, forced den owners to become "very secretive in conducting the business," according to the deputy sheriff. The people of Deadwood did not mind "such crimes as gambling," he admitted, but they took action against opium smoking due to concern with "how quickly it would rob a man of all semblance of manhood."[76]

\* \* \*

Dens were public, but proprietors sometimes limited their service to those they knew. Some den owners provided letters of introduction to their customers who would be traveling so they would be welcomed in dens in other cities. When one smoker left New York City for a trip upstate, for example, a man who ran his regular den gave him the address of a "laundry" in Syracuse, with credentials that looked like "an ordinary wash ticket," according to reporter Allen Williams. He visited the den, smoked there, and gave his ticket to the proprietor, who gave him a new address and ticket to use in Buffalo, his next stop.[77] To diehard smokers, access to the network was crucial. When George Appo and a friend could not find a den in Lafayette, Indiana, Appo recalled, "we had to leave that town."[78] Finding a den wherever one went, however, became easier over time. Around 1880, H. H. Kane interviewed theater folk and traveling salesmen, whose work kept them on the road. They told him that there was "hardly a town of any size in the East, and none in the West, where there is not a place to smoke and Americans smoking."[79] Williams met another smoker who concurred. "It's a poor town now-a-days that has not a Chinese laundry," the man told him in 1883, "and nearly every one of these has its lay-out."[80]

The fact that opium smoking was usually hidden unnerved many people, because it reinforced the notion that the practice was disreputable while making it difficult to ascertain just how widespread it was. The raucousness of saloons also bothered people, but the spaces and users were conspicuous. The public could therefore know, to a significant extent, the locations, scope, and nature of the impact of drinking. In accounts of overseas opium use, habitués sometimes ingested the drug outdoors in broad daylight. American opium dens, meanwhile, tended to be located in underground rooms that people could visit only if they had a connection. The smoking took place "down in the cellars, under the sidewalks," said William Brooks, who wrote about San Francisco's Chinatown.[81] Some saw the dens' seclusion as indicating the users' concern with public opinion and, therefore, as a sign of concern with their reputations. In his 1860 account of his trip to California, *New York Tribune* editor Horace Greeley wrote that a Chinese immigrant who smoked opium was "never so devoid of self-respect as to be seen drunk in a public place; even for an opium debauch, he secludes himself where none but a friendly eye can reach him."[82] Others were concerned that usage could be hidden and yet rampant. In *New York's Chinatown* (1898), journalist Louis Beck noted that opium joints existed in houses that looked "much like the rest." Even at night, he added, most pedestrians would not notice that the basement was lighted "while all the rest of the house was wrapped in gloom."[83]

Journalists, doctors, and police chiefs shared stories of their own opium smoking without reservation, apparently because such usage, if it were done to further knowledge, would be accepted. Reporter Allen Williams explained that for no more than a dollar, a patron could enjoy "a perfect ease of body, brain, and conscience." Upon smoking opium, he stated, the user "knows not fear, and wants nothing."[84] Thomas F. Byrnes, who headed New York's police department from 1880 to 1895, also tried it, though his experience ended unpleasantly. Initially, he enjoyed a "delightful dreamy half sleep, languidly knowing all that was going on around me, but caring for nothing." Then, however, he became restless and saw horrible images that reminded him of harpies from Dante's *Inferno.* "I . . . went home with all my nerves in a state of protest," he added, and never smoked opium again.[85] Dr. Kane found opium smoking appealing because he could enjoy "a certain element of good-fellowship, a pleasure in doing with some degree of secrecy that which the law forbids, and upon which the masses look as something mysterious."[86] He also sought to understand the drug thoroughly. He discussed it with doctors and police chiefs, became acquainted with about fifty opium smokers, treated two habitual users, made hours-long, daily visits to an opium joint, smoked opium "in small quantities and to excess," and invited habitués to his home, where he would "freely question and experiment upon them."[87]

The advent of flash photography in the late 1880s made it possible for reporters to capture images of dens and to share them with the public.[88] Such pictures became popular in part due to widespread American curiosity about Chinese immigrants' lives. In an 1891 periodical focused on travel and recreation, for example, W. I. Lincoln Adams noted that photographs of the Chinatowns in San

Francisco and Los Angeles were "the only 'flash' pictures of the Chinese smoking opium, sleeping, eating and engaged in other characteristic occupations in their own haunts."[89]

The images of the dens became part of the genre of "exposure journalism," which drew attention to social ills. Proprietors and customers tended to dodge photographers—certainly because they did not want to be captured in that way, perhaps because they considered it intrusive to be photographed while going about their business or because they feared legal repercussions, and likely a combination of these. Regardless of their reasons, their efforts to cloak the practice, such as operating in basements and barring photographers, heightened outsiders' perceptions that their actions could not withstand public scrutiny. Literally, these reporters saw a benefit in shedding light on the practice. In 1888, a writer for *Harper's Magazine* suggested that pictures of a den would be revelatory for everybody, including the den's inhabitants, because the "miserable occupants had never seen their own filth before."[90] This suggested the belief that smokers never thought about what they were doing. While some members of the public likely regarded the pictures as drawing attention to a social ill, others were probably just interested in getting a glimpse of a den.

Capturing images of illegal smoking was a considerable challenge, so when photographers accomplished the feat, some magazine articles focused on their process rather than on the dens themselves. In 1892, for example, a writer for *Californian Illustrated Magazine* bragged that the pictures accompanying the article were "the first interiors of these dens ever shown or likely to be." He explained how difficult it was to get the pictures, because the inhabitants objected strongly. The photographer had snapped the pictures "amid yells, oaths, threats and shrieks," and many smokers left or hid before the picture was taken. Some of the photographer's confederates chatted with the smokers while the photographer lurked outside. He and his assistants then rushed in, shot the picture, and left. The image captured four smokers. One was standing, while three looked at the camera with surprised expressions.[91]

What was not photographed was as important as what was. A handful of photos from the era feature white den patrons—white women sleeping or "sporting" types for whom opium smoking was a rebellious pastime—and some journals published sketches depicting white people in dens. The number of these images, however, is dwarfed by the number of images of Chinese and Chinese American smokers. Photographs of Chinese Americans in opium dens not only reinforced the notion of them as habitués but also supported the mistaken notion that they were the *only* habitués. Most habitual drug users in nineteenth-century America were native-born women, but they hid their habit. In 1910, Dr. Hamilton Wright would erroneously assert in a report to Congress that there was "nothing to show that up to 1860 there was a serious misuse of opium or

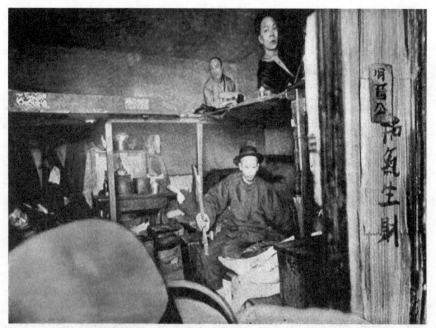

*Flash Light Photograph* An Underground Den
Smokers starting up, on upper and lower levels, alarmed at the flash light—Smoker with hat on is half
stupefied —The hat in the foreground represents Detective Cox who guarded the door
while the flash light man and photographer did their work

*Figure 7.2.* "An Underground Den" from "The Opium Den Pictures—How They Were Taken," *Californian Illustrated Magazine,* May 1892. Opium dens were typically secluded establishments, and they garnered popular interest. With flashlight photography and the element of surprise, reporters provided audiences with images of the dens and presented such photojournalism as a public service. Courtesy of Google Books.

other habit-forming drugs in this country, bar the practice of opium smoking by the Chinese."[92]

In the fall of 1881, Dr. H. H. Kane warned readers of *Harper's Weekly* that opium smoking was becoming popular with native-born Americans and that the habit was damaging and unbreakable. Drawing on his extensive research on the topic, Kane acknowledged that a smoker would initially feel "at peace with himself and all the world" after smoking a pipe. He also conceded that chronic drinking was worse than opium smoking, for both users and those around them. But smoking also presented dangers. Kane stated that the practice's pleasures were eventually replaced by "a demon who binds his victim hand and foot." The user soon smoked only to avoid withdrawal and would experience physical problems, memory loss, and resistance to "continued mental effort." About four thousand Americans smoked opium, most of them daily, and their numbers were growing. Imports of the drug were on the rise, and few of the new customers were Chinese. Opium dens existed in "every town of any importance" in America, and there were always at least some white customers present. Kane's second article in the series included an illustration that indicated the practice's increasing popularity. In the image, eight young white men are in a windowless opium den, most of them sleeping or drowsy and smoking. The Chinese keeper of the den is bringing the opium layout to a customer who is still sitting up and has perhaps just arrived. The customers appear unconcerned with the outside world or the passage of time. In the image, the only one who is industrious is the Chinese attendant. Because he is providing a habit-forming drug, the image could have had a sinister connotation for white readers. In one sense, it depicted white customers at leisure, attended by a nonwhite servant. In another, the image of the den, with its service clearly in demand, suggested that native-born young men were privileging the habit over their work and other responsibilities.[93]

* * *

Many native-born Americans believed that Chinese immigrants could not become truly "American"—that their primary allegiance would be to their native land. Some criticized them for sending some of their earnings back to their

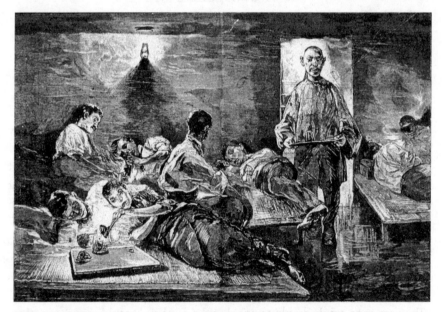

*Figure 7.3.* J. W. Alexander, "American Opium-Smokers—Interior of a New York Opium Den," *Harper's Weekly,* October 8, 1881. Americans initially associated domestic opium smoking with Chinese immigrants on the West Coast. By the early 1880s, opium dens existed in all US cities and white smokers were among the clientele, despite laws that had been passed to combat the practice. Courtesy of the National Library of Medicine, ID 101392816.

families, for example, rather than spending it domestically. Some were not convinced that the Chinese were assimilating even when they seemed to be doing so. In *How the Other Half Lives* (1890), journalist Jacob Riis doubted the sincerity of Chinese immigrants who appeared to embrace American culture. He believed that when a Chinese immigrant converted to Christianity, he only did so "as he puts on American clothes, with . . . an ulterior motive."[94] Writer Thomas J. Vivian believed that a Chinese immigrant would remain "forever an alien" due to his "impenetrable reserve."[95] Many were similarly skeptical, and the practice of opium smoking was an aspect of Chinese immigrant culture that appeared to signify that cultural divide.

Nowhere was the perception of Chinese immigrants' foreignness more overt than in the tours of Chinatowns in San Francisco and New York, excursions that took middle-class, white Americans to the districts' restaurants, theaters, houses of worship, and opium dens.[96] Visitors could hire a guide at any of the larger hotels, though journalist George H. Fitch recommended hiring an "intelligent detective" who knew the area thoroughly, or a Chinese guide, to ensure that they would see the dens. These tours appealed to those who were sympathetic to the Chinese immigrant community as well as those who were not. In an article for *Cosmopolitan* magazine, Fitch explained that the former wanted to confirm "that John Chinaman has been libeled," while the anti-Chinese visitor wanted "to be shocked by the Oriental depravity that he has heard so much about."[97] Meanwhile, visiting the dens could give them an experience akin to what Bayard Taylor had experienced in Damascus, or what Richard Robert Madden felt as he sat among Constantinople's *Theriakis*: to be in the midst of a fascinating setting without being a part of it. Many tourists had a "desire to see the racially abject," as historian Barbara Berglund has observed.[98] Architectural historian J. Philip Gruen concurs, stating that many sought to reinforce their "moral superiority over those they visited."[99] Some said that in Chinatown, they felt as if they were no longer in America. In 1883, the Reverend O. T. Gifford insisted that anyone who visited San Francisco's Chinatown would be struck by "the power of Chinese civilization to change an American city." While there, he insisted, it was as if "you have passed through the earth, and are upon the opposite side."[100]

Some enjoyed watching raids of opium dens, as long as they were assured that they were in no danger. In 1905, as a writer for the *Syracuse Post-Standard* reported, a large police raid began near Mott and Pell streets in New York when several "big 'Seeing Chinatown by Night' automobiles," filled with tourists, were in the vicinity. The female tourists at first feared that they would be arrested but were assured that would not happen. The reporter considered them lucky: they "got a bargain counter quantity of excitement for their fare."[101]

\* \* \*

When white, middle-class Americans expressed concerns about the dens, they tended to focus not on how opium smoking affected the smokers but on how it affected themselves. There was an inclination to let Chinese men smoke as long as they kept to themselves. There was some concern when members of the white underworld took up the practice. When fellow members of the white middle class took it up, however, especially middle-class youth, opposition increased. And when newspapers suggested that Chinese men lured youth to the dens, opposition was further heightened, though many of these allegations turned out to be false.

The white American "sporting class"—prostitutes, criminals, and the like—began patronizing opium dens in significant numbers in the 1870s, enticed by the novelty and entrancement that opium smoking could provide.[102] In 1896, Stephen Crane explained that "cheap actors, race track touts, gamblers, and the different kinds of confidence men" smoked opium, and that the practice had become widespread.[103] In his history of the New York Police Department, Augustine Costello concluded that the white underworld had embraced the practice because they were "ever on the lookout for a new sensation," especially when an old sensation had lost its thrill. "The lower order of theatrical people" and members of the "demi-monde," he wrote, found opium smoking to be "a new and agreeable substitute for whiskey."[104] The practice also might have enhanced the daring image that they wanted to project. In 1891, ethnographer Stewart Culin surmised that "people who are best defined by the word 'fast'" were most inclined to pick up the pipe and that they "take considerable pride in the practice of this form of dissipation."[105]

While some commentators were opposed to any white patronage of opium dens, others expressed concern only when the usage extended to white youth. In 1879, the staff of the *Memphis Daily Appeal* urged the police to close one of the city's dens as the customers included "fast white men and lewd white women."[106] And in 1894, the *San Francisco Chronicle* reported that opium smoking in the city had reached its "most serious phase" because the practice had "secured a hold upon the lower and more depraved classes of whites."[107] According to New York chief of police George Walling, the police would raid a den once they learned that it admitted white patrons, even those who were "degraded white" smokers.[108] Others, however, did not mind if members of that class chose to smoke. In 1877, a reporter for the Eureka, Nevada, *Sentinel* stated that patrons of the town's dens were "men and women who have lost all self-respect" and "gamblers and lewd women." Although he did not care about them, he worried that youth were taking up the practice as well. If the sporting crowd "were the only ones who gave themselves up to the drug," he stated, "it might be well enough not to interfere, but in Eureka," he lamented, "it has become fashionable among the boys to learn the habit." They bragged about how much they could smoke, and their parents could not rein them in. "A heavy hand should be laid on them," he advised, "for out of such material graduates the criminal element."[109]

As dens opened outside of vice districts, some "respectable" white Americans became more inclined to partake. San Francisco police officer James Mahoney spoke about this trend in an 1881 interview. A few years earlier, he explained, most white users had been "hoodlums and prostitutes." Then, many "clean" dens opened up "in respectable portions of the city." As a consequence, he believed that white usage would "gradually extend up the social grade."[110] His prediction was accurate. In Philadelphia in the early 1880s, for example, Kate Chisom ran an elegant "opium parlor," and she stated that her customers included "'some of the wealthiest ladies in the city,'" according to the *New York Times*. Its hiddenness was key. Her business suffered when one woman who stayed there told the customers' husbands "that their wives came to my house to smoke opium," Chisom rued.[111]

Soon, wealthy white New Yorkers could patronize sumptuous opium joints in the most affluent parts of town, apparently without the risk of arrest. ("Joint" often referred to a den with white patrons and perhaps a white owner.[112]) Elite joints featured paintings, carpets, and chandeliers and provided expensive, ornate layouts for their customers' use—far different from the spare wooden bunks in other dens. They also offered private rooms, so notable customers could slip in and out unseen.[113] Stephen Crane recalled a "palatial" joint on 42nd Street where an "occasional man from Fifth avenue or Madison avenue would have there his private layout." He added that some patrons' names "are not altogether unknown to the public."[114] In 1882, a reporter for the *Brooklyn Daily Eagle* visited such a joint. In addition to the proprietor, he relayed, "The attendants are also white, and there is not a single Chinese about the den, all the frequenters . . . being white and the majority of them Americans." It was within "five minutes' walk of one of the most fashionable neighborhoods in New York," he added, and "a stone's throw from one of the richest and best attended churches." The joint's proprietor had opened the business to cater to New Yorkers "who are always ready for something new in the way of dissipation." His earliest customers were stockbrokers, though many others were members of the "fast set." Other white-owned dens opened around this time, because such enterprises were profitable.[115] Some dens with white proprietors had Chinese customers, but they tended not to be posh joints. When New York policemen raided a white woman's joint in 1884, five of the smokers were Chinese. The building, however, had "small, poorly ventilated rooms," and its interior resembled a prison, according to a writer for the *New York Times*.[116]

Other wealthy smokers patronized dens whose clients were of different races, classes, and levels of "respectability." In 1881, Dr. Leslie Keeley noted that some "richly dressed ladies" would go to "subterranean opium 'joints'" and smoke alongside social "outcasts."[117] Opium smoking sometimes broke down barriers between people who otherwise had little to do with each other. A reporter for the *New York Times* wrote that a smoker would lie alongside people to whom, before he began smoking, "he would not condescend a nod on the street."[118] In 1877, a writer for the *Enterprise* of Prescott, Arizona, stated that patrons of the dens on Granite Street ranged from "some of our leading citizens down to the lowest harlot who plies her vocation on that street."[119]

The interracial dimension, however, was often paramount, due to some whites' concerns with the possibility of interracial sexual relationships. Dr. H. H. Kane asserted that a woman who smoked opium would find that her "sexual appetite . . . sometimes approaches to frenzy, the woman losing all modesty."[120] In 1880, a writer for the *Salt Lake Tribune* reported that a black woman had been arrested at a local den, then stated that "her skin was not half as dusky as the souls of these young white men who could so far forget themselves as to lie down with her in a Chinese opium hell."[121] There was considerably more concern when a Chinese man was in a potentially compromising situation with a white woman. Many believed that "otherwise chaste white women" might "forget themselves" upon smoking opium and could be willing to have sex with nonwhite men.[122] Some perceived this as a challenge, not just to white people as a race but to white men, specifically. On one occasion, police in San Francisco found "white women and Chinamen side by side" under the effect of opium. In the police department's report to the state legislature, the author stated that he found such a sight "humiliating . . . to any one who has anything left of manhood."[123]

Some Chinese and Chinese American men did marry white women. In some cases, these couples ran opium dens.[124] The white women were usually Irish, German, or Italian members of the working class. Chinese American journalist Wong Chin Foo asserted that these women married "well-to-do Chinamen" who adopted American ways and treated their wives well. He maintained that the women were better off with these husbands than they would be with "men of their own nation."[125] (At the time, many states banned interracial marriage, but Wong was writing about New York, where no such law existed.)[126] Many white Americans opposed interracial marriage because they saw miscegenation—the mixing of races—as sullying what they regarded as a pure Caucasian race.[127] In 1910, Dr. Hamilton Wright would play on the widespread white sentiment against interracial marriage as he pushed for national legislation regulating drug use. In a report to Congress, he said that one of the "most unfortunate phases" of the smoking habit was the "large number of women" who were "living as common-law wives of or cohabiting with Chinese" in American Chinatowns.[128]

Extensive press was devoted to opium smoking by white youth. Opium and morphine habitués typically became habitual users when they were middle aged, but opium smokers could be much younger. According to reporter Allen Williams, most female visitors to New York's opium dens had not yet turned twenty-one.[129] Nevada historian Mary McNair Mathews said that patrons of opium dens were "girls and boys from twelve to twenty."[130] Some authorities took action in the 1870s when the practice became entrenched among "the younger class of boys and girls, many of the latter of the more respected class of families," as Dr. G. B. Harris of Virginia City, Nevada, described them. At that point, Virginia City passed an ordinance in an attempt to ban use. A subsequent law that threatened violators with imprisonment appeared to curb the spread of the habit.[131]

Occasionally, reporters blamed white youth for becoming inured to the drug. In 1881, a correspondent for the *New York Tribune* reported that many California youth were patronizing the dens. "California children are very precocious," the reporter explained. "They seem to have an exaggerated desire to indulge in everything which is forbidden."[132]

Many writers, however, accused Chinese den proprietors of luring white youth to dens and giving them opium. In 1877, a writer for the *Daily Territorial Enterprise* (Virginia City, Nevada) stated that the men, "with the cunning of devils," had "learned how to appeal to the turbulent passions of youth" and thus entice them to partake of the vice. He blamed the Chinese immigrants for "killing self-respect in the minds of young men" and for "taking away all sense of shame from the hearts of young women."[133] In 1879, a writer for the *San Francisco Post* expressed a similar view. Using a term that referred to a generic Chinese immigrant, he asserted that "Johnny Comprador had impoverished our country, degraded our free labor and hoodlumized our children. . . . He is now destroying our young men with opium."[134] In the *New York Sun*, Allen Williams wrote that the dens were "drawing in recruits for the host of opium victims from among the inhabitants of the neighborhood who are not Chinese."[135]

Many commentators accused Chinese men of giving opium to young girls and then raping them, but most allegations were exposed as false, some espoused by advocates for Chinese exclusion who had an incentive to lie. In 1873, the *New York Times* reported that Chinese men took in young white girls because of the men's interest in them. When the journalist visited a den, he saw a white girl, whom he described as "handsome but squalidly-dressed." His Chinese guide explained that she was hungry, and they had given her food—and also that he liked her. As the reporter quoted him, "Chinamen always [have] something to eat, and he like young white girl." The reporter added that many "young white girls" smoked opium and that they "sell their souls for the sustenance of their bodies."[136] In 1897, a grand jury in San Francisco reported that "white girls between the ages of 13 and 20 are enticed into these dens, become regular habitués, and are finally subject wholly to the wishes of the Chinese visitors."[137]

Many were skeptical of such stories. Some members of the Chinese American community stated that these articles unfairly smeared their community. Wong Chin Foo criticized newspapers that had implied "that all the Chinese in the city were guilty of . . . ruin[ing] the innocent children of their neighbors." He wished they would name those who were guilty, rather than making a "sweeping assertion" that indicted everyone.[138] Others, meanwhile, doubted the stories' veracity. In 1883, for example, a priest and some young men from his parish believed that several young girls were staying at a New York opium joint and sought support to shut the business down. Wong said that "respectable Chinamen" would help in "breaking up any joint where girls were found." He added, however, that the Chinese community had "no knowledge that such places have been conducted in the guise of opium shops." A representative of the Society for the Prevention of Cruelty to Children agreed with Wong. He did not believe the stories with regard to "the decoying of girls of tender years into the joints" and said he would give fifty dollars to anyone who could prove him wrong.[139] In his history of New York's police force, Augustine Costello noted that there had been many reports of "Chinamen dragging young girls into their dens and stupefying them with the drug" but that such stories were "untrue and without foundation." He quoted a police captain who acknowledged that opium smoking "makes sad work of them"—the Chinese men, that is—but who also insisted that "the Chinamen are one of the most harmless classes of dwellers in New York."[140]

The accusations against the Chinese men fit into a pattern in which marginalized men were accused of using drugs and assaulting white women. In his 1886 work *The Conflict of Races*, for example, Dr. Washington Ryer included a news item about a Boston girl named Nellie Gately who had gone to a laundry to pick up an order when she was "seized by Chinamen, who thrust a lighted pipe into her mouth and compelled her [to] smoke until she became unconscious." Ryer was quoting Gately's account of what happened. The veracity of the account cannot be confirmed, but the story bolstered Ryer's anti-Chinese invective. His motivation is suspect, as he wrote *The Conflict of Races* to criticize the press "east of the Rocky Mountains" for what he regarded as an unfairly sympathetic depiction of Chinese immigrants and Chinese Americans, and to persuade the federal government that the Chinese and white Americans could never live together in harmony.[141] Samuel Gompers, president of the American Federation of Labor, also claimed that Chinese immigrants posed a threat to white girls. In 1902, while he was pushing for renewal of the Chinese Exclusion Act, he stated that there were Chinese laundries in California where "tiny lost souls" were forced to "yield up their virgin bodies to their maniacal yellow captors."[142] Like Ryer, Gompers presented the most extreme version of the scenario in order to intensify anti-Chinese sentiment.

Many similar assertions were revealed to be lies. In 1883, a young female opium smoker told a judge that the Irish wife of a Chinese man had been "dosing children with opium concealed in candy." In 1883, Allen Williams wrote in the *Brooklyn Eagle* that Chinese immigrant men sold candy laced with opium, thereby giving children "an insatiable longing for the drug." He added that they then brought "little girls" to the dens and "brutally maltreated" them.[143] He later reported, however, that the stories were lies that some people had spread "to provoke an Irish crusade against the heathen." He concluded that the allegations were "preposterous," but they had had the desired effect. "Crowds of young 'hoodlums,'" he reported, had thrown stones through the windows of Chinese immigrants' homes. Williams poked more holes in the anti-Chinese allegations. Because rumors circulated that Chinese immigrants carried weapons, Williams pointed out, it was odd that when their homes were vandalized, they did not "massacre their enemies" in response. He suggested that the Chinese might be too accepting, as they paid their rent faithfully despite being charged "enormously high rents for the wretched houses in which they live." He added that the anti-Chinese rumors could be dangerous. Had the false rumor of the opium candy circulated "more rapidly," he pointed out, it could have resulted in the Irish "exterminating the yellow heathen."[144] Tension often existed between Chinese American and Irish American communities, since they competed for working-class jobs. There was also antagonism because, as John Kuo Wei Tchen has pointed out, "demonizing racial 'others'" was a way that a marginalized group could improve its own standing.[145]

Some white workers accused Chinese immigrants of immoral behavior in order to remove them as job competition, a tactic that has been used repeatedly and that, when used, has frequently accompanied anti-drug legislation. Time and again, groups of workers face competition from marginalized laborers who are willing to work for lower wages. The response, as sociologist Kathleen Auerhahn has observed, has often been to concoct a "moral panic": to accuse members of the marginalized group of immorality linked to drug use and to advocate drug laws to try to control that group. These occurrences tend to correlate with times of major social disruption. White and Chinese immigrant workers, for example, competed for jobs during an economic depression. As a consequence, "conditions were ripe for the scapegoating of the Chinese," according to Auerhahn. Baseless "moral panics" and concern with economic competition also provide important context when understanding the temperance movement and support for later measures restricting sales of cocaine and marijuana.[146]

Concern with drug use by middle-class white youth spurred passage of a drug law that was the nation's first—excepting measures pertaining to alcohol—when San Francisco officials banned opium dens in 1875. At their meeting, members of the city's board of supervisors discussed the fact that several dens in the city had an exclusively white clientele, and their regular customers, rather than consisting solely of the "vicious and depraved," included youth who had "respectable parentage" as well as "young men engaged in respectable business avocations," according to a reporter for the *San Francisco Chronicle*. Members of the Health and Police committee warned that opium smoking could become prevalent if nothing were done, and they advocated passage of an ordinance to close the dens. The committee then approved a measure by which a person who visited or ran a den could be fined up to five hundred dollars and imprisoned for up to six months.[147] Similar legislation elsewhere made the concern with white involvement more apparent. In 1887, Idaho's legislature approved a measure that "every white person" who ran or patronized an opium den would be guilty of a misdemeanor.[148] By 1896, twenty-two states and territories, in all regions of the country, had made it illegal to keep an opium den. As historian Ronald Hamowy has noted, those who advocated the laws did so "to protect whites from what was commonly regarded as a loathsome Oriental vice."[149]

Laws barring opium dens and requiring prescriptions for opium, however, did little to lessen use of the drug. Laws against dens "facilitated police harassment of the Chinese," according to sociologist Marion Goldman.[150] In an 1886 case, for example, a Chinese man was arrested in Oregon for selling opium. US district judge Matthew Deady, who ruled on the case, stated that support for the law could have derived not from concern with opium smoking per se but from anti-Chinese sentiment. "Smoking opium," he pointed out, "is not our vice." Instead, he added, the legislation was perhaps enforced "more from a desire to vex and annoy the 'Heathen Chinee' . . . than to protect the people from the evil habit."[151] And as Richard Davenport-Hines has noted, the laws that western states passed between 1877 and 1890 were the first to "criminalise users rather than to regulate substances."[152] Outlawing opium dens, however, could achieve only so much. When Virginia City, Nevada, banned them in 1876, most dens reopened after a raid within a few days or weeks, and new ones opened in neighboring towns that lacked prohibitory laws. Because of the demand, intensified by addiction to the drug, a government could not simply legislate the dens out of existence.[153]

Sometimes, raids moved opium smoking into private homes rather than ending the practice altogether. In the early 1880s, police in San Francisco closed the city's Chinese-run dens where most of the customers had been white. Former smokers then smoked in homes. The police could gauge the extent of smoking by tracking "the number of whites who come into Chinatown for opium," as Officer James Mahoney explained. He believed that raids increased the popularity of opium smoking. Most white smokers, he noted, had been "hoodlums and prostitutes," because few "decent" people were willing to visit Chinatown's "filthy" dens. After the raids, however, there were many "clean rooms . . . in re-spectable portions of the city" where someone could go to smoke. "Schoolboys and clerks," he added, who would never have patronized a Chinese den, were "finding out the respectable places and learning to like the habit."[154] Stephen Crane saw a similar trend in New York. Initially, he explained, there had been two "colonies" of opium smokers: one in Chinatown, and the other in the vice district. Reforms, he added, had divided these colonies into "something less than 25,000 fragments." Although some could assume that reform efforts had succeeded, due to opium smoking's lack of visibility, the practice "retired to pri-vate flats," where it would be even more difficult for authorities to end it.[155] The crackdown on opium dens helped make it a habit that was available primarily to the wealthy, as Wong Chin Foo noted. A person had to be "indolent and rich" to be an opium smoker, he insisted in 1888, due to the time that the habit took and the expense of the layout.[156] Some smokers, of course, could afford more elaborate setups than others. Around 1900, millionaire J. J. Vandegrift, who had made his fortune in oil, built his estate, Vancroft, in what is now Wellsburg, West Virginia. The mansion included an opium den, which was decorated with Turkish-style couches.[157]

The focus on opium smoking significantly shaped perceptions of domestic drug use. Because Chinese immigrants' opiate use was more visible than that of white laudanum habitués, many Americans regarded opium smoking through the lens of race rather than regarding it as a form of relaxation akin to drinking alcohol. Also, they were not inclined to comprehend habitual use as a disease. According to William White, a longtime researcher in the field of addiction treatment, "The creation of America's first 'dope fiend' caricature slowed the per-ception of opiate addiction as a medical disorder and injected the issue of racism into the public perception of opiate use."[158]

\* \* \*

When American journalists began to write about domestic nonmedical drug use, they tended to overlook the many native-born Americans who had become opium habitués, since their consumption could be difficult to distinguish from medical use and they could conceal their plight, sometimes even from family members. Many compulsive users, meanwhile, wanted to forgo their use but did not know how. Public silence on the topic could help them to hide their habit, but it also obscured paths to recovery. In the late 1860s, however, doctors and former habitués would begin to publish books and articles that addressed large-scale domestic habituation. The works would end users' feelings of isola-tion, provide possible methods of treatment, and spur a discussion regarding such use.

# A Public Problem, 1867–1905

Some American journalists had focused on Chinese immigrants' opium smoking because it was a comparatively conspicuous form of domestic, nonmedical drug use and there was significant anti-Chinese sentiment in the United States. Beginning in the late 1860s, however, public discussion also focused regularly on compulsive drug use among native-born Americans. Dr. David Cheever addressed it. In the *North American Review* he observed that for a long time, Westerners had not regarded drug habituation as a problem among themselves. They had "been accustomed to regarding the Oriental nations as a race of opium-eaters," he wrote, while "we have congratulated ourselves that such vile habits did not concern us of Europe or America." Thomas De Quincey had shown that habitual use was a problem in England, and Cheever noted that it was becoming more prevalent in the United States. Advances in transportation and industrialization had ushered in a "busy world of competition," he explained, and some sought a narcotic to help them endure the increased intensity of everyday life. The topic of domestic drug habituation would soon explode in the popular press.[1]

Cheever asserted that middle- and upper-class Americans were more susceptible to illness than were members of the working class or people in countries with less technological advancement. According to the doctor, members of the "lower orders of creation" were typically healthy, while sickness was more common among "civilized" people—those whose work, like his own, was primarily mental. "We think, and we exhaust," he explained; "we scheme, imagine, study, worry, and enjoy, and proportionately we waste." In an effort to "restore the equilibrium," they would drink coffee or tea, smoke tobacco, or opt for something stronger.[2] Cheever was not alone in believing that well-to-do Americans deserved more license than others to use psychoactive substances. Many members of the middle class would use this perceived dichotomy—between an exhausted middle class and a robust working class—to justify their own nonmedical drug use while denouncing that of others as indulgent.

*Habit Forming.* Elizabeth Kelly Gray, Oxford University Press. © Oxford University Press 2023.
DOI: 10.1093/oso/9780190073121.003.0009

* * *

On a Christmas Day in the 1860s, New York physician and opium habitué Horace Day decided to visit a doctor to help him end his drug use. He had tried on his own but found the process agonizing. Reduced doses brought stomach pains, a "prickling sensation" all over, and "constant perspiration of icy coldness" along his spine, he later recalled. He could write only by steadying one hand with the other. On that day, loath to walk in the cold, wet weather, he opted for an omnibus. He stood on "the step of the carriage"—the only available spot—but doubted he could hold on for the half-hour-long journey. "You look very pale, Sir; I am afraid you are sick," said an Irishwoman inside the carriage, who offered him her seat. Day accepted the offer, and two men helped him to the spot. When he reached his destination he headed for his doctor's office but then walked past it, fretting that his case was likely "beyond human aid."[3]

While aboard the omnibus his weakened condition attracted attention, but it appears that his fellow passengers only saw an ailing man; they likely did not realize that he was a habitual drug user, weak from withdrawal. Day, however, would recount that morning's events—and his ultimate success in ending his use—in *The Opium Habit: With Suggestions as to the Remedy* (1868). The work helped draw public attention to the topic of domestic habitual drug use.

At the time he wrote, nonmedical drug use in the United States was increasing. Between 1867 and 1877, the American population grew by 10 percent while the amount of opium that was imported increased by 70 percent.[4] A druggist in Albany, New York, recalled that in the 1850s, he made laudanum "by the gallon." When he was interviewed in 1881, however, he was "prepar[ing] it by the barrel."[5] Using import statistics, David Courtwright has estimated that by the mid-1890s, the addiction rate in the United States was as much as six times what it had been in 1842. The substantial population growth of those decades makes the increase in use more striking still. While there were no more than 10,875 American opium habitués in 1842, there could have been as many as 313,177 opiate users, including opium smokers, in the nation by the mid-1890s. Soon thereafter, the rate of usage began to decline.[6]

The late 1860s brought a surge of publications by doctors and habitués about domestic drug use, thereby elevating the topic in the public consciousness while making the case that addiction was a curable disease rather than a failure of will. Habitués emphasized how intractable addiction could be, and by writing about their experiences, they helped readers to better understand their own condition and gave advice to those who were drug-dependent in learning how to treat it. Some doctors believed that addiction should be regarded and treated as a physical disorder. Many physicians considered the white, middle-class morphine users who constituted a large segment of the addicted population to be good candidates for treatment and cure. The focus on medical treatment gave doctors a role but also opened the door to charlatans, who advertised quack cures to a national audience.

Like Cheever, many authors of works on the topic were white and middle class, and they regarded members of their group as justified in using drugs for restorative purposes; they theorized that they alone suffered the stresses associated with modern times, and that no other sources of anguish existed. Poverty, prejudice, and unhealthy living conditions were widespread at the time, but many writers implied that people whose work primarily involved physical labor—that is, people of color and members of the working class—were immune to the era's challenges and therefore would have no need for relief. The result was a tendency to excuse the use of drugs by middle-class white people, asserting that for them it was therapeutic, while condemning such use by others as a self-centered indulgence.

* * *

In the late 1860s and 1870s, several decades after morphine was first isolated, the hypodermic administration of the drug came into widespread use.[7] The delivery of morphine by syringe, which replaced an earlier tablet, enabled patients to avoid "the unpleasant gastrointestinal effects associated with the oral administration of opium," as attorney Jeffrey Clayton Foster has noted.[8] Scottish physician Alexander Wood, the inventor of the syringe, had mistakenly assumed that a person could not crave an injected drug, only a swallowed substance.[9] In reality, however, injected drugs had the highest likelihood of leading to addiction, and doctors were now using injection frequently.[10] They gave opium and morphine to patients with chronic respiratory disorders, such as asthma or bronchitis, or infectious diseases, such as syphilis. They also used morphine to treat women with gynecological ailments; as a consequence, morphine habitués were disproportionately female. Other aspects of morphine use also led to high rates of habituation. Many doctors, for example, left morphine at patients' homes to be administered as needed since they were typically located some distance from the doctor's residence. Unsupervised use could lead to excessive use. Meanwhile, doctors liked to use morphine because patients and their families appreciated the quick relief that it provided.[11] "Of all methods ever devised for the relief of pain and suffering," Dr. Henry Gibbons asserted in 1869, "no one is so prompt and effectual as the injection of morphia into the cellular tissue. At the touch of the hypodermic syringe," he continued, pains "vanish as if by magic."[12]

Gibbons, however, wrote his book *Letheomania* not to praise morphine but to urge physicians to use it only when necessary due to the high risk of addiction. A patient who was administered the drug would seek "the same source for relief" again, he cautioned, and could likely become "the spell-bound slave of the enchantress!" In the early 1860s, for example, he had treated a man who had endured head pains for more than two years. A morphine injection produced "almost complete relief in from three to five minutes." The next morning, however, the patient told Gibbons that "the pain was returning, and he wanted to be 'stuck' again," the doctor recalled. Over time, the duration of each injection's effects on a patient would diminish, thus leading to more frequent dosing. Some patients began to self-medicate. One who suffered from neuralgia, in which there is intense pain along nerves, was so delighted with morphine's efficacy that he bought himself a syringe—both morphine and syringes could be purchased without a prescription. Four years later, the man's neuralgia was gone, but he was giving himself at least six injections per day.[13] Compounding the problem, morphine was often a component of proprietary medicines—drugs typically sold under a trade name—which added to American consumption of the drug.[14]

Other physicians also warned their colleagues that morphine injections could lead to dependency; habitual use had become prevalent among people who could afford medical care. In 1869, a writer for the *New York Herald* reported that it was "generally agreed" that opium use in America was increasing and that doctors were prescribing opiates frequently. The journalist suggested that in part, the extensive use could be attributed to a "prevalence of nervous diseases among American men and to the fact that morphia is one of the easiest palliatives that can be prescribed."[15] In 1875, Dr. Charles Cranmer deemed doctors "reckless" who prescribed morphine and opium "for every simple ache or pain." He had seen a microcosm of the problem in Saratoga, New York, where he could name at least a dozen opiate habitués in proximity to his office. Town druggists backed up his assertions.[16] In 1877, Dr. S. F. McFarland implored fellow physicians not to teach patients or their patients' friends or relatives how to administer morphine. Once they had been given the drug this way "for any considerable length of time," he warned, "they will seldom discontinue it, and will soon be inquiring where they can get 'one of those things.'"[17]

For various reasons, morphine use would diminish later in the century. Some doctors recognized that they had overused it and began administering it more sparingly, while medical students were cautioned about its risks.[18] Some states began requiring a doctor's prescription for morphine sales. Use also sometimes dropped due to diminishing need. David Musto has suggested that the market reached a point where everyone who was "environmentally or biochemically disposed to opiates" was using them, and demand consequently leveled off.[19] In some cases, the advent of vaccinations obviated the need for morphine by keeping people healthier.[20] And some people encouraged others to endure a degree of discomfort rather than use it. A writer for the *American Agriculturist* suggested in 1878 that widespread morphine use had derived from "ignorance of danger." The writer pointed out that while morphine quelled pain, it cured nothing, and he insisted that people should instead learn from an early age to "bear pain heroically."[21]

* * *

Books and articles addressing morphine habituation were among the many writings about domestic drug use that were being published at the time. Horace Day's *The Opium Habit* was the first book presenting the issue as a social problem. It and subsequent works replaced long-standing silence on the issue. Dr. Alonzo Calkins's *Opium and the Opium Appetite* and Dr. George Miller Beard's *Stimulants and Narcotics; Medically, Philosophically, and Morally Considered* were both published in 1871.[22] Popular magazines also began to report on the topic more frequently. Cheever's article had appeared in 1862, but the Civil War likely delayed more extended attention to the topic. An article penned by Fitz Hugh Ludlow had appeared in an 1867 issue of *Harper's Magazine*, and in 1874 the *Atlantic Monthly* published James Coulter Layard's account of his experience as a morphine habitué.[23] The medical community also increased its focus on the issue. In 1870, doctors interested in the treatment of addiction formed the American Association for the Study and Cure of Inebriety and seven years later began to publish the *Quarterly Journal of Inebriety*. The society regarded the condition as a curable disease and wanted governments to respond with treatment, not criminal penalties.[24] Before publication of these works, American habitual users suffered and circulated in a society that was largely unaware of their condition. Most Americans, when they thought about habitual drug use, had regarded it as a foreign problem. One writer who reviewed Calkins's *Opium and the Opium Appetite* anticipated this, cautioning his readers that while "We are apt to think ourselves far from this danger," the American public was consuming opiates at a pace that surpassed population growth, based on evidence from druggists and other witnesses to the great extent of nonmedical use.[25]

The issue became conspicuous in other ways as well, such as through public confessions, revelations in court trials, and newspaper advertisements for fraudulent addiction cures. Those whose stories were reported were typically white and well-to-do. In the fall of 1880, for example, the Reverend W. F. Camp, a well-known Methodist minister in Missouri, confessed in a St. Louis temperance meeting that he had become "an inveterate opium eater" after first using the drug thirty years earlier. When he had been mysteriously absent earlier that year, he admitted, he had been in an inebriate asylum.[26] A few years later, many newspapers reported on the divorce case of Frank and Grace Deems, a couple who had been part of New York society.[27] Each accused the other of morphine habituation. Grace denied it; Frank acknowledged his past dependency but insisted that he had recovered. Journalist Charles J. Rosebault stated that the case received so much attention because the Weemses "had been reared in pious homes, and both are well educated, refined and intelligent." "Both, however, are undoubtedly opium fiends," he surmised, "and it is this discovery that has so greatly astounded nearly everyone."[28] The large volume of newspaper ads for treatments for opiate addiction indicated that many habitués were seeking relief. In 1877, a writer for the *Medical and Surgical Reporter* found their prevalence "startling." Because the ads were published to reach "slaves to the drug who have the wish to stop," the writer concluded that the entire number of users must be considerable.[29]

Fiction writers and early filmmakers included American habitués in their stories. Edward P. Roe's bestseller *Without a Home*, published in 1881, was the first American novel in which hypodermic morphine dependency was central to the story.[30] In the work, a Confederate veteran first takes the drug to help treat a "painful disease," and his use becomes habitual. Problems resulting from his addiction lead to the premature deaths of the man, his wife, and one of their daughters.[31] Kate M. Cleary was a habitué, and she conveyed the anguish of withdrawal in her 1900 short story "The Boy's Mother."[32] At one point in the story, an invalid begs for more morphine:

> Give it to me—give it to me! My God, I'll go crazy if you don't. The point of the needle is broken off? What do I care? You can tear my arm in pieces—only give it to me! Just a little bit of morphine—you can take my rings for it, Jane! Here—here! Only a few grains! Then I'll be still—so still.[33]

Writers of adventure stories and pulp fiction published works such as *Old Tramp, the Hermit Detective; or, Tracking the Opium Smugglers of San Francisco* (1896) and *The King of the Opium Ring* (1905), in which a "crafty" Chinese man runs a smuggling ring. He later abducts a young white woman and tells her boyfriend that "no white man shall ever see her face again." The story "Hop Lee, the Chinese Slave Dealer; or, Old and Young King Brady and the Opium Fiends" appeared in the detective story magazine *Secret Service* in 1899.[34] Soon thereafter, with the advent of movies, more than two hundred silent films were made "featuring addicts, peddlers, and smugglers," as Dr. Stephen Kandall has pointed out.[35]

Many who wrote on the topic sought to emphasize that domestic drug addiction was a much more extensive problem than people realized. In a review of Horace Day's *The Opium Habit*, a writer for the publication *Old Guard* asserted that "few persons have any notion what huge amounts of opium are consumed in this country as a mere stimulant."[36] In 1883, Dr. H. H. Kane agreed that "few"

realized "how common a practice it has become in these days of hurry, excitement, nervous strain and tension" for people to use "dangerous narcotics." Non-
users frequently encountered users, albeit unwittingly. They were "constantly
jostling them in the street, being waited upon by them at tables and in stores,
meeting them in society, . . . being married, doctored, ay, even buried by them."[37]
There was also a lack of knowledge about the intensity of addiction. In 1885,
a writer for *Popular Science Monthly* asserted that only a "small portion of the
general public" comprehended "the strength of this 'habit,' and of the great difficulty, or impossibility, in most cases, of unaided cure."[38]

With modernization, stronger drugs were reaching a wider audience, thus
leading to increased use and more habituation. Drugs before the 1870s were
"simple and tried remedies," as historian Lorine Swainston Goodwin has
observed.[39] Pharmaceutical companies, however, began to isolate, produce,
and sell more and more drug alkaloids, which are the components that affect
users. In isolation, those alkaloids are more potent and predictable in their
effects than the drugs are in their unrefined state. Morphine, for example, is
an alkaloid of opium, and doctors who had access to morphine could provide
pain relief with more certain outcomes than they could with opium or laudanum. American use of cocaine, an alkaloid of the coca plant, began in the
1870s. Heroin, which was synthesized from morphine, became commercially
available in the late 1890s. As historian David Musto has noted, manufacturers
became "increasingly adept at exploiting a marketable innovation and moving
it into mass production, as well as advertising and distributing it throughout
the world."[40]

Other innovations facilitated the "advertising and distributing" aspects.
Before the 1870s, people primarily bought medicine from people they knew—
local sellers who had to provide acceptable goods in order to stay in business.
Lowered postal rates, the transcontinental railroad, and the penny press then
helped to create a national market.[41] These changes "amplified the menace of
narcotic addiction," as historian Timothy Hickman has observed. Drugs that
were stronger than the narcotics available to previous generations were reaching
more customers than would have been possible before.[42] And with this commerce, there was no personal connection between buyer and seller.

* * *

The public attention gave people who used drugs habitually the opportunity to
refute popular notions about their use, such as the idea that they could, by and
large, end their use with willpower. In 1868, a habitué told readers of *Lippincott's
Magazine* that telling a user to summon willpower to end his usage would be
as effective as "tell[ing] a man to will not to die under a mortal disease."[43] In an

1876 account of habituation, a pious Civil War veteran stated, "I believe the appetite destroys the will as firmly as I do that God exists."[44]

Some habitués believed that willpower should be sufficient, and they stated publicly that they regretted their lack of productivity. One opium user in Stockton, California, for example, admitted to a reporter in 1883 that he regarded himself as "good for nothing." He admitted that the drug gave him "the only hours of pleasure I know." He was certain that he could not end his use, and he blamed himself. "I am like 'most all the other fiends," he stated. "I have stuck to the thing so long that I have not the moral courage left to stop using it." He predicted that he would face "a good and deserved punishment" after his death. The reporter regarded the account as a valuable cautionary tale. The man's comments also demonstrated that a drug "fiend" who sustained his habit could be remorseful and remain keenly aware of his failings but simply see no way out. Meanwhile, however, he left unchallenged the mistaken notion that willpower should be sufficient to end his use.[45]

For others there was a growing understanding of the nature of addiction, including the concept of drug withdrawal. In 1869, a doctor wrote to the *Medical and Surgical Reporter* explaining that he had been taking morphine for about five years and that he felt miserable if he did not take it. "To neglect taking it destroys all appetite," he wrote, "and leaves me in a most miserable condition, which seems intolerable." The journal's editor informed him that the problem was "by no means uncommon." He then explained that the man's pains resulted from his stopping use of the drug—what would later be dubbed withdrawal. The "unpleasant sensations you experience on quitting the drug," he explained, "are more owing to the loss of it than to any disease." The editor recommended that he spend $1.50 on a copy of *The Opium Habit*.[46]

Some who shared their stories described the misery of trying to end their use. Horace Day, for example, felt "burning, tinglings, and twitchings . . . just beneath the surface of the skin over the whole body." The feelings were "so strange," he explained, that the user wants "to scream, and strike the wall, the bed, or himself, to vary them." Then, "a violent diarrhea sets in."[47] In 1895, recovering morphine habitué Henry Cole quoted the recollections of another user and insisted that "innumerable persons" had experienced the same. The man endured "cold chills" followed by "hot flashes," and "pains which pierce and sting like poisoned spears . . . all over the body." He had felt "as if a pack of sharp-toothed, hungry wolves were gnawing and tearing" at his stomach.[48]

Some doctors conveyed how intense drug addiction was by writing about some morphine users' injection scars and the broken needles inside their bodies—indicators that, apparently, nothing could make them quit. An abscess could appear when a morphine habitué used a dirty needle to inject the drug. Many users, however, continued to reuse needles, according to a St. Louis physician, even if they knew that "every injection is sure to be followed by an abscess."[49] In *Drugs That Enslave* (1881), Dr. H. H. Kane included a photograph of a male habitué. The image was taken shortly before the man died, and his body was covered in abscesses. Kane wrote that other patients of his were "quite as badly scarred."[50] Some habitués tried to avoid such visible marks, but the intensity of their addiction led to degrading behavior. "Mrs. B.," for example, was a twenty-five-year-old New York morphine user, whom Dr. Alonzo Calkins characterized as being "of delicate habit." To avoid telltale scars she administered the drug rectally, with a glass syringe. And because she needed it "several times in the day," she sometimes took it while away from home. The locations she chose were out of the way but by no means private. She told her doctor that they included "a side-room in a broker's office, or a nook in a secluded street."[51] What else could explain such behavior but intractable addiction? Other habitués had difficulty removing the needles from their bodies after injecting. In 1871, a thirty-year-old seamstress spent the last five months of her life at the New York State Lunatic Asylum. She had self-administered morphine hypodermically for about four years. At the asylum, doctors removed almost three hundred subcutaneous rusted needles and parts of needles from her body.[52]

Some habitués described their own degradation. In his memoir, D. F. MacMartin recalled using water from muddy streams to prepare his morphine injections and breaking off a needle in his right arm that eventually came out

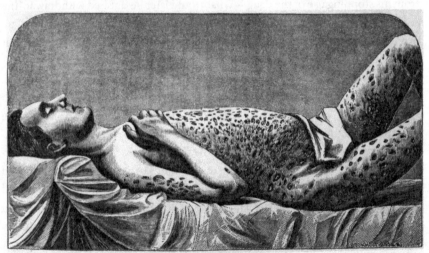

RESULT OF SUBCUTANEOUS INJECTION (see p. 71).

*Figure 8.1.* "Result of Subcutaneous Injection" from Dr. H. H. Kane's *Drugs That Enslave* (1881). According to Kane, many habitués who injected morphine were badly scarred, like this man, typically due to the use of dirty needles or a dirty solution of morphine. Many such scars would have been covered by clothing. Courtesy of Google Books.

of his right calf. He once went swimming and a "wine bum," upon seeing his abscesses, said, "This is the tattooed man from the Barnum & Bailey circus!"[53] When Annie Meyers craved cocaine but had no money for it, she thought of a way she could get some. "I . . . took a pair of shears and pried loose a tooth which was filled with gold," she recalled in *Eight Years in Cocaine Hell*. With "the blood streaming down my face and drenching my clothes," she pawned the filling for eighty cents.[54] Shocking stories had the potential to attract attention and provide a cautionary tale to readers. Some recovering habitués wanted to warn others about addiction, but other compulsive users derived satisfaction instead from shocking their audiences. Henry Sanford, for example, bragged to a reporter that doctors had once told him "they had never heard of any one who took so much morphine" as he did.[55] He also conveyed that due to his addiction, he cared about nothing but his drug. "I would kill my own father in a minute, if I could get enough for one dose," he admitted.[56]

As in earlier eras, some people worried that discussing nonmedical drug use, even while focusing on its dangers, could lead people to try it. In 1892, Dr. Leslie Keeley expressed concern that "after reading these unwise and most dangerous books, or articles, upon the opium habit," college students would decide "to procure the 'drug' and test upon themselves its magic power! They, too," he lamented, "desire to dream dreams and see visions."[57] And they might disregard the risks when doing so. Each user initially tried a drug assuming "that in his case there is no danger of forming a habit," Dr. Frederick Heman Hubbard suggested in 1881, and then some of them would keep taking it.[58]

Doctors' and habitués' publications, however, also had the potential to change popular understanding, and some commentators recognized this. One reviewer noted that Day's *The Opium Habit* showed "to what degree a man can become the slave of habit, and what extraordinary means are necessary to accomplish his freedom."[59] In 1882, other reviewers regarded Hubbard's *The Opium Habit and Alcoholism* as an effective warning. They hoped it would be read by those who are "accustomed to stop every pain with paregoric, laudanum, chloral, morphine, etc., [and] to all who are inclined to the use of the hypodermic syringe."[60] Some of the effects were evident. Dr. H. H. Kane "transformed the medical debate regarding opium" by publishing extensively on the topic and thereby educating the public on the dangers of opium habituation, as urban historian Timothy Gilfoyle has noted. Kane's writings helped to bring about an 1882 law that banned opium smoking in New York state.[61]

Habitués probably read these works eagerly, as they were desperate for information about their condition and its treatment. Before the late 1860s, to better understand their plight, American users might have had few options beyond reading a forty-year-old copy of Thomas De Quincey's *Confessions of an English Opium-Eater*. When Fitz Hugh Ludlow's essay about drug use had been published in *Harper's Monthly* in 1867, the piece "brought him hundreds of letters from all parts of the country," according to a friend of his.[62] And when Horace Day published *The Opium Habit*, he wanted to show fellow habitués that recovery was possible and thereby motivate them to "escape from the thick night" that surrounded them. He knew they were eager for information about effective treatment, and he could empathize. He recalled that in *Confessions of an English Opium-Eater*, De Quincey had included a table that showed his daily progress in reducing his doses of laudanum. Day had "read and re-read" that page, seeing it as a how-to guide, and he suspected that "hundreds of opium-eaters" were as familiar with it as he was.[63]

Despite the new openness on the topic, however, many users still tried to keep their practice secret, as the stigma remained. In the late nineteenth century, much of the medical community embraced the notion that inebriety was a disease, but much of the public remained unsympathetic.[64] One woman in upstate New York bought opium from a pharmacy ten miles from her home to hide her habit from her neighbors.[65] William Rosser Cobbe changed his routine whenever he believed that someone had discovered his secret. He stopped buying from a "good-natured and honest Greek fruit-seller," he recalled later with regret, because Cobbe misinterpreted the man's smile as a sign that he had figured out that Cobbe was drug-dependent. And Cobbe avoided an office building where "the elevator boys seemed to stare the knowledge from their inquisitive eyes."[66] Habituated members of the professional and upper classes often sought to hide their usage. A reviewer of Day's book stated that "the lawyer, the minister, [and] the literary man" "deliberately" opted for opium, because it allegedly provided a boost to the intellect but also because of "its convenient secrecy."[67] And a journalist in Colorado in 1880 explained that "fashionable women" consumed opium in the form of McMunn's Elixir. It enabled them to enjoy a "giddy round of evanescent pleasure" without "exciting the gossip" that could result from drinking champagne.[68]

In many cases, the habit was not hard to hide. Like Horace Day on that rainy Christmas morning, habitués encountered people who might notice them but were unlikely to guess their secret. A writer for Chicago's *Daily Inter-Ocean* explained that this was because their behavior was far different from that of heavy drinkers. Opium habitués did not "reel down the streets," he wrote in 1874. Instead, they tended to opt for "a quiet siesta in the solitary recesses of their chamber."[69] Even those who observed closely could miss the signs. In 1884, a New York doctor admitted that those who told him of their addiction included people "whom I should not have suspected," and that some had been able to hide their dependency "for considerable time, from their nearest friends."[70] Late in the century, patients who injected morphine could have the supplies delivered to them. In 1897, the Sears-Roebuck catalog sold a kit that included a syringe, two needles, two vials, and a case for $1.50. Although the intended customers were country doctors, sales were not limited to them.[71] Secrecy, however, made the practice seem more sinister. As Edward Roe observed of morphine dependency in *Without a Home*, "The very obscurity in which the vice is involved makes it seem all the more unnatural and repulsive."[72]

\* \* \*

Doctors had been responsible for most American habituation. In the mid-1860s, a doctor gave his patient "Patrick D——" a morphine injection to treat acute foot pain. The doctor showed Patrick's wife how to administer the injections and did not warn them to limit use of it. Less than two years later, Patrick was giving himself up to twelve morphine injections per day. "He has ruined me," he said of the doctor; his friends encouraged him to sue.[73] In 1883, drug wholesaler Charles Edward French wrote slyly in his diary, "I have found out M D means: 'more drugs.' "[74] In 1885, a reporter for the *Denver Rocky Mountain News* provided the physicians' perspective. Opiates were among "the most valued agents" to a doctor, he explained, in a world of "pain and suffering, disappointment and sorrow, a world where disease is more likely to baffle the physician than otherwise."[75] William Rosser Cobbe, however, deemed it "incomprehensible" that doctors used opium so frequently, when they must be aware of "the weakness of humanity," he stated in *Doctor Judas* (1895).[76] Although some habitués began using opiates on the recommendations of friends and family members, and some used more than their doctors had advised, doctors' administration of opiates was the biggest factor leading to opiate addiction.[77] In 1896, Dr. F. W. Comings informed members of the Vermont Medical Society that doctors were likely responsible for 90 percent of such cases.[78]

Some doctors and habitués recognized cases of addiction belatedly, because the concept was unfamiliar. In the late 1870s, a doctor in North Carolina reported to Dr. H. H. Kane that he had "used the hypodermic syringe between 2,500 and 3,000 times in a period of eighteen months" on one patient—an average of four or five injections per day—"and so far see no signs of the opium habit."[79] When Missouri physician W. D. Wilhite discussed morphine addiction with fellow physicians in the early 1880s, he learned that they knew "little of the magnitude and power of the habit of opium-eating." Wilhite learned firsthand. He had begun taking morphine in 1870 to treat rheumatism. When he stopped using it, he experienced withdrawal, but he initially thought the pain was neuralgia, which affects the nerves. "The fact was," he admitted, "I did not realize the magnitude and power of the enemy I had to fight."[80] A Civil War soldier from Madison, Wisconsin, was given morphine as a painkiller during the war and continued using it in increasingly larger doses, but not until he read Fitz Hugh

Ludlow's article in *Harper's Weekly* was he "awakened to the fact that he was a confirmed opium eater," according to Dr. Leslie Keeley.[81]

Some physicians regarded ongoing drug use as a vice and maintained that habitués could end their use through concerted effort and with limited medical support. In an 1885 medical guide, Dr. E. R. Squibb and his sons insisted that opium habituation was "a vice," not "a bodily disease." "Almost as well," they scoffed, "might they expect to cure lying or stealing." In their opinion, people needed only "moral courage" to end their usage and perhaps a doctor's assistance early on.[82] Dr. Charles Earle believed that addiction resulted solely from long periods of "intemperate" use rather than from medical doses. He therefore concluded that opium habituation was a "vice," and he believed that doctors should emphasize habitués' responsibility for their predicament. His view, however, was not the dominant one. When he wrote, in 1880, he acknowledged that "the majority of the profession" disagreed with him.[83] There is a consensus that doctors' advice led to the vast majority of cases of addiction at the time. In 1902, Dr. T. D. Crothers deemed it "very dangerous" that doctors had taught their patients how to self-administer morphine. "This practice," he observed, "undoubtedly made many morphin[e] victims."[84]

The widespread belief that someone who was addicted could end his use by summoning willpower had demoralized habitués who sought treatment. In 1895, William Rosser Cobbe recalled meeting with a doctor who believed that inebriety was a vice and that there was, therefore, no medical cure for it. Instead, the doctor stated, the habitué could end his use "only by the exercise of the power of the will." Cobbe insisted, however, that opium deprived the user of willpower. The doctor asserted that a habitué was a "sinner" and should pray, but Cobbe believed that every opium habitué had already tried that. He himself had prayed "all the hours," from morning to night. Most disheartening was the message that this doctor would provide no help. "His words," Cobbe wrote, "were as the knell of death to the condemned criminal, who knows that every hope of pardon has departed forever."[85] Some habitués who were turned away by doctors resorted to "quack cures," one physician later rued, and then stopped searching for a cure altogether and tried to live their lives as best they could.[86]

Around 1880, however, the problem was being "medicalized," as many doctors asserted that addiction was a curable illness that anybody could contract. German physician Eduard Levinstein contended that it was a medical issue rather than a moral one, and his writings influenced popular views of the problem.[87] His book was published in 1877 as *Die Morphiumsucht* and came out in English the following year as *The Morbid Craving for Morphia*. In the work, he made the case that excessive morphine use led to a "diseased state of the system."[88] His book was pathbreaking, according to social scientists Terry M. Parssinen and Karen Kerner, because he was "describing a new disease" that he linked to the user's body, not the mind. This, they maintain, paved the way for doctors to both regard it and treat it "like any other disease."[89]

Other doctors were also concluding that addiction was a disease, based on their work with habitués. Dr. S. W. Gould of Argos, Indiana, wrote in 1878 to support the disease theory. He had worked with many "so-called opium eaters" in his twenty years as a physician. Early on, he had believed that habitués could end their use with willpower and that a patient who did not do so had a "want of resolution." Experience, however, convinced him otherwise. One patient tried to end his thirty-year-long morphine habit. He could reduce the amount he consumed, but after a certain level, he "suffered beyond mortal endurance," Gould recalled. "He ached in every joint, his head, to use his own words, was bursting."[90] In 1910, Dr. George Pettey also pointed to the suffering of those who tried to quit. If it were a "mere vice," he asked, could ceasing use cause a "severe intestinal colic, nausea, vomiting, diarrhœa, labored and deficient heart action, rigors, cold, clammy sweats," and possibly death? He believed that the habitué's reaction should "convince any one that there was a real pathological condition present."[91]

Many doctors in the 1880s had an extra incentive for regarding addiction as curable: they had decided that curing wealthy habitués would be easy and profitable. Doctors tended to believe that people whose use began with a doctor's prescription could be cured.[92] Therefore, it followed that treating professional and elite habitués would not be difficult and that it could be lucrative.[93] Regarding addiction as a curable disease also enabled physicians to defend these users by explaining "why so many intelligent people could not abandon the habit," historian H. Wayne Morgan has speculated.[94] Meanwhile, treating their condition as curable also enabled doctors to challenge charlatans who sold proprietary medicines. Physicians' interest in treating cases of addiction would drop in the early twentieth century as the demographics of drug users changed to a younger and poorer group whose use had not begun by consulting a doctor.

Doctors recommended various forms of treatment, but there was extensive support for decreasing doses at a brisk pace, as opposed to a cold-turkey approach or a more gradual diminution of doses.[95] Many regarded the immediate cessation of use as cruel. In 1884 C. H. Hughes, a doctor in St. Louis, insisted that abruptly withdrawing a habitué's opium supply would "unmask a battery of Horrors which many constitutions can not endure." He advocated that authorities provide opium to habitués who were in jails, almshouses, and mental hospitals.[96] Dr. David Paulson, who worked at the sanitarium in Battle Creek, Michigan, said that administering gradually smaller doses of an opiate worked, but "it takes a while and is challenging." He preferred rapid withdrawal with physiological support, though he admitted that this process would, in its early stages, require constant attention to the patient.[97] Dr. Joseph Parrish recommended reducing the dose by two-thirds early on, and then reducing it "by inconsiderable fractional differences," while ensuring that the patient had baths, plenty of rest, a healthy diet, and medicine.[98]

Some recommended treatment in sanitaria because professional staff treated patients more strictly than family members would, but such stays could be lengthy and expensive—another sign of some patients' affluence. A writer for the *Medical and Surgical Reporter* believed that an inpatient approach was the "only reliable means of escape" from addiction.[99] Dr. Kane explained that treating habitués at home rarely worked, because relatives would succumb to the patient's "pitiful pleadings" for the drug. In a sanitarium, on the other hand, the staff would search the person's possessions for hidden morphine and would enforce doctors' orders.[100] In 1891, Dr. E. W. Mitchell agreed, stating that "strangers have far more control than relatives or friends."[101] Others pointed out, however, that managers of sanitaria had a financial incentive to draw out the recovery process, since the cost correlated with the length of the stay. And after passage of the 1914 Harrison Act, some sanitaria took advantage of an exemption in the law and supplied their residents with drugs rather than treating them.[102]

Some compulsive users were able to end their usage. In a letter to his doctor, a former habitué stated that by summoning "indomitable persistence," he had been "delivered from . . . the horrible nightmare that weighed upon me." The physician had had about forty similar cases in the previous ten years, and a third of them, as far as he could tell, were "permanent recoveries." Some former habitués asserted that religious devotion had enabled them to end their use. One woman in the 1860s, for example, had consumed opium on an almost daily basis for years. She claimed that she ended her use easily after she became active in the Methodist Church.[103] Dr. T. D. Crothers said that some could stop using it if they saw a compelling reason to do so. One woman did it because she concluded that "addiction was an unpardonable sin," he wrote. Another was miserly, and his wife emphasized the expense of the habit. He ended his use, Crothers wrote, "without any discomfort."[104]

Meanwhile, the notion that addiction could be cured opened the door to many others, including charlatans. Advances in industrialization, urbanization, and transportation had created a nationwide market for these sellers of proprietary medicines, who took advantage of the lack of personal connections between buyer and seller. A lack of conscience also made it possible. At the dawn of the twentieth century, drug manufacturers did not have a "decent regard for the health of the Public," journalist Mark Sullivan has observed.[105] Their products were not patent medicines, because they were never patented. To have done so would have required revealing their composition. Manufacturers avoided this so people would not discover, for example, that substances that could supposedly end opiate habituation contained opiates themselves.[106] Instead, many dishonest dealers registered only a trade name.[107] For a time, mountebanks could sell dangerous or ineffective products with false advertising yet remain within the law.[108]

Their ads capitalized on habitués' "desperation, shame, and gullibility," as Stephen Kandall has pointed out, and they were supported by glowing testimonials.[109] Samuel B. Collins, for example, billed himself as "Dr. S. B. Collins," although he had no medical training.[110] He promised to provide "a speedy and a sure relief for the Opium Eater . . . without pain and without inconvenience" and claimed to have already cured many.[111] Fitz Hugh Ludlow told Collins that he would promote his treatment if it worked and encouraged him to patent it, or at least to let him know what it contained. In 1872, Collins accused Ludlow of trying to steal his formula and grow rich from it.[112] Collins, however, had a different reason for keeping the composition secret: in 1876, a study revealed that it contained morphine.[113] In 1896, Dr. Basil M. Woolley advertised his remedy with ads promising "OPIUM And Whisky Habit cured at home without Pain." He offered to all interested parties free copies of *The Opium Habit and Its Cure,* a pamphlet with testimonials from doctors and others who claimed to have benefited from his treatment.[114] A muckraking reporter, however, established that Woolley's elixir "consists in 1.9 grains of morphin[e] per teaspoonful dose, to be repeated four times a day." The journalist maintained that the world "would be a better place" if Woolley were in jail.[115]

The public long remained unaware that the nostrums were dangerous or ineffective because almost all publications refused to run stories condemning them. Proprietary medicine companies protected their profits by including a clause in their advertising contracts stating that they would stop buying space in a periodical if the state in which it was published banned the manufacture or sale of proprietary medicines, a ploy that the Women's Christian Temperance Union discovered. The ads provided an important source of revenue, as their numbers attest. As a result, editors and publishers had a strong incentive to avoid steps that could lead to the passage of such legislation.[116] In the early twentieth century, muckrakers would expose these companies, and the 1906 Pure Food and Drug Act would put most of them out of business.

\* \* \*

Americans' reactions to the dangers of chloral hydrate in the later nineteenth century suggest that few considered regulating habit-forming medicines, even when their improper use could be fatal. Germans had synthesized the drug in the 1830s, and in the 1860s, doctors discovered that it was effective as a sedative and did not appear to have side effects. Use of the drug helped to usher in the era of modern psychopharmacology, in which drugs that are used to support mental health are produced by scientists rather than having a natural origin.[117]

Chloral hydrate was promoted in America as a safe sedative in the early 1870s. Professor John Darby predicted that Americans would switch from laudanum to chloral hydrate because, he asserted, it provided opiates' benefits with none of their problems. The staff of *Scientific American* agreed. Although opiates provided "ease and quiet," they also caused "Headache, sickness of the stomach, [and] loss of appetite." Chloral hydrate, on the other hand, appeared to produce "refreshing sleep" even for those experiencing "the most excruciating pains" and to do so without unpleasant consequences.[118]

Soon, doctors and others were warning the public of the risk of habituation to this drug, which occurred primarily within the middle and upper classes. According to Dr. H. H. Kane, ending the habitual use of chloral was, for the most part, easier than ending the use of an opiate. With that said, some who used chloral hydrate for an extended time developed a "morbid craving" for it and experienced effects that were more severe than the effects of morphine. Kane added that chloral habitués were "usually of the educated class, as is the case with opium." Drawing on a survey conducted around 1880, Kane reported that most female chloral users were married and suffered from "painful uterine complaints." Most of the men were alcoholic; they likely saw it as a substitute for alcohol. Some habitués first took it out of curiosity, and others hoped it would help them as they coped with "family troubles, business failures and the like."[119] A writer for the *New York Times* in 1876 noted that "chloral-punch" became "an 'institution' in the drinking-saloons of New-York scarcely a year after its introduction to medical practice."[120] By the 1880s, the habit had reached such a point that some life insurance companies were asking applicants if they used chloral. It was popular not only with insomniacs but also with "persons who are irritable and excitable and broken down by late hours and dissipation," according to a writer for *Demorest's Monthly Magazine*.[121] In 1895, recovering habitué William Rosser Cobbe stated that chloral habitués were not "in the crowded tenement houses or in the cottages of the toiling masses." Instead, it was "an intellectual and aristocratic potency, offering solace only to brain workers and those who have pushed fashionable dissipation to its extreme limit."[122]

Overdoses posed another serious risk. In 1872, Dr. I. A. Watson of Groveton, New Hampshire, reported that he had given several doses of chloral hydrate to a patient who almost died as a result, and fatal overdoses had occurred. He recommended that everyone use "the utmost care" in prescribing it, and he was especially concerned when the drug was in "unskilled hands."[123] In 1875, the *Los Angeles Herald* reported that an excessive dose could kill the user "as instantaneously as a flash of lightning."[124] In 1876, a writer for the *Ladies' Repository* implored readers to avoid chloral hydrate. Although it had been "hailed as the great hypnotic, or sleep-giver," the Germans, who had discovered it, had since concluded that it was "a destructive poison."[125]

Despite the dangers of chloral hydrate, however, commentators tended to encourage consumers to consult with doctors about it rather than calling for it to be regulated. In 1871, for example, a writer for *Harper's Bazar* warned readers to avoid "free use" of chloral hydrate due to its "dangerous properties," which could include "convulsions and death." The columnist stated that the "masses" had embraced the drug as "a sort of panacea" but criticized public experimentation with it, since even "the most intelligent physicians" only partially understood it. The writer implored consumers to consult doctors: like "other powerful drugs," chloral should be taken only "upon the prescription of a competent physician."[126] The writer did not suggest restricting access to the drug. Doctors also highlighted the value of consulting with a member of their profession, either to avoid dangerous nostrums or to focus on the underlying complaints that caused the "pain and sleeplessness" that would-be consumers endured. In such cases, taking medicine stifled the symptoms but did not solve the problem.[127]

Much of the population, however, would continue to experiment with remedies. In Burlington, New Jersey, Dr. Joseph Parrish reported that some people took a variety of drugs to procure ease. They "alternate between morphia, chloral, whiskey, and the bromides," he explained, "with the result of rest and composure from each in its turn."[128] Others saw the same thing. In 1890, a writer for the *Christian Advocate* observed that many Americans "are always dosing themselves. A new remedy is advertised, and they try it." The writer considered such people to be gullible, as they assumed that new products would help them, even though they did not know what they were taking.[129]

Such experimentation was possible, of course, because the drugs remained widely available. In 1878, Dr. Orville Marshall of North Lansing, Michigan, reported that in his state, it "would not be difficult for a lunatic or a child to obtain at the drug stores all the opium he called for, provided he told a plausible story and had the money to pay for it."[130] Recalling his time out west, pharmacist Louis Weiss wrote that druggists would sell "strychnia, arsenic, laudanum, or any other poisonous drugs . . . to any one that pleased to buy, and no questions asked."[131] And when habitué Henry Cole broke his syringe in an Albany hotel room late one night, he worried that he would have difficulty replacing it, but his concerns were baseless. There and in other cities, he "never experienced any more difficulty in obtaining the drug than in buying the most harmless thing." Someone directed him to a druggist, who told Cole "that he had twelve opium patients to whom he daily administered the drug."[132]

\* \* \*

Drug habituation was extensive among the middle and upper classes in the late nineteenth century, and many maintained that the intensity of modern times exhausted the professional classes, thus making a resort to drugs necessary, for restorative purposes. In 1893, the American Association for the Study and Cure of Inebriety (AASCI) described the people who were most susceptible to drug use. They included "business and professional men, who have broken down from overwork, worry, and irregularity of life." These men were exhausted by "the rushing, grinding civilization of to-day" and "the struggle for position, wealth and power." Such men typically had "the highest talent and genius" but were prone to "inebriety and its allied diseases." To the AASCI, these people were patients. "In this class," they wrote, "the use of alcohol, opium, or any other narcotic is often more of a symptom of exhaustion and debility, for which rest and medical care are essential."[133]

Alongside this notion was a widely believed corollary: that manual labor was not taxing, and because those who performed it would remain physically and mentally healthy, they would never need a tonic. Dr. Leslie Keeley expressed this prevalent view when he wrote, "The laborer in the field, at the anvil, or in any other mere physical pursuit" had no grounds for drug use. Without it, a member of the working class would still awaken the next morning with "clear eye, clear head, hearty appetite and vigorous strength."[134] Dr. George Miller Beard agreed, insisting that "nervous diseases" were rare among "muscle-workers," whom he deemed to be in "the lower orders in our great cities."[135] This perspective implied that the only possible source of adversity for people was the work that they did and that physical labor could not take a toll. Some concluded that drug use by members of the working class, therefore, could not be restorative and must be self-indulgent. Because these workers were "supposedly free of the commercial and cultural strains of modern life," their use was criticized, as Timothy Hickman has pointed out.[136]

Some asserted that "geniuses" were most inclined to be inebriates. In 1879, a writer for the *Philadelphia Press* suggested that this correlation existed—that the most intelligent people were the most likely to end up as opium habitués. "Like alcoholic drunkenness," he surmised, "its prey is chosen from the gifted, the intellectual and the most admired for wit and fancy."[137] In 1893, the AASCI asserted that the people who were susceptible included those with "a constant tendency to exhaust themselves, as, for instance, in case of extraordinary mental or physical genius." Such people—including "many of the so-called great men of the world"—appeared to need drugs for restorative purposes.[138]

Beard believed that the innovations that helped to define modern America taxed the energies of the middle and upper classes and that their enervation constituted an ailment, which he called "neurasthenia." He believed, for example, that Thomas Edison's inventions made "constant and exhausting draughts on the nervous forces of America and Europe."[139] He saw Samuel F. B. Morse's telegraph, which had connected the nation in the 1840s and 1850s, as providing additional pressure.[140] He also included the nation's political system and penny press, leadership opportunities for women, and challenges to traditional Protestant Christianity. All these, he insisted, "are so many additional lamps interposed in the circuit." He did not suggest, however, that neurasthenia afflicted everybody. Members of the working class had "little education," he stated, and little ambition: they were exempt because they were "not striving for honor, or expecting eminence or wealth."[141] And Dr. Anna Hayward Johnson specified in 1881 that it was "adult Americans of the upper and middle classes" who "live on the principal, not the interest, of their strength."[142] The concept was influential, as the diagnosis was used until the 1910s to explain why some users had become habitués.[143]

Popular publications, when addressing the addictive drug use of the times, also noted that many habitués were middle and upper class. In 1900, a writer for the humor magazine *Puck* asserted that almost everyone had "some favorite 'bracer' to-day that he or she takes habitually." Worse still, people were relying on advertisements, rather than doctors, for medical advice. The writer deemed such drug use "a greater evil to-day than intemperance in alcohol." In the accompanying cartoon, customers clamor to buy tonics at the "Killem' Quick Pharmacy." The establishment is open all night. The counter is crowded with bottles of opium, cocaine, and other dangerous substances, and a syringe is in a glass case. Children are among the clientele. A frustrated saloon keeper observes the pharmacist waiting on customers and complains, "I can't begin to compete with this fellow." Users could justify their use of elixirs as therapeutic in nature, while such an explanation could not apply to drinking in a saloon. The customers are white and affluent: a man in the foreground wears pinstripes and gloves and carries a walking cane, and the woman behind him wears an elegant outfit, including a necklace and muff.[144]

Some people associated drug use with "civilization" and thereby presented drug habituation as a mark of distinction for the United States and western Europe. In 1871, Dr. Beard asserted that of all the people on earth, those in the "most enlightened, the most progressive nations" used drugs "in the greatest abundance and widest variety." Those nations were the United States, Great Britain, and Germany. He insisted that a nation's level of "enlightenment" correlated positively with how much its population indulged in drugs. The "semi-civilized" populations in some Asian and Latin American nations, he stated, "use some varieties to considerable excess." And "purely barbarous races and tribes," he continued, had only one or two drugs to choose from and rarely used them excessively. "Africa," he wrote, "seems to use less

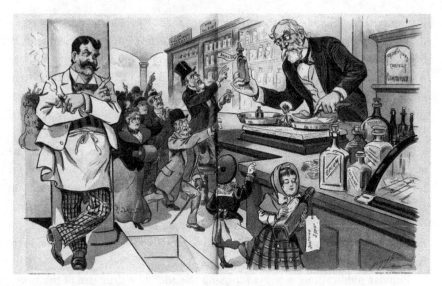

*Figure 8.2.* Louis Dalrymple, "The Age of Drugs," *Puck,* October 10, 1900. The customers are white and well-dressed. Their worried expressions as they offer money to the pharmacist suggests they are habitual users—that they are eager to purchase their drugs before he runs out of them. At the time, many writers regarded members of the middle and upper classes as particularly susceptible to addiction. Courtesy of the Library of Congress, LC-DIG-ppmsca-25463.

than any other continent." Beard explained this pattern by stating that "advanced civilization" required men to do intense mental work, and they coped with the resulting "cares, toils, and pressures" by using a variety of drugs. He, however, saw a problem with this: the "most enlightened" nations, he stated, had some citizens whose work was primarily manual. Beard suggested that this created a perilous situation in which people who had no real need for the drugs had access to a variety of them. "The poor, and ignorant, and idle classes," as he put it, lacked the "moral force and elevation" to use the drugs moderately. As a result, they would "fall into the habit of indulging in them to enormous excess."[145]

Some doctors agreed with Beard that "nervousness" prevailed extensively in America, that it was unknown in nations that were neither industrialized nor urbanized, and that many Americans used drugs to relieve their anxiety. In 1888, Dr. Edward P. Thwing stated that "barbarians are not nervous" and maintained that this was because they were free from the trappings of civilization. Among them,

stock quotations are unknown; telephones and telegraphs; daily newspapers, with all their crowded columns of horror and crimes, are not thrust upon them; and the shriek of the steam engine does not disturb their mid-day or their midnight sleep.

He asserted that looking at a watch "when an appointment is near, sensibly accelerates the heart's action and is correlated to a definite loss of nervous energy." Every "advance of refinement," he summed up, was paid for "in blood and nerve and life."[146] This strain could lead to widespread drug use. Writing in Chicago in 1894, Dr. W. F. Waugh characterized extensive use of opium in America as "the price we pay for our modern civilization."[147]

Others associated compulsive opium use with refinement and emphasized differences directly along racial lines by suggesting that white people were the most vulnerable to opiate habituation. When describing opium use in the United States in 1877, for example, a writer for the *New York Times* maintained that the "negro and Indian races" were "exempt" from the habit. "From a social standpoint," he wrote, "the higher and more cultivated classes . . . furnish the largest number of opium-takers."[148] Racist ideas shaped these suppositions whether the focus was national or international in scope. In 1881, Dr. D. W. Nolan suggested that "the Caucasian" might have a particularly "delicate nervous organization" that could "render him more susceptible to the deleterious effects of narcotic stimulants than is the Chinaman or Hindoo."[149] And in 1885, a writer for the *Memphis Avalanche* reported that the opium habit was "most injurious to the Caucasian race, as it attacks the brain first." He stated that "the Mongolian" fared better with opium than did white people, and "the African seems to withstand its effects best of all."[150] Such beliefs led some to conclude that white people who were addicted deserved sympathy for their condition, due to their unusual vulnerability, while nobody else was entitled to such support. As Timothy Hickman has observed of America at the time, "The relatively safe haven of victimhood was often denied to Chinese immigrants and to African Americans because they were allegedly free from the strains of modern economic and social competition." If they were using drugs, white commentators tended to criticize their behavior as a failure of self-control, based on the assumption that they led carefree lives.[151]

The tendency to criticize drug habituation among marginalized Americans, of course, ignores the fact that there were many types of adversity, especially those linked to poverty and prejudice, that would not have afflicted the white middle class. In the late 1880s, about 40 percent of industrial workers lived below the poverty line.[152] Some lived in tenements that had narrow and "foul-smelling" courtyards and "steep rickety stairs," journalist Allan Forman reported in 1888. He warned that in the event of a fire, the buildings would be "perfect death-traps."[153] The era's recurring economic depressions led to high rates of unemployment. After the Panic of 1893, for example, unemployment reached 18.4 percent.[154]

Meanwhile, as labor historian Brian Kelly has pointed out, African Americans between the Civil War and 1900 experienced a "staggering descent from high optimism to despondency."[155] After the end of Reconstruction, in 1877, white southerners established segregation laws in an effort to erase freedmen's gains, and as late as 1910, 90 percent of African Americans still lived in the South.[156] Although white southern men asserted that black men threatened white women, "in practice, it was white men who . . . targeted black homes," as historian Richard White has observed. White people believed they could still control "black lives and politics," and they resorted to violence, including murder, when African Americans challenged that control. Chinese immigrants and Chinese Americans faced prejudice and violence because they competed with white workers for jobs and because many native-born Americans regarded them as unable to assimilate. According to White, "in the 1890s, the United States was less egalitarian" than it had been immediately following the Civil War.[157] Many who wrote about the restorative potential of certain drugs, however, focused only on the challenges faced by those in the white middle class.

Occasionally, some would point out that all people dealt with challenging situations and that it was unsurprising that they would use intoxicants to help them cope. In *The Opium Habit*, Horace Day acknowledged that opiate use was common among women who were "obliged by their necessities to work beyond their strength."[158] In 1883, Dr. A. P. Meylert noted that women in the "poor under-class" who drank or used narcotics had often been "driven to intemperance by poverty, sorrow or abuse."[159] In 1886, Philadelphia physician James Wilson stated that opium had great appeal to "the overworked and underfed mill-operator."[160] And in 1893, the AASCI acknowledged that "all business and professional activity" involved "constant strain and excitement." This, they added, affected everyone, "From the poorest laborer to the millionaire and professional man."[161] Some expressed concern that those who indulged in habitual use were often those who could least afford to do so. In 1879, writers for the *American Socialist* criticized the fact that "the poorer classes" everywhere "subject themselves" to practices that make them poorer, including "luxuries" such as opium use.[162]

Immigrants from Europe rarely became habitual opiate users. This was partly because many preferred alcohol, but some suggested it was because their lives were more relaxed than those of the "American type." In 1880, Chicago physician Charles W. Earle wrote that it was unusual to find German or Irish immigrants using opiates, since Germans found solace in beer and the Irish found "relief from their troubles" in whiskey. He added, "It is very rare to find a poor Bohemian or Swede habitually taking any kind of an opiate."[163] In 1871, Dr. Alonzo Calkins agreed that "almost to a man," Irish and German immigrants did not use opiates habitually.[164] Also, they might be underrepresented because

European immigrants were disproportionately robust men—a category that, in general, produced few habitués.[165] An 1888 study in Boston revealed that drugstores in the "aristocratic quarters" dispensed opiates most frequently and that the pharmacy with the "lowest proportion" of opiate prescriptions was in a neighborhood "among poor Italian laborers."[166] And in 1916, Charles W. Towns claimed that of the "thousands of drug-users" he had known, he had "never seen an Italian, a Hungarian, a Russian, or a Pole," and he had only seen "four cases of drug-taking by Hebrews." He contrasted their lives with those of people whom he designated the "American type." Members of the latter group lived "under pressure," he wrote, "always going to the full limit, or beyond," and were there-fore "peculiarly liable to disorders that lead to the habitual use of drugs."[167]

* * *

Despite the ready availability of drugs, the number of American habitués began to decline as the twentieth century drew near. Soon, however, the nation's foreign-policy goals would oblige the federal government to enact drug-control legislation at home, and young, marginalized men would emerge as the nation's most visible group of habitual drug users. In these changed circumstances, the US government would, for the first time, consider regulatory measures.

# Federal Regulation Begins, 1875–1914

In the late 1860s many publications began to focus on native-born Americans' drug dependency, but there had been no efforts at the federal level to regulate habit-forming drugs, despite the dangers resulting from their untethered availability. In his essay for the *North American Review*, Dr. David Cheever noted one concern: while many Americans used opium, many more ingested it unknowingly. Opium was "used secretly in patent medicines and quack preparations, to an enormous extent," he reported. In any medicines to treat spasms or pain, including neuralgia, as well as "for cough-mixtures, diarrhea-mixtures . . . and 'soothing syrups,'" he explained, "opium, in the form of morphine, laudanum, or paregoric, is the sine qua non." He lamented that "those very remedies which are advertised and puffed as free from opium or paregoric, and hence adapted to the tenderest infancy, often contain large amounts of this drug."[1] Consumers would continue to buy those products for decades, but as the United States entered the twentieth century, Progressive Era legislation would begin to regulate drugs at the federal level. These proprietary preparations would be among the first to receive this oversight with passage of the 1906 Pure Food and Drug Act.

\* \* \*

In the late 1890s, a detective at Marshall Field & Co. caught Annie Meyers, a white and well-to-do member of Chicago society, trying to shoplift "costly silks and expensive pocket-books" from the store. Meyers had become addicted to cocaine in 1894 when she took it to treat a bad cold, as she recalled in her memoir, *Eight Years in Cocaine Hell*. She turned to shoplifting because her habit cost ten dollars a day, a burdensome amount at the time. When the detective caught her, he took her to the manager's office:

*Habit Forming.* Elizabeth Kelly Gray, Oxford University Press. © Oxford University Press 2023.
DOI: 10.1093/oso/9780190073121.003.0010

The manager said, "If we let you go will you keep out of the store?" I answered, "Gentlemen, excuse me while I take a blow of my cocaine," as I had to take it about every five minutes. They asked me to show them again, and several different times, while there, how I took it. The manager spoke kindly to me, saying, "Poor unfortunate woman, God has been merciful to me and I will be merciful to you. You are free."

The detective ordered her not to return to the store, but she did so, and he caught her again, this time stealing a pair of fur gloves. Once again, he brought her to the manager's office. The subsequent exchange suggests the manager regarded her more as a likable if addlepated woman than as a drug-addicted thief. "'Do you know the value of these gloves, Mrs. Meyers?'" he asked her. He and the detective then "laughed" when she learned that she had grossly underestimated their cost and, thus, would have sold them illegally for far less than she could have gotten. She offered to let them search her for additional merchandise, but they declined and let her go. This facilitated her theft. "I still had about $25 worth of goods on me," she admitted, "and sold them for $10."[2]

Although Meyers endured some public reproach—her thievery was reported in the newspaper, and she served time in jail—her race and upper-class status minimized the legal consequences that she faced. When she admitted to the manager of Rothschild's department store that she had stolen about two thousand dollars' worth of merchandise from his store, for example, he also declined to press charges on the condition that she not return.[3] She was arrested at a third store and ended up in court, where she begged the judge, "in the language of a woman of culture, to deal kindly with her," according to a newspaper reporter for Chicago's *Inter-Ocean*. She promised to stay away from department stores. Her pledge worked; the judge suspended her fifty-dollar penalty.[4] Even so, the scope of her crimes was extensive. In 1899, the *Inter-Ocean* reported that the "prominent society woman" had become a "confirmed shoplifter," and she served thirty-seven days in jail. She later published her memoir to provide a cautionary tale to those who had never used cocaine and an inspirational story to habitués who regarded recovery as impossible.[5] Her willingness to reveal her identity and share her story provides another example of the shift in public discourse, as some former habitués concluded that being open about addiction would help in addressing the problem. Again, however, her race and class status protected her, and the opportunity to present her own story allowed her to garner sympathy.

State governments and the US government passed anti-drug legislation in the early twentieth century, and many supporters of such measures saw it as facilitating control over marginalized groups, especially people of color who allegedly menaced their white neighbors. Proponents of new laws sometimes mentioned problematic drug use by white members of the so-called criminal classes, but the focus was on members of other races.[6] A 1909 law, for example, barred sales of peyote mushrooms, which were associated almost exclusively with Native Americans, who supposedly threatened whites in the vicinity. Dr. Hamilton Wright, who advocated passage of the 1909 Smoking Opium Exclusion Act, admitted that he hoped it would impel many Chinese American users to leave the country. And in 1914, the Harrison Narcotic Act outlawed the nonmedical use of cocaine and opiates. Some proponents suggested, falsely, that cocaine use had led African American men to assault white women sexually.

The passage of national legislation was facilitated by the changing demographics of domestic habitués, but it responded to international considerations. The United States annexed the Philippines in 1898 and sought to reduce opium use there. To do this, it pursued cooperation from other nations. The need to show American commitment on the issue to a global audience overwhelmed traditional domestic belief that drug regulation was a matter for states rather than for the federal government. Domestic considerations, however, shaped support for the bills. Most significantly, well-to-do white women who were habituated to morphine were passing away. This group, who had inspired compassion, were supplanted by young men of marginal circumstances who began using drugs such as heroin for pleasure-seeking purposes. Like others, they sought solace in drugs, but they received little sympathy.

National legislation removed drugs from soda fountains and mail order warehouses and concentrated control of them with doctors, pharmaceutical companies, and the US government. These changes, however, also established two classes of people who were addicted: those whose use was medical in origin would be treated like patients, and others, if they could not end their habitual use, would have to break the law in order to sustain their access. Frequently, users' race and class, rather than the nature of their habituation, determined the response that they received.

* * *

Cocaine came from South America's coca plant, and coca leaves had long suppressed users' appetites while renewing their energy. In 1860, a writer for the *American Journal of the Medical Sciences* had characterized coca leaves as the alternative to "tea, coffee, betel, tobacco, haschisch, and opium" for the people of Bolivia, Chile, and Peru.[7] There, the leaves helped agricultural workers and others with arduous jobs to get through their days. They were useful to "the porter who carries the mail, and accompanies the traveller over the roughest roads," and to "the Indian who works half naked in the silver and quicksilver mines," the writer explained. Employers often provided coca to their laborers in addition to wages.[8] The cocaine alkaloid had been isolated in 1860.[9] By the

1870s, the pharmaceutical company Parke-Davis was doing research on coca, and American researchers were advertising it.[10]

In a medical context, Americans used cocaine as an anesthetic and as a treatment for ailments including sinus problems and opiate addiction. Before the advent of cocaine, general anesthetics such as ether and chloroform were doctors' only options, but with cocaine, a patient could remain awake during surgery, and there was a greater chance that the procedure, especially eye surgery, would be successful. Physicians also discovered cocaine's ability to clear clogged sinuses, and cocaine-based nasal sprays were widely used to treat conditions including hay fever.[11] The use of cocaine to treat morphine habituation derived from the theory "that narcotics were antagonised by stimulants," as Richard Davenport-Hines has explained. Dr. John Pemberton, the inventor of Coca-Cola, first took coca to treat the morphine habit that he contracted following the Civil War.[12] By the 1890s, however, the medical community recognized the switch from morphine to cocaine as a harmful one.[13]

In the 1880s, many regarded cocaine as an aid to productivity, in part because it could enhance alertness and cognitive skills. Dr. Walter Woodman in Portland, Maine, for example, suffered from insomnia, and one night after injecting the drug, he felt awake enough "to read understandingly a very abstruse book." He added that his cocaine use did not lead to "disagreeable after-effects."[14] Another doctor also found that cocaine use gave him "a desire for brain work" and that, after taking some, he would "pass the greater part of the night reading and writing on professional topics, experiencing a keenness of perception and a mental vigor greater than normal."[15]

At the turn of the century, many African American men used cocaine to sustain themselves as they worked tough jobs for long hours, and they did so with their employers' sanction, and even with their involvement. "Under the influence of cocaine," a pharmacist explained in 1895, "capacity for labor is augmented, and the need of sleep much diminished."[16] Cocaine enabled stevedores in New Orleans to load and unload steamboats for as many as seventy consecutive hours, "without sleep or rest, in rain, in cold and in heat," a writer for the *New York Sun* explained in 1902. Long hours and a job well done meant extra income, and many employers provided cocaine as part of the wages. Men who built levees along the Mississippi River—"where the work is hard, and the conditions of life and work unfavorable," according to the *Sun* writer—also adopted the practice, as did men who picked cotton on plantations. Picking cotton was not as demanding as unloading cargo, but planters faced a labor shortage. Both workers and employers, therefore, saw advantages in the increased productivity that cocaine made possible: workers increased their pay, and employers solved their labor-shortage problems. One "big planter" kept cocaine on hand, the writer added, and gave it to his workers "just as he was accustomed in the past to issue

rations of whiskey." Some workers in Mississippi made access to cocaine a condition of their employment.[17]

Workers in other regions of the country also used cocaine to enhance their
performance, sometimes at the behest of those they worked for. An employer at
a Connecticut silk mill, for example, gave workers a "menthol and cocaine spray"
so they would not be bothered by the dust that the work generated. Employees of
textile mills in Lewiston, Maine, also received cocaine from those who oversaw
them. In 1894, Dr. C. P. Ambler reported that cocaine use had become "very
common" in "some portions of the far West, especially in the mining regions,"
due to its stimulant effects. Commissaries in many Colorado mining camps, for
example, sold cocaine for a time, as it seemed to help exhausted employees restore their energy. And in 1903, engineers in Pittsburgh bought it when they
worked overtime to help them stay awake.[18]

Many white, middle-class Americans used cocaine-laced drinks as a restorative after a strenuous day. Some relaxed with "coca wines" such as Vin Mariani.
Angelo Mariani had developed the drink—a combination of red wine and coca
leaves—as a cure for depression while living in Paris in the 1860s. Later in the
century it became popular in America. A wineglass of Vin Mariani contained
just under 25 milligrams of cocaine and, in 1903, the company recommended a
glass of it with each meal.[19] America's middle class also drank Coca-Cola, which
originally contained about 8.45 milligrams of cocaine per serving. For matters
of comparison, a line of cocaine would contain about 50 to 75 milligrams, and
snorting it would give the user a "pleasurable 'rush,'" Dr. Steven Karch notes.
Cocaine has a greater impact when inhaled than when it is consumed in a drink.
Nonetheless, as writer Mark Pendergrast points out, the cocaine in Coca-Cola
could have had an effect "when combined with the 80 milligrams of caffeine"
that the original drink also contained.[20] Few, however, saw this as a problem. In
the late nineteenth century, Americans tended to regard cocaine as a beneficial
medicine, tonic, and aid to productivity.

* * *

In the early twentieth century, there were successful challenges to the proprietary drug industry. Women had organized to challenge these businesses in the
1880s because they saw the products as a threat to society's safety, and several
magazines later ran articles about the industry's fraudulent practices.[21] Freelance
journalist Samuel Hopkins Adams, for example, exposed the industry's misdeeds
in a series of articles that appeared in Collier's magazine from 1905 to 1907. He
revealed that most of the products were ineffective, and many were dangerous.[22]
"Gullible America," he warned, was spending $75 million annually on proprie-
tary medicines that contained "huge quantities of alcohol, an appalling amount

of opiates and narcotics, [and] a wide assortment of varied drugs ranging from powerful and dangerous heart depressants to insidious liver stimulants." To Adams, those who sold false cures for drug addiction were the worst of the worst, since they took advantage of "human wrecks" who were desperate for help. He had ordered many of the products and then had them tested. "In every case," he reported, "the 'remedy' sent me to cure the morphin[e] habit has been a morphin[e] solution."[23]

Passage of the Pure Food and Drug Act in 1906 dealt a blow to the industry, since it required companies that participated in interstate commerce to list their products' ingredients on the packaging. The package also had to accurately list the quantity of alcohol and opiates present.[24] The law revealed that almost all alleged treatments for drug addiction "are simply the drug itself in concealed form," as Adams explained.[25] The substances were not outlawed, but the exposure had a significant effect. Within a couple years of its passage, sales of proprietary medicines containing opiates dropped by between 25 and 50 percent.[26] Catarrh powders, such as the one that Annie Meyers used, were no longer manufactured. And due to its cocaine content, Vin Mariani could no longer be sold in New York, Chicago, and Philadelphia, and throughout Massachusetts.[27]

\* \* \*

Many Mexicans immigrated to the United States in the early twentieth century, and early sources erroneously identified marijuana use with Mexico and with violent behavior. In the late nineteenth and early twentieth centuries, Mexicans came to the United States to help meet the demand for labor in the West that followed the arrival of railroads and to escape the violence of the Mexican Revolution. Some smoked cannabis, but the press exaggerated both the extent of their use of it and the drug's hazards.[28] In 1897, some California papers reported on "a weed called the mariguana," the effects of which were reportedly more powerful than opium.[29] In 1900, a Redlands paper stated that marijuana was a "Mexican herb" and that a person, on smoking it, "wants at once to kill everybody and anybody."[30] Subsequent articles also associated marijuana with Mexicans and reinforced the idea that its users became violent and unrestrainable. A Santa Barbara paper, for example, reported that a Mexican laborer had been "seized with a fit of insanity" after smoking it. He "made a murderous assault upon his wife with a knife," the *Independent* reported, stabbed a policeman who responded to the scene, and then attacked those who pursued him.[31] Newspapers in other states carried similar stories.[32]

One of the false ideas that such stories conveyed was the notion that America's marijuana users were, overwhelmingly, Mexican immigrants. Mexicans were among the customers for it, buying it for medical or pleasure-seeking purposes.

White and black Americans, however, were also using it, and the drug was selling in parts of the country where few, if any, Mexican immigrants lived. In 1915, for example, officers in the juvenile court of Portland, Oregon, learned that teenaged boys were buying cannabis at drugstores and using it for nonmedical purposes. About a dozen had become addicted. Historian Isaac Campos suggests that the popularity of marijuana use grew because Americans were increasingly smoking it rather than eating it, since that method of ingestion was less likely to produce the negative consequences of excessive use. Usage also could have increased because some people sought new options after restrictions were imposed on alcohol, opiates, and cocaine.[33]

Although many Americans perceived Mexico as the main source of marijuana imports, this was not the case. By the early twentieth century, when some Americans and Mexicans were experimenting with the drug, American drugstores had been selling cannabis for medical purposes for decades. Reginald Smith, who worked for the Department of Agriculture's Bureau of Chemistry, concluded that most of the cannabis in America had come from India and that pharmaceutical companies were selling it in many parts of the United States. In the 1910s, the company Parke Davis was an especially successful distributor.[34]

Many people came to associate marijuana use with violent, crazed behavior because its use can lead to erratic conduct and because some Mexicans were loath to defend its use. Researchers have noted that the degree of social acceptance of the drug can affect the user's behavior—that panic reactions, for example, are much more likely if a person uses marijuana in an environment where its use is condemned as opposed to a setting where it is accepted. Isaac Campos suggests that few questioned allegations that marijuana use led to violence because marijuana users in Mexico were primarily marginalized people, and the "small class of literate elites" who wrote on the subject held them in disdain. The resulting sensational stories provided content for US newspapers.[35]

Readers were led to conclude that marijuana use led to violent behavior, but many such stories were unsubstantiated. In 1913, for example, the El Paso Herald ran the article "Crazed by a Weed, Man Murders," which stated that "Marihuana, that native Mexican herb which causes the smoker to crave murder, is held accountable for two deaths." The assertion that drug use caused the man's rampage, however, was based solely on witnesses' suspicions. Nobody had seen him use marijuana, and his identity was unknown, but bystanders stated that, "unmistakably," he had been "smoking the native opium, 'marihuana,'" based on their observations of his violent behavior, as the paper reported. The assumption that the drug was to blame contributed to a "vicious and misleading circle" of reasoning about it, as historian Bob Chessey has pointed out.[36] Meanwhile, defendants sometimes attested that marijuana use caused violent behavior, but there is reason to question their assertions as well. Law professors Richard

J. Bonnie and Charles H. Whitebread concluded that "desperate defendants" saw the value of attributing their acts to marijuana use. Having been caught red-handed, they "sought mitigation of their penalties" by blaming their behavior on a drug that supposedly inspired violence.[37]

California outlawed marijuana in 1913, but this move resulted partly from opposition to another marginalized group, the Sikh community. In 1911, California was home to a community of fewer than three thousand Sikh immigrants, most of them agricultural workers who had arrived in San Francisco from India's Punjab region. They faced prejudice from opponents of Asian immigration, including local politicians who played to nativist sentiment as well as those who saw them as providing unwelcome job competition. Henry J. Finger, a longtime member of the state's Board of Pharmacy, was slated to go with Hamilton Wright, the United States Opium Commissioner, to the International Opium Conference. In a letter to Wright, he presented the Sikhs as a threat. Many "Hindoos" had been moving to California, he wrote, and they wanted *Cannabis indica*. He characterized them as "very undesirable" and feared they would be "initiating our whites into this habit." He added, "Can we do anything in the Hague that might assist in curbing this matter?" There was little support for the idea of controlling the international traffic in cannabis, so Wright recommended that Finger work with California's legislature. Evidence of drug use by the state's immigrants from India, however, is sparse.[38] When a Hindu man in California stole a watch in 1913 and blamed his behavior on inadvertent marijuana use, for example, the case made the papers due to its novelty.[39]

The association of marijuana use with violence did facilitate the passage of anti-marijuana legislation that appeared to establish a means of control over Mexican immigrants. "Once the potential of marijuana legislation for suppressing the migrants was realized," Martin Booth has observed, "other cities and districts were quick to imitate it."[40]

\* \* \*

State restrictions on drug use would extend to a cactus called peyote, which some Native Americans consumed in religious ceremonies and which white Americans learned about in the latter half of the nineteenth century. In the 1890s, Native Americans in the southern plains ate peyote, also known as mescal buttons, for its "medical and psychologic properties," according to ethnographer James Mooney. A mescal button has prickles and is about one to three inches in diameter.[41] Peyote ceremonies typically began on a Saturday night and ended at noon the next day. In them, men would gather around a fire in a tipi and would pray, sing, and eat. After the opening prayer, each man would consume four mescal buttons, and they would eat more peyote after midnight. As Mooney explained, they regarded peyote as the "incarnation of a deity," something that could both cure ailments and give users access to "the glories of another world."[42]

Peyote appeared to be effective as an appetite suppressant and to have curative potential.[43] Many Native Americans found it effective in treating consumption, now known as tuberculosis, an ailment for which there had been no known cures.[44] Two doctors who studied it in the mid-1890s concluded that it could also treat abdominal pain, depression, chronic coughs, and neurasthenia. Part of a mescal button "the size of a pea," for example, relieved the cough of a man with chronic bronchitis, and a second dose enabled him to get a good night's sleep. Another man had endured neurasthenia for six months, but three mescal buttons relieved him of his "bodily and mental fatigue," according to the physicians.[45] Although some doctors maintain that peyote can help treat mental illnesses and alcoholism, its status as a Schedule I drug limits study of its medical efficacy.[46]

Around the turn of the century, some researchers maintained that peyote use was safe and that it elicited positive visions. Mooney observed peyote use many times and saw no evidence of negative effects.[47] In the 1890s, two doctors in Washington, D. C., tested it on six white men. One participant acknowledged that under its influence, negative thoughts could bring negative visions, but he also reported experiencing greater pleasure than he ever had before—a "high ecstatic state in which our exclamations of enjoyment become involuntary," as he later described it. The subjects, the doctors summed up, experienced visions that "ranged from ill-defined flashes of color to most beautiful figures, forms, landscapes, [and] dances."[48] In 1902, English physician Havelock Ellis reported in *Popular Science Monthly* that mescal buttons could help the user to see beauty in "the very simplest things."[49] And a study in the mid-1890s included a participant who admired Robert G. Ingersoll, a lawyer known for his support of agnosticism. Under peyote's influence, the man believed that he could see "angels in the streets of gold." He said, "I wish I could talk with Ingersoll just for a minute: I could convince him that there is a heaven. I see it."[50]

Some agents for the U.S. Bureau of Indian Affairs pressed for a ban on peyote, however, on the theory that its use was dangerous and that users might threaten the white population. In 1886, United States Indian Agent J. Lee Hall believed that peyote use was injurious and was becoming more widespread, and he suggested to the commissioner of Indian Affairs that it "be made contraband."[51] Two years later his successor, E. E. White, stated that "white people living in the vicinity of the Comanches . . . were becoming alarmed for their safety," due to the hallucinations that peyote inspired. He provided little evidence of the dangers of its use. Nonetheless, he sought to persuade the Comanches to limit their use and to end it altogether when their supply ran out.[52] In 1909, William E. Johnson, the chief special officer of the Bureau of Indian Affairs, sought to stop the peyote traffic on the grounds that it was an intoxicant. To this end, he reported that he had bought and destroyed "the entire visible supply at Laredo, Texas, amounting to about 200,000 peyotes."[53] The agents did not always succeed in suppressing use. In 1907, the superintendent for the Cheyenne and Arapaho Agency tried to outlaw peyote at the Oklahoma Constitutional Convention. He failed, however, as members of the Kiowa, Comanche, Plains Apache, and Cheyenne tribes also attended and defended the use of mescal buttons, and members of the legislature found them persuasive. The Comanche Quanah Parker, for example, spoke in defense of peyote use, and he bore no negative effects from his use of it. The legislators considered him to be witty and intelligent, and they were impressed that he was a successful cattleman.[54]

Some who wrote about the use of peyote erroneously assumed that all psychoactive drugs affected users in similar and censured ways by spurring lascivious sexual behavior, addiction, and a lack of productivity. Journalist Gertrude Seymour, for example, stated that women who were not "originally given to immorality" were sometimes "tearing their clothes" at peyote ceremonies. She also believed that peyote use correlated with a lack of productivity. She stated that Native American men who were Christians were more than twice as likely to be "self-supporting" than were those "in mescal organizations."[55] In 1889, Agent W. D. Myers wrote that peyote use led to addiction in much the way that the "morphine, opium, or alcohol habits" affected white people.[56] And in 1915, Mrs. Delavan L. Pierson, a missionary's wife, stated that peyote users cared about nothing but their drug. The "peyote-eater," she wrote, "becomes an idle, worthless member of society, [and] loses all interest in improving his grant of land, and will sacrifice anything, however dear, to obtain the sacred bean."[57]

There was little evidence to support criticisms of peyote, and even some critics acknowledged its appeal and the fact that it was safer than other drugs. Peyote has never been proven to be addictive, and there are strong indications that it is not. Members of the Native American Church, in which peyote use is a sacrament, typically consume the drug only at peyote ceremonies. The ceremonies occur at most once a week, and sometimes they are not even held once a month. People who are addicted to a drug would typically require much more frequent use of it.[58] According to sociologist Benjamin Kracht, arguments about peyote were often "based on rumor and hearsay," and lobbyists against the drug in the 1910s depended heavily on "false accusations and stereotypes."[59] Historian Alexander Dawson asserts that extensive scientific evidence attests to peyote's "relative harmlessness."[60] Pierson, who was critical of the drug, acknowledged that peyote did not cause users to become violent.[61] Seymour, another detractor, recognized that it was less dangerous than morphine and cocaine, and she quoted a doctor who stated that peyote use was appealing because it had "so much to charm and so little to excite or disgust." She also acknowledged that some peyotists attributed opposition to their practice to religious competition rather than the dangers of use: "They can't drive the red people with an iron rod to join their churches."[62]

Indeed, much of the opposition came from missionaries because the Native American Church competed with Christianity. The Native American Church, which was not formally established until 1918, had adherents by 1890 and attracted many more due to peyote's therapeutic effects.[63] In 1915, Pierson had stated that Native American youth were not attending church because they "have been lured away by the peyote habit."[64] In 1917, Colorado, Nevada, and Utah outlawed peyote possession. A conviction for possession could lead to a month in jail.[65] Some of these laws likely derived from accounts suggesting that peyote use was addictive and debilitating. Before the measure's passage in Utah, for example, a widely reprinted article characterized the drug as having "enslaved the Indians of the Uintah basin and reservations elsewhere."[66]

It is reasonable to conclude that many officials and missionaries opposed peyote use not because they deemed it dangerous to users but because it was an obstacle to assimilation. Kracht has observed that peyote was not associated with dangerous drugs until "non-Indians" discovered it, and they objected to it because they regarded it as detrimental to the Native Americans' "assimilation into mainstream American society."[67] Dawson agrees that opposition arose because Native Americans' use of peyote challenged officials' authority— that it "disrupt[ed] the performance of power"—because peyote users were demonstrating that they did not fully acquiesce to the circumstances in which they lived.[68]

* * *

Many white people in the early twentieth century accused African Americans of using cocaine recklessly, but their rate of cocaine use was higher than others' due to work-related considerations and because their medical options were limited. In 1903, druggists E. G. Eberle and Frederick T. Gordon suggested that black Americans did not consider the risks when they used drugs—that "the negroes . . . give little thought to the seriousness of the habit forming."[69] And in 1919, Dr. Thomas Blair characterized the "American Negro" as "seemingly, a willing addict." "Some of the negro labor camps in the South simply breed addicts," he suggested. "The men work about four days in the week and 'celebrate' the rest of the time," he stated, the "celebrations" involving cocaine or opiate use.[70] Blair did not consider that many workers were introduced to cocaine by their employers, who gave them the drug to sustain their productivity, and that this could lead to habitual use. Also, due to poverty many were susceptible to illness, but they lacked the means or opportunity to see a doctor. Some then opted for proprietary medicines, many of which contained cocaine. Also, some could have used cocaine to help them to endure life's challenges. Oftentimes, local officials monitored African Americans' liquor consumption closely. Because alcohol was not easily accessible, some could have opted for cocaine instead.[71]

Meanwhile, white physicians, who would have been the most familiar with cocaine's risks, were also among those who became unwittingly addicted. When Dr. Charles Bradley was chronicling his addiction for readers of Chicago's *Inter-Ocean* in 1887, he explained that when he experimented with cocaine, he "never realized the insidious and dangerous nature of the drug until I tried to discontinue its use." The reporter noted that it was surprising that a man who was "intelligent, accomplished and a trained physician" would become addicted.[72] Other doctors at the time also became addicted to cocaine and, as a result, suffered serious mental illness.[73]

Many news stories suggested that cocaine use made African Americans violent. In 1900, for example, a paper in Lake Providence, Louisiana, reported that two "negro levee women" had gotten into a fight. One was a "cocaine fiend," and she stabbed the other. According to the reporter, "It is said that when she is partly under the influence of this drug that she is a regular demon."[74] In 1907, the *New York Times* reported that a black man in Arkansas was "crazed by cocaine" and had "shot seven white persons." He was then surrounded and killed.[75] There was never any proof that cocaine had played a role in this incident. In 1909, several newspapers reported that a black man named Everett Royster had shot three men in Richmond, Virginia. Some included headlines such as "Negro Was Crazed by Cocaine." According to the *Baltimore Sun*, although the police believed that cocaine use "drove him into his murderous frenzy," it was only a theory: "Royster was either crazy or 'doped,'" the reporter stated.[76]

Others challenged the notion that cocaine typically made African Americans violent or that it had a negative effect solely on their population. In 1900, a writer for the *Journal of the American Medical Association* noted that many African Americans used cocaine but stated that its effects varied. Some became "quarrelsome, some hilarious, some morose," he wrote, "and many are happy and indifferent."[77] And some cocaine users who became violent were white, including physicians. In 1888, a Pennsylvania paper reported that a doctor who had been addicted to cocaine had become a "raving maniac." While aboard a train he had "assaulted and nearly killed the attendant," and he was then taken to a mental hospital.[78] Another doctor, a "hard working, conscientious, and skillful physician," switched from opium to cocaine and became "irritable, quarrelsome, [and] impetuous," according to Dr. D. R. Brower. He began "carrying a pistol and frequently brandishing it in public places, threatening vengeance" on anyone who would question him, "a perfect terror in his neighborhood."[79] The selective highlighting of stories, however, disproportionately focused on cocaine use and African American violence. As historian Douglas Flowe has observed, "Media descriptions of cocaine users depicted African Americans as incurable fiends, and whites as unfortunate victims caught in the clutches of a harmful substance."[80]

Asa Candler, who had secured ownership of the formula for Coca-Cola, had the coca extract removed from the beverage in 1903 in response to the widely held belief that cocaine use led to African American violence. He was reacting to a "wave of anti-black drug panic," according to Michael Cohen, an American Studies scholar. This decision could partly explain why the soft drink endured. When white supremacists blamed race riots on "pinches of cocaine sold in whiskey shots," Cohen observed, nobody could blame Coca-Cola.[81]

When addressing Congress in the 1910s, proponents of national drug legislation perpetuated a false theory that many white Americans would believe: that cocaine use gave African American men "superhuman strength" and impelled them to rape white women. Dr. Christopher Koch, for example, vice president of Pennsylvania's State Pharmaceutical Examining Board, shared his belief that "the colored people" who used cocaine "would just as leave rape a woman as anything else."[82] Dr. Hamilton Wright, in a report to Congress advocating national legislation to control the drug, claimed, "It has been authoritatively stated that cocaine is often the direct incentive to the crime of rape by the negroes of the South and other sections of the country."[83] Wright had attended the International Opium Commission in Shanghai as part of the U.S. delegation.[84]

Koch and Wright almost certainly derived their comments from a widely cited article that was grounded in racist assumptions and that alleged, without evidence, a connection between African Americans' cocaine use and sexual assaults. The article appeared in 1909 in *Everyday Life*, an obscure, short-lived magazine owned by Chicago publisher George H. Currier.[85] Currier had financed a commission and appointed it to investigate the claim that half a million Americans were addicted to cocaine, and he published their conclusions in his periodical.[86] In one of the articles, the authors—commission members Charles W. Collins and John Day—quoted at length the writings of Harris Dickson, a Mississippi judge whom they characterized as "a close student of the race problem."[87] In his writings, Dickson advocated racist ideas. In other articles that he wrote in 1909, he insisted that permitting black suffrage would lead to unstable governance and that African Americans were inherently unhealthy and therefore likely to die off.[88] Collins and Day quoted Dickson's assertion that African American men in the early twentieth century were less healthy than they had been when enslaved because "drunkenness, *cocaine*, dissipation and immorality are at work." Collins and Day also quoted this assertion of Dickson's, which would be widely quoted:

A man who deliberately puts cocaine into a negro is more dangerous than he who would inoculate a dog with hydrophobia. This deadly drug arouses every evil passion, gives the negro superhuman strength, and destroys his sense of fear. Yet the steamboat negro and the levee negro will not work without it.[89]

Many newspapers reported on the commission's conclusions. The articles often quoted the Currier Commission's lie linking black men's cocaine use with cases of rape.[90] According to Collins and Day, "Cocaine now ranks with whisky as the chief provocative of rape and its consequent lynching bee in the South." Although Collins and Day do not appear as authorities on the American drug problem in other sources or settings, some newspapers characterized them as having "expert" knowledge of the topic.[91]

Dickson, the man they had quoted extensively, did not just share his ideas about African American men's cocaine use in the pages of *Hampton's Magazine*. A few months after he penned that article, he wrote to Hamilton Wright and told him that cocaine use was "quite common" among "the lower orders of working negroes." He also insisted that the men demanded it from their employers, rather than acknowledging that employers supported such use and some advocated it. This could have heightened white people's perception of cocaine as a drug that needed to be regulated, if African American men were insisting that they be given it regularly.[92]

Collins and Day did not refer to specific incidents in which African American men had committed rapes while under the influence of cocaine, and it is reasonable to conclude that they knew of none. Among the articles published in early twentieth-century newspapers, a few vague stories suggest a possible link between the availability of cocaine and African American men's subsequent assaulting of women, and in one case a black man blamed his cocaine use for the attempted rape that he had committed.[93] A search of American newspapers from 1899 to 1910, however, reveals not a single story in which an African American man used cocaine and then committed a rape or was alleged to have done so, let alone the torrent of such cases that Koch, Wright, and the Currier Commission described.[94] It is a noteworthy silence given the era's racism, which often led to false allegations; numerous charges of African American men as rapists; and assertions that cocaine use spurred African American violence. Given the support for national legislation restricting cocaine use, however, racially charged arguments for drug legislation appear to have been effective, regardless of their veracity.[95] They were not only used when the focus was on cocaine. When prohibitionists sought to garner white southern support for going dry, many warned their audiences that black men's drinking could lead to violence, even though African Americans had few problems with alcohol in comparison with society at large.[96]

* * *

The move toward national legislation advanced in 1898 when, following the Spanish-American War, the United States annexed the Philippines and sought to end opium use there. Spain had allowed Chinese residents to smoke opium but forbade the practice among native Filipinos.[97] To supply the market, Spain had rented out "opium farms" to the highest bidder. The winner enjoyed a monopoly on opium production and sales, and Spain received revenue. Other colonial powers in Asia used a similar approach. In many parts of the continent, "opium addiction balanced colonial budgets," according to historian Anne Foster.[98]

Rather than preserving the Spanish system, the United States tried to control the opium trade with high tariffs, believing that would discourage use. The administration hoped the extra cost would put opium use beyond the means of the ordinary Filipino or Chinese worker.[99] This approach was paternalistic, and it derived from a false premise regarding the incentives for use of the drug. The American commissioners were assuming that workers used opium for pleasure-seeking purposes rather than acknowledging the considerable extent to which they used it as a medicine.[100] Also, Brigadier General Charles Whittier warned that a high tariff would lead to an increase in smuggling. He was in charge of customs, and his successor agreed and noted that the Philippines' extensive coastline would be difficult to patrol. Upon assuming control, however, U.S. leaders opted for a tariff and did not prohibit opium use by Filipinos.[101] Smuggling increased, and despite the high tariff, annual opium imports more than tripled between 1899 and 1902. In 1904, a writer for the Quaker journal the *Friend* noted that "the use of opium is spreading to native Filipinos to an alarming extent."[102]

The increase in usage led some to advocate a return to the farm system, but missionaries defeated the idea. William Howard Taft, the islands' governor-general, liked the farm system option. He regarded opium smoking as primarily social in nature, surmised that its effects were no worse than the "liquor habit," and believed that the arrangement would work well and generate revenue. In 1903, however, he explained to Secretary of State Elihu Root that American churchgoers would not accept an arrangement that sanctioned opium smoking.[103] Charles Fahs, for example, who was active in the Methodist Episcopal Church's Missionary Society, wrote to President Theodore Roosevelt that the United States should not "duplicate the disgraceful record of Great Britain" by accepting and profiting from opium use. He did not care how "difficult" it would be to enforce prohibitory laws.[104] A writer for the Baptist *Watchman* agreed, stating in 1904 that "the government has no right to plan for a revenue from this traffic, [which is] so hurtful to the people."[105] Taft appointed a committee to study the matter. He accepted their recommended plan: a government monopoly on the drug, allowing opium sales only to those with a doctor's prescription, and free treatment for habitués.[106] Habitués would have three years to end their use and would then lose legal access to the drug.[107]

The United States decided also to pursue international cooperation to limit drug traffic, both to address the situation in the Philippines and to improve relations with China. In 1906, the Protestant Episcopal bishop of the Philippines, the Reverend Charles H. Brent, had persuaded President Roosevelt that such cooperation was necessary to end opium smuggling in the Philippines.[108] Soon thereafter, China began an earnest effort to reduce opium smoking within its borders. International cooperation was crucial for the Chinese to realize their goal. As writer Rosa Pendleton Chiles would observe, "No country can protect itself singly against a trade as insistent and remunerative as the opium traffic in its present monstrous proportions."[109] Meanwhile, relations between the United States and China were strained. After passage of the 1882 Chinese Exclusion Act, which barred the immigration of Chinese workers to the United States, China had placed an embargo on American manufactures. American efforts to combat China's opium problem, therefore, was a "no-lose proposition for the United States," as David Courtwright has observed, since assisting China could reopen such a lucrative market.[110]

The United States invited countries with Asian possessions to a conference in Shanghai to discuss international opium policy, but some American officials were embarrassed that their nation had no federal legislation of its own regulating drugs.[111] This was addressed by passage of the Smoking Opium Act in 1909, which allowed opium imports "for medical purposes only."[112] Hamilton Wright targeted smoking opium because such a ban would be relatively uncontroversial and, consequently, could be approved quickly. Smoking opium had no real medical value, and it was "identified with the Chinese, gamblers, and prostitutes," as Courtwright noted.[113] Time was of the essence; *Outlook* magazine would title its article about the legislation "Congress Acts in the Nick of Time."[114] Wright hoped that the measure would also impel Chinese Americans to emigrate elsewhere. In a 1908 letter to President Roosevelt, he had predicted that the measure would "work a certain hardship to all Chinese habitués and might cause the emigration of a large number of them, a result to be devoutly hoped for."[115] The measure passed, but some congressmen opposed it, due to the consequent loss of revenue. Between 1870 and 1899, for example, the United States had reaped almost $18 million from the tariff on smoking opium, three times what it made from the importation of medical opium.[116]

The decisions of the International Opium Commission were not binding, but those in attendance did agree on certain principles, such as the need to respect other nations' drug laws.[117] The U.S. representatives were Wright, long-time missionary Charles E. Tenney, and the Reverend Brent, who headed the

delegation and served as chairman of the conference.[118] Participants included
the United States, several European nations, China, Japan, Siam, and Persia.[119]
The nations agreed to work to end opium smoking domestically and to close
opium dens in parts of China that they controlled.[120] The United States asked
countries in which opium was produced to monitor their markets and to
ban exports to countries where it was outlawed.[121] These resolutions were,
however, as David Musto points out, "merely recommendations." Because
the gathering was a commission, it could not make binding decisions, and
participating governments did not have to ratify its resolutions.[122] Despite
this, as historian Lars Seiler put it, the commission revealed that there was a
shared "understanding about the nature of opium's effects on global economic
and political process."[123]

The United States could easily support many of these conditions, since it
did not benefit from the opium trade; other countries, meanwhile, were deeply
invested and reluctant to surrender their profits. Great Britain, for example,
wanted to keep producing opium in India for the China market, and Persia and
Turkey also depended heavily on opium sales.[124] Several governments were,
therefore, willing to cooperate to fight smuggling, but they were not in favor of
prohibiting opium use.[125]

* * *

Before the government at any level began restricting access to habit-forming
drugs, people with drug-dependent spouses began making the case that sales to
such people should be forbidden. In 1867, a husband in Watertown, New York,
sued a druggist who had, for months, secretly sold laudanum to his wife despite
knowing that the practice was "impairing her health," as a judge on the state's
Supreme Court later wrote. The druggist knew that she consumed it "as a beverage"—that is, not for an accepted medical reason—and, as her habit progressed,
she could no longer manage the household or take care of the couple's two children. The defendant pointed out that selling laudanum was legal and asserted
that the woman had bought it of her own volition. The Court, however, ruled
that the druggist's actions "contributed largely to the injury complained of" and
that he was therefore liable.[126] In similar cases elsewhere, courts also tended to
side with the family member when there was evidence that the druggist knew
the customer's use was habitual.[127]

Because cases involving people who were habituated to drugs were still novel,
some people who sought help found the existing laws to be insufficient, and
some states saw the need for new legislation. Since the 1820s, for example, the
state of Illinois had accepted a spouse's habitual drunkenness as grounds for divorce. In 1889, a woman sought to divorce her husband, a habitual morphine

user, by making the case that the drug's effects closely resembled drunkenness. The Illinois Supreme Court rejected the argument, as the justices concluded that "drunkenness" could result only from alcohol consumption.[128] Even so, many states adopted new laws or revised old ones. In 1872, Kentucky's General Assembly passed a law permitting the institutionalization of people whose "excessive use of opium, arsenic, hasheesh, or any drug" had rendered them "incompetent" to manage their own affairs if two "respectable" people would sign affidavits attesting to the circumstances.[129]

In the late nineteenth century, many states and municipalities began passing laws to restrict sales of habit-forming drugs. In 1875, the city of San Francisco, in an effort to combat opium smoking, outlawed the owning and patronizing of opium dens.[130] Although the measure applied to everybody, city leaders were responding to reports that "young men and women of respectable parentage" were visiting the dens, according to the *San Francisco Chronicle*. Members of the board feared that if no action were taken, the practice would become more widespread.[131] In 1881, the state of California adopted the measure. By 1896, twenty-two states and territories had banned opium dens. While half these laws were passed in the West, some states in the Midwest, South, and Northeast had also approved such statutes.[132]

Many states began requiring prescriptions for some drug purchases, but the effectiveness of this patchwork of laws can be overstated. In 1889, for example, the territory of Montana began mandating prescriptions for the purchase of cocaine, opium, or morphine. By 1900, nine other states had passed similar laws for some of these drugs, most often cocaine. By 1914, the year in which national legislation was passed to regulate sales of cocaine and opiates, thirty-five states and territories already required a prescription for their purchase, and another dozen had a law pertaining just to cocaine. Despite this, there were "no effective legal impediments to purchasing either cocaine or opiates throughout the country," as historian Ronald Hamowy has noted. In general, those who broke the law either were not caught or, if they were, faced only a small fine. Meanwhile, customers could buy proprietary medicines or beverages with cocaine, such as coca wines and the earliest version of Coca-Cola.[133]

Meanwhile, regulations at the state level varied; the laws consequently relocated parts of the drug market while stymying efforts to address the problem effectively. Reformers in New York, for example, believed that their efforts to restrict drug access were confounded by comparatively lax laws in neighboring New Jersey.[134] People in states with few regulations, meanwhile, dealt with unwelcome customers. Just before the Harrison Act became law, Vermont's *Middlebury Register* supported a state bill that would restrict drug sales. Similar legislation was already on the books in neighboring New York and Massachusetts, and those laws had "driven a great many 'dope fiends' to this State," the writer explained, to buy their "deadly drugs" at Vermont pharmacies. Surely, he added, the Green Mountain State did not want to become "the mecca for those addicted to the opium and morphine habits."[135]

An additional problem was interstate commerce. Sellers frequently shipped drugs out of state "to the consumer, peddler, or any other irresponsible party," lamented Lyman Kebler, who worked for the government's Bureau of Chemistry, predecessor of the Food and Drug Administration. He pled for national legislation. "District and state laws are violated daily," he wrote in 1909, "for want of a satisfactory Federal law regulating the shipment into interstate commerce of these pernicious products."[136] Still, few regarded restrictions on drugs as a federal matter. Enforcing laws would require police involvement, a matter traditionally reserved to the states. Consequently, many members of Congress saw the approach as unconstitutional.[137]

\* \* \*

At the turn of the century, the number of Americans addicted to drugs had begun to decline, due to the decreasing medical need for the pharmaceuticals and doctors' increasing wariness of them, and the perception of the "typical" American user was changing. The number of habitués had peaked at around 250,000, in the mid-1890s. Many women who had been habituated to morphine were passing away and fewer were developing an addiction because of state laws that restricted access to morphine and doctors' growing aversion to prescribing it. Advances in vaccinations and the advent of the germ theory of disease, meanwhile, helped to keep people healthier.[138] Also, opium had long been the world's most effective pain reliever, but in 1899 a scientist at Bayer discovered that aspirin relieved pain, and the company would market it widely by 1915. This lessened the demand for opiates.[139]

Increasingly, habitués were young, marginalized men whose use began for pleasure-seeking purposes rather than from medical need. Henry Cole, for example, began his morphine use in 1873. He admitted that he was part of the "fast" scene, frequenting places such as "the gambling house, the drinking palace, the racetrack, and the brothel." His group sought "sensual pleasures only, and excitement and dissipation," without dwelling on the consequences.[140] Sixteen-year-old George Fromme bought catarrh powders with his friends. His mother had him arrested in 1907, after she discovered that he had pawned his new suit in order to buy the drug. According to the *Times* reporter, Mrs. Fromme responded in this way because she had seen the consequences of addiction. Her husband, the reporter explained, "had acquired the liquor habit and had then deserted her."[141]

One drug of choice of the young men was heroin, which Bayer introduced in 1898 as a cough suppressant. The company chose the name from the German word *heroisch,* which means "large" or "powerful," and they presented it as non-addictive, perhaps because morphine habitués became addicted more quickly than did heroin users.[142] Nonetheless, it was about three times stronger than morphine, and some doctors asserted that it was at least as effective a painkiller as morphine while lacking morphine's negative side effects.[143] While morphine had been used to treat a variety of ailments, heroin was promoted mainly to treat respiratory disorders.[144] In 1900, for example, the *Medical News* reported on its effectiveness in treating "acute and chronic bronchitis, and pneumonia."[145]

The new users' disdain for social norms was a departure from previous habitués' interest in society's approval and helps to explain the condemnation of their usage. Users in previous generations sought to hide their dependency; even smokers in dens that were technically public sought to obscure the practice. These users, however, who were in their late teens and early twenties, seemed brazen. In 1913, the paper reported that the area surrounding a Boston drugstore where heroin was sold had become known as "heroin square," an indication that the use was not furtive. And subcultures were forming. Earlier that year, four young men had been arrested in the Bronx for their heroin use. In court, one stated that "scores of young men" in their neighborhood "were addicted to the heroin habit" and that they shared the drug with their girlfriends.[146] The open use by a younger group without the semblance of medical need or signs of contrition helps to explain why they received little sympathy.

Many of these youth, however, used their drugs for the same reason that middle-class white women had taken morphine: to alleviate gloom and to have a good experience. These young men realized that heroin "provided powerful euphoric and calmative effects and began sharing it in poolrooms and dance halls," as historian Caroline Acker has noted. When some sought treatment later on, the reasons they gave for their usage resembled the reasons of habitual users of morphine. One said the drug "makes me feel normal," while another admitted that "sometimes a gloomy day would get me started using again."[147] One schoolboy told a woman at Chicago's Hull House that using cocaine made him feel "as if I was going up in a flying machine." Another felt "as if I was a millionaire and could do anything I pleased."[148] Around 1900, a twenty-year-old in Pittsburgh explained to his doctor that he became addicted to cocaine because using it made him feel, if only for an hour, "as if I was Andrew Carnegie."[149]

As the popular perception of habitués switched from well-to-do female morphine users to young men of the lower class using morphine, cocaine, or heroin, support for anti-drug laws increased. By the 1910s, young men of the lower classes who used morphine or heroin had become "increasingly conspicuous," according to David Courtwright. As a consequence, the public became more and more inclined to regard opiate addiction as "an underworld phenomenon."[150] The shift facilitated the passage of legislation. As sociologist Patricia Erickson has observed, it is easier to enact legislation regarding a substance when its users are "a small, low-status part of the population." Since the law would not affect most people, non-users are often indifferent to it.[151]

* * *

After the meeting at Shanghai, Dr. Hamilton Wright wanted the United States to pass legislation to control drugs at the federal level so the nation would be in an unassailable position as it asked other nations to do the same.[152] The first effort was the Foster Bill, which did not become law, due to its strict scrutiny of prescriptions and sales.[153] The measure, which was introduced by Congressman David Foster of Vermont, would have tracked all sales of "opiates, cocaine, chloral hydrate, and cannabis," including minute quantities of the drugs and proprietary medicines that contained them. Under its strictures, druggists and manufacturers could sell these drugs only to customers with a prescription, they would have to record all transactions, and they would face stiff penalties if they neglected to do so. Druggists saw the measure as burdensome. Brooklyn pharmacist William Muir explained that, for example, a druggist would have to record every time he sold a corn cure, since they contained cannabis. Others pointed out that the law could destroy their careers, as a clerical error could re-sult in a fine of $500 or a year in jail. Because of the hardship that it would have placed on routine drug sales, the Foster Bill did not pass.[154]

Its successor, the Harrison Narcotic Act, was less cumbersome than the Foster Bill.[155] As with Foster, a prescription would be required to buy opiates and cocaine, and doctors could write prescriptions only for people with le-gitimate medical needs. Also, doctors and pharmacists would have to register with the government and keep track of what they sold. Bookkeeping, how-ever, would be simpler. While the Foster Bill included cannabis and chloral hydrate, the Harrison Act did not.[156] Sales of proprietary medicines with mi-nute amounts of the drugs did not need to be recorded. Furthermore, the tax itself was nominal.[157] The measure passed in December 1914 and went into effect on March 1, 1915.[158] David Musto has suggested that the public supported the measure because it seemed like "a routine slap at a moral evil."[159] The legislation received little attention at the time, because it competed with greater concerns, including World War I. As a writer for the *Chicago Tribune* explained, many had assumed that the law's main purpose was to generate rev-enue, and people were focused more on the economy and "the uncertainties of the war."[160]

To increase support for the Harrison measure, advocates inflated the ex-tent and danger of drug use in America and played to racist beliefs. Wright and other advocates exaggerated "the number of addicts and the criminal menace they posed," as David Courtwright points out. Although rates of addiction in America had begun to decline in the late 1890s, for example, Wright distorted the data in 1910 to suggest that it was still climbing.[161] He inaccurately blamed Chinese Americans for the opium problem, saying the country "had become contaminated through the presence of a large Chinese population," and he and others blamed cocaine use for inciting African Americans to violence.[162] In 1914, for example, Dr. Edward Huntington Williams stated that cocaine use caused even "hitherto inoffensive, law-abiding negroes" to commit a "large proportion of the wholesale killings in the South during recent years."[163] Due to the pervasiveness of racist stereotypes, few white people questioned these claims.[164] Such allegations appear to have bolstered white southern support for the legislation. South Carolina senator Ben Tillman said that he backed the legislation, for example, because drugs were "causing so much trouble among the negroes." He referred to a story of cocaine-inspired violence that he had read about.[165]

Tillman's and his colleagues' support for the legislation is noteworthy. Most southern states banned cocaine many years before they prohibited "opium, morphine, or heroin, the drugs of choice for most white addicts in the South," according to Michael Cohen.[166] The determination to control the black population was intense. When Tillman mentioned that he had read about cocaine-inspired violence, he was referring to killings in Harriston, Mississippi, in 1913. He did not mention that the news articles that reported the violence also reported that the young black men deemed responsible, brothers Walter and Will Jones, had been lynched. In the climate of the time, a judge from nearby Fayette felt comfortable admitting to the press that he had led the lynch mob.[167]

* * *

Late in 1911, soon after the failure of the Foster Bill, the next international conference convened at The Hague with the purpose of making international agreements that would be binding. While thirteen nations had attended the Shanghai conference, thirty-four sent representatives to The Hague. Participating nations agreed to restrict to medical use the manufacture, use, and sale of opiates and cocaine. Two subsequent conferences were held to give all countries the opportunity to sign and ratify the convention, which went into effect in 1914.[168] Some were excessively optimistic as to what its impact would be. A writer for *Outlook* predicted that with the signing of the agreements, "the use of vicious drugs will be regulated from one end of the globe to the other."[169] The onset of World War I halted the anti-opium momentum. The last Hague conference ended on June 25, 1914, and Archduke Franz Ferdinand was assassinated three days later.[170] Drug production would escalate to address military needs.[171] In

1919, however, ratifying the 1912 convention became a condition of the Treaty of Versailles.[172]

\* \* \*

Passage of the Harrison Act, meanwhile, was one of many signs that doctors were abandoning the field of drug treatment, as the law furthered that split. Many physicians had supported the act in part because they saw it as a way to remove the competition that they faced from purveyors of opium-laced home remedies and also because of their increasing pessimism regarding addiction and low regard for habitués.[173] The *Quarterly Journal of Inebriety* folded in 1914, and the American Association for the Cure of Inebriates dissolved in 1920. Many historians attribute the loss of support for curing addiction to the demographic change regarding those who were addicted. The new users were "unattractive as medical clients," as anthropologist Marcus Aurin has noted.[174] There were several reasons for this. For one, drug use was increasingly associated with immigrants or people who were otherwise marginalized, including African Americans, Chinese Americans, and underemployed white transients. And some saw their usage as threatening the white middle class, either because members of the middle class might then take up the habit, or because of a growing belief, propagated by members of the medical community, that drug use inclined users "toward insanity and crime."[175] But if the Harrison Act deprived these habitués of their drug, and the medical community would not help them to end their addiction, it was unclear where they were to turn.

Some suggested that outlawing drugs would not cause suffering, because users would either end their use effortlessly or would find an alternative source of their narcotic. In 1914, for example, Dr. C. B. Pearson wrote about a "prominent" morphine habitué who had made eleven attempts to end her use. He suggested that her twelfth try succeeded because it was the last one that she could afford. Pearson considered it "evident" that the woman "could have succeeded at any of her previous attempts had she wished to."[176] In 1920, Dr. Frederick H. Hubbard agreed that removing the drug supply would prompt a relatively easy cure. "If the addicts cannot obtain a supply of their drug, they will reform, and not a fatality will be recorded," he predicted in the *Journal of the American Medical Association*.[177] Charles Towns, the author of *Habits That Handicap* (1916), provided a different reason that the Harrison Act could be implemented without inconveniencing anyone. The "under-world," he insisted, "will always be able to get its drugs."[178] Towns claimed to have discovered an effective treatment for drug addiction—a treatment that he kept secret. Many people believed him, however, thinking perhaps that if a cure existed, there was no need to think twice about banning nonmedical access to drugs.[179]

Others considered such views absurd; habitués would suffer. Before passage of the Harrison Act, many doctors had routinely written prescriptions for people whom they knew were addicted.[180] Druggist Albert Doerschuk explained the consequences of depriving users of their drugs. "After the habit is once acquired," he explained, "the system craves the drug very much as the body craves food." Without it, the habitué would endure a period of suffering akin to "natural starvation."[181] John Harrison Hughes, who was recovering from addiction, was appalled by the Harrison Act and the distorted beliefs that had led to it. He insisted that lawmakers knew "no more" about opium's effects on habitués "than a goose does about God." He believed that legislators passed it because of negative perceptions of pleasure-seeking users. From their limited contact "with Chinese opium-smoking joints, or with 'hop-heads' and 'coke-fiends' of the tenderloin districts," he wrote, they mistakenly concluded that all drug use was pursued for pleasure. "And yet," he added, "they essay to make laws on the subject!"[182]

Some advocated maintenance programs, which would provide habitués with free doses of their drug. Just before passage of the Harrison Act, Dr. C. E. Terry of Jacksonville, Florida, made the case for such programs, like the one he oversaw. Maintenance programs had many advantages: they deprived druggists of an excuse for illegal sales, made drugs difficult to obtain illegally, and helped to ensure that habitués would be in touch with health officers. Terry considered it "inhuman" not to allow users to have the drug and insisted that "any effective prohibitive legislation must provide for the free treatment of existing users."[183] Some maintenance programs opened when the U.S. government was considering options for federal legislation. The one in Jacksonville was established in 1912, and many enrolled. Some participants were transients rather than Jacksonville natives, but there was significant demand for the program, in part because opiate addiction was more widespread in the South than in other regions.[184] The Tennessee Narcotic Act of 1913 allowed habitués to receive opiates, both to minimize suffering and to prevent the establishing of an illicit market.[185] Some recognized the precarious situation for habitués. Although the editorial board of the *Chicago Tribune* believed that the Harrison Act was necessary to curb addiction, it also stated that "everything should be done to carry victims over to safety and sanity."[186]

Some had maintained that the Harrison Act would not bar maintenance, and its parameters were initially unclear. When a morphine habitué lamented in March 1915 that she had lost access to her drug due to the Harrison Act, the surgeon general assured her that the purpose of the law was to gather information and that she would still be able to get morphine from her doctor.[187]

Still others opposed the act because they believed it would drive the traffic underground rather than eliminating it. They were correct, but many others overlooked the complexity of the problem and the need for a nuanced response. Some refused to consider responses that allowed the continuance of any ongoing habitual drug use. Concerns with the creation of an illicit market were "overcome by the conviction that compromise should not be made with unquestioned evils," as David Musto wrote.[188] Illicit sales did result, with habitués paying dearly to compensate sellers for participating in the risky commerce. When the Harrison Act was passed, Violet McNeal and her husband were using morphine and cocaine. The law made it harder, but not impossible, for them to get the drugs. After passage of the law, she recalled, "We were paying thirty-five dollars a dram for stuff that had cost sixty cents in any drugstore" beforehand. One druggist refused to sell her morphine, but he told her where he kept it and said she could leave money on the counter and take it. "He would report the theft to the police," she explained, "but would profess not to know the thief."[189]

# Conclusion

## The Hydra Emerges

The Harrison Narcotic Act went into effect in 1915, the year that Dr. David Cheever died. At first, it was unclear whether the measure would change the ways that people bought addictive drugs or prevent anyone from getting them, or if it would serve solely as a measure to gather revenue and information. A few years after the law's passage, a pair of Supreme Court decisions regarding it would bar habitués from legal access to drugs unless they suffered from an intractable ailment other than their addiction.

Because the law was passed when the number of medical habitués was dwindling, and because its interpretation permitted maintenance only for those with serious illnesses, the Harrison Act solidified a division that many had long endorsed. Officially, the law sanctioned compassionate treatment for those who took drugs to manage ailments while cutting off those whose use had no accepted medical basis. The policy, however, disregarded the fact that any drug-dependent people, when deprived of their supply, would find it challenging if not impossible to end their use and to avoid a relapse. Therefore, the law brought misery to those who had no accepted medical excuse for their use. Many other Americans might not have minded the fact that non-medical habitués suffered, and some likely regarded their pain as a just punishment for their past choices. They might have had second thoughts had they considered that a large illicit market would soon develop to serve these users, which would spur an increase in property crime. Also, many assumed that white, middle-class drug users were blameless and that other people—people who were poor, or working class, and people of color—began their use to seek pleasure. Repeatedly, these assumptions resulted in sympathetic treatment of white, middle-class users and a dismissive attitude toward others, regardless of the origin of their drug use. Unfortunately, many users who were poor or were people of color were taking the drugs for medical reasons, to assuage pain.

*Habit Forming*. Elizabeth Kelly Gray, Oxford University Press. © Oxford University Press 2023.
DOI: 10.1093/oso/9780190073121.003.0011

\* \* \*

Soon after the Harrison Act was passed, some people pointed out that cutting off the legal drug supply would leave users vulnerable and would thus aid illicit markets. A couple of months before the measure went into effect, Dr. Donald McCaskey warned that people who were addicted would turn to crime if necessary to get their "favorite drug." Such a person would "lie, beg, borrow or steal to attain his end," he insisted, and "the quicker we recognize this fact, the better."[1] A few months after the law went into effect, a writer for *American Medicine* agreed that the law put habitués in "a precarious condition," because they had few legal ways to maintain their habit. Doctors were leery of helping them—understandably, the writer maintained—since "honest mistakes" could get them in trouble. This concern had also led many druggists to stop selling narcotic drugs. As a consequence, a drug habitué was "forced to become a law-breaker," the writer explained, as he sought his drug from underworld sources. McCaskey acknowledged that drug users could seek help from the police but predicted that they, like other officials, would show "no sympathy," because they did not understand "what drug addiction really is."[2]

The legislation was toughest on the poorest users. In 1915, New York police lieutenant Henry Scherb, head of the city's "dope squad," described the impact of both the Harrison Act and the Boylan Law, a state law akin to the Harrison Act that had passed the previous year. Wealthy users could still get cocaine and heroin from "dope doctors and fake-cure places," Scherb explained, but the "poorer people"—"the men and women we call the 'bums'"—were panicking, because they had purchased drugs from peddlers but could no longer do so. On passage of the laws, the police had begun watching these sellers closely, and they found it difficult to replenish their supplies. According to a writer for the *New York Times,* the restrictive legislation had put "hundreds of habitual users of heroin and cocaine" in a "pitiful state of craving and suffering." Hospitals provided some relief.[3] Many, however, regarded the difficulty that poorer users faced as a feature of the legislation, not a glitch. Drug policy analyst David Musto maintains that the Harrison Act passed because it was directed primarily "at a social subgroup viewed as a menace to society."[4]

Implementation of the act was disorganized because doctors' approaches often clashed with broadly held assumptions regarding the nature of addiction and how to treat it. Pharmacists were caught in the middle. A druggist in Helena, Montana, for example, received six prescriptions for cocaine in the spring of 1915 but did not know if he could fill them legally. Revenue agents told him the prescriptions were for "excessive amounts," but the doctor who wrote them defended them. The druggist was skeptical of the revenue agents' views, since they were "neither lawyers nor physicians," but he wanted clarity with regard to the law. As he explained in a letter to the U.S. attorney general, he sought a "clear-cut answer and not a vague one that will still leave us to our own opinions and the resulting friction with different inspectors." The attorney general deferred the question. In May 1915, the Treasury Department asserted that prescriptions for someone who was addicted should show a "reduction of the quantity prescribed from time to time," because that would signify "the good faith of the physician in the legitimate practice of his profession."[5]

Medical authorities on the topic insisted that treating addiction presented a complex challenge and that it was unrealistic to expect that users could simply taper off their usage. "This is not really a 'bad habit,' like biting one's nails," a writer for *Current Opinion* asserted of morphine dependency in 1915. "It is a vicious circle in the chemistry of the body."[6] The author of an editorial for *American Medicine* agreed that addiction was a disease and should be treated as such. "The drug addict is sick, with a pathology as definite as that of any other toxic disorder," he explained. Addiction was "not a police or a penological problem," he insisted. It was "a medical problem purely and exclusively."[7]

Interpretation of the act was also contentious because it provided a potential opportunity for the federal government to exercise police powers, a power that the US Constitution had reserved to the states. Relevant state laws, however, had done little to improve the situation. In 1919 Cornelius F. Collins, a New York judge, lamented the apparent absence of a remedy. Drug addiction, he wrote, existed "to a deplorable extent throughout this country." Because of the scope of the problem, the impact of each state law was limited. Meanwhile, he added, "The Federal Government has no police power." It could only address the issue by focusing on aspects such as interstate commerce and using its power of taxation.[8] Because police powers resided with the states, "any law that looked like the exercise of that sort of authority was constitutionally suspect," as historian Kurt Hohenstein has pointed out. It was for this reason that the Harrison Act had been crafted as a tax measure.[9]

In 1916, the Supreme Court regarded the Harrison Act as a revenue measure, asserted that police powers were reserved to the states, and allowed doctors to prescribe maintenance doses of an opiate. They heard the case of Jin Fuey Moy, a Pittsburgh doctor who had prescribed a maintenance dose of morphine to a habitué. The Department of Justice had asserted that Fuey Moy had acted in bad faith, on the grounds that the Harrison Act forbade ongoing drug maintenance except for patients with serious medical conditions, such as cancer.[10] Yet the Supreme Court saw the law as more limited in scope and sided with Fuey Moy by a 6-2 vote. (One justice had passed away before the decision, and his successor had not yet been confirmed.)[11] The justices concluded that the Harrison Act merely provided a way to gather revenue and information and that it did not bestow "regulatory power over suppliers and consumers of the drugs," as historian Timothy Hickman has explained. They also decided that it was legal for people who were addicted to possess narcotics, as long as they received them through proper channels, since they were not required to register. In writing for the majority, Justice Oliver Wendell Holmes stated that the Court would have "grave doubts" regarding the law's constitutionality if it were more than a revenue measure. If it were construed as "a police regulation to suppress the traffic in opium and other drugs," Holmes explained, it would be unconstitutional.[12]

Four years later, however, the Court ruled that the federal government could regulate doctors' prescriptions. In these cases, the doctors had prescribed opiates on a scale that Fuey Moy had not. San Antonio physician Charles T. Doremus was accused of providing drug habitués with heroin and morphine tablets. He was not treating them as patients but instead was merely keeping them supplied.[13] The district court had sided with Doremus, asserting that the Harrison Act encroached on states' police powers and was therefore unconstitutional. Nonetheless, the Supreme Court ruled that although the law was a revenue measure, it could not be declared unconstitutional simply because it would "accomplish another purpose" in the process, in the words of Justice William R. Day. In writing for the slim 5-4 majority, Day also suggested that one of Doremus's patients, who received five hundred heroin tablets, could have sold some of them without paying the tax and that it was reasonable for Congress to try to prevent such occurrences.[14] The four dissenters regarded the law as infringing on states' police powers—as an "attempt by Congress to exert a power not delegated" to it, in the words of Chief Justice Edward Douglass White.[15]

The same day, the Court issued its decision in the case of *Webb et al. v. United States,* ruling that a doctor could not provide maintenance doses of a drug to a patient unless it was done in a way that would bring about a cure. W. S. Webb, a Memphis physician, had routinely prescribed doses of morphine to habitual users, and druggist Jacob Goldbaum had filled the prescriptions. The case focused on whether maintenance was allowed, but the circuit court of appeals had emphasized the scope of their arrangement: Webb prescribed as much morphine as his patients wanted, and Goldbaum bought thirty times more morphine than did the typical druggist. The circuit court had ruled against the men. In its certificate to the Supreme Court, the lower court asked whether a registered doctor could provide a habitual user "with morphine sufficient to keep him comfortable by maintaining his customary use." The Supreme Court split as it had in *Doremus.* Again writing for the majority, Justice Day replied that such practice was forbidden. "To call such an order for the use of morphine a physician's prescription," he wrote, "would be so plain a perversion of meaning that no discussion of the subject is required."[16] These rulings made doctors "increasingly reluctant to treat addicts," as physician Stephen Kandall has noted.[17] It also made it illegal for doctors to treat addiction in any way other than curing it, at a time when few authorities on the topic believed that a cure existed.[18]

When the Court issued its decisions, there was growing recognition that the largest cohort of drug users was much younger than previous habitués had been, and they were more likely to have begun their use without medical need.[19] In the 1910s, as one study in New York City noted, habitual drug users tended to be young white men who began their use due to "Bad Associates."[20] Sara Graham-Mulhall, who served in New York's Department of Narcotic Drug Control, also saw the generational divide. Overwhelmingly, she asserted, middle-class and elderly habitués "become addicts through self-medication." Meanwhile, about 90 percent of drug users younger than thirty began their usage not to treat an ailment but as a result of "bad association and home environment."[21] As members of the older cohort passed away, society would increasingly identify addiction with these younger, poorer, male " 'sporting' addicts," as David Courtwright has observed.[22]

The Court's lack of sympathy for habitués also came at a time when fears of communism and the possible ramifications of domestic unrest elicited support for rigid judicial authority. Many Americans were shocked at the Bolsheviks' success in overthrowing the Russian tsar in 1917, and they feared subversion at home. As a consequence, they "turned their backs on the liberalizing reforms of the preceding era" including maintenance programs for habitual drug users, according to drug policy analyst Ethan Nadelmann.[23] Although the link between drug addiction and support for communism might seem farfetched, some drew connections between them. In 1919, Dr. Thomas Blair reported that many members of the Industrial Workers of the World (IWW) in California had "become industrial outcasts from indulgence in alcohol and narcotics."[24] At the time, many Americans regarded the organization as "the American version of bolshevism," historian Patrick Renshaw has observed.[25] In 1920, a committee appointed by the American Medical Association saw both communism and drug addiction as responses to inequitable conditions. In their report on the drug problem, they explained why "social misfits" turned to political activism and drugs. Society offered these people little: an outdated educational system and monotonous child labor early on, then more unfulfilling and unappreciated work. Such a person might conclude that he was "a victim of conditions far more far-reaching than his individual life. When he becomes organized and vocal," the writers continued, "society awakens to the fact that he is an I.W.W., a bolshevik, or what not." And if he could not improve his conditions, "he will seek out something to forget his woes," such as drugs.[26]

Fears of domestic threats were exacerbated by concerns that the population of addicted Americans would soon increase significantly. Late in 1917, committees focusing on "drug evils" in New York City worried that "thousands of soldiers will come back from the front addicted to the use of drugs" that they initially took for medical reasons, a *New York Times* reporter explained.[27] In 1919, staff at the Treasury Department had mused that the impending onset of Prohibition would lead some drinkers to switch to other drugs. As they explained in their report on the drug traffic, "Drinkers will seek a substitute for alcohol and . . . opiates and cocaine will be found to be most satisfactory for this purpose." The cause and effect were evident in parts of the South that had already gone dry.[28] The pattern had also appeared in response to the Maine Laws.

Meanwhile, others inaccurately estimated that there were as many as a hundred thousand addicted people in New York City and at least a million nationwide. These figures were derived from investigations conducted in 1917 and 1918.[29] The numbers suggested that it was a problem of enormous scope and that the consequences of the Supreme Court forbidding maintenance could lead to high levels of criminality and death.[30] As a result, after the Supreme Court's decisions, forty-four maintenance clinics opened in the United States to provide people who were addicted with doses—albeit diminishing doses—of their drugs.[31] Initially there was support for these programs.[32] The actual number of Americans who were drug dependent, however, was much smaller than believed. The number of American habitués in 1900 was likely closer to 200,000 than a million.[33] And when New York's Worth Street Clinic opened in 1919, fewer than 7,500 showed up seeking help.[34] Surely, some stayed away to avoid making their dependency known. Even so, it was clear that the earlier estimates had been far off the mark.[35] Early in 1920 Dr. S. Dana Hubbard, New York's acting director of the Bureau of Public Health Education, acknowledged that "the enormous numbers of drug addicts supposed to exist, in this vicinity at least . . . are mythical and untrue."[36] Not long after the clinics opened, the Narcotic Division of the Prohibition Unit of the Treasury Department decided to close them. They would allow maintenance only for people who were elderly or who suffered from an incurable disease.[37]

Doctors tried to treat habitués who had visited clinics by addressing illnesses that had led many of them to use drugs in the first place. Some clinic directors considered it crucial to treat underlying illnesses before trying to wean a patient from a drug. Dr. Willard Butler, for example, regarded addiction as "a continuing response to pain," as David Courtwright has pointed out. In his Shreveport, Louisiana, clinic, Butler noticed that most users also suffered from syphilis, tuberculosis, or another illness. If the malady were not treated, Butler surmised, relapse would be almost inevitable. He therefore divided his patients into two groups: those who were incurable, most of whom were elderly and bedridden, and those who suffered from an illness that, once treated, could put them in a position to end their drug use.[38] In a 1919 report on the drug traffic, a Department of the Treasury committee acknowledged that many addicted people who were in private hospitals and sanitaria suffered from diseases including "nervous troubles," venereal diseases, cancer, and "insanity." Others suffered from lung diseases including tuberculosis.[39]

Some reduction plans did work, such as switching some heroin users to morphine. In 1920, Dr. Arthur Braunlich reported on the success of such efforts. Although the first few days without heroin were a "nightmare" for patients, he explained, within a few days they became accustomed to the less powerful drug. "Very few complained," Braunlich reported, and several "expressed their happiness at the change." This, however, involved switching from a strong opiate to a weaker one rather than requiring abstinence.[40]

Clinics were less successful when they required patients to taper off the use of their drug without substituting another. The staff at New York's Worth Street Clinic, for example, disbursed doses that were often far smaller than the amounts to which the users were accustomed. The doses were then reduced over time "in accordance with the decision of the United States Supreme Court," according to Sara Graham-Mulhall. When users experienced withdrawal despite the doses, many resorted to forgery and theft to get money to buy more of the drug. Someone who was relapsing might steal "pocketbooks, [or] fountain pens," Graham-Mulhall recalled, "any small saleable object that he could lay his hands upon." Drug peddlers lingered nearby to meet the demand. The city had hoped to keep track of drug users, but many disappeared when they could no longer receive maintenance doses and did not choose to go to the hospital. "We lost sight of thousands of addicts," Graham-Mulhall admitted, and "the socalled reduction method failed to cure any addicts."[41]

Advocates of maintenance clinics faced a challenge, as many people saw little difference between "dope doctors," who wrote prescriptions for any paying customer, and physicians or clinics providing maintenance doses to patients. Members of the former group paid little attention to the dosage, instead caring only about profit. One doctor in New York, for example, did not meet with patients. Instead, he left partially open a basement window, into which his patients would drop registration cards—identification cards that some clinics required. When the doctor was arrested, he was writing prescriptions and had a pile of forty-five cards. Doctors in the latter group, meanwhile, met with each patient, established that the person was addicted, and kept track of the person's usage. The maintenance program in Jacksonville, Florida, became a national model. Dr. Charles Terry, the city's health officer, believed that any legislation restricting drug access should also provide free treatment to habitués. "To deprive them of their supply alone would be inhuman," he explained, and few could afford to stay at a private hospital or sanitarium. He found that doctors could gain patients' trust through "repeated visits and kindly treatment."[42] Some doctors applauded such arrangements. In 1915, Dr. Donald McCaskey had emphasized the importance of a method involving "actual, efficient, personal contact of the physician with the dope user." It was important, he added, that doctors regard their patients with "intelligent, kindly sympathy." Many authorities, however, did not see providing maintenance doses as legitimate medical practice.[43]

Few doctors were prepared to treat cases of addiction because medical schools gave limited attention to the problem, and some of the information they did provide was outdated. When Charles Terry attended medical school at the turn of the century, as he later recalled, the faculty mentioned opium's addictive potential only in "the most casual manner." Twenty years later, he was dismayed to learn that medical training on the subject had barely advanced. On average, medical schools spent two hours on the subject, and some did not address it at all. Responses to a questionnaire in the late 1910s showed that only one of thirty-seven medical schools taught that addiction was a disease, while the others characterized it as a vice or merely a habit. Also, few medical students saw or treated an addicted person; some only observed an "occasional case seen in the insane asylum or jails." Newly minted doctors, Terry lamented, were "almost totally unprepared to treat this condition." He believed that this helped to explain why the medical profession had "refused to seriously consider the matter" and doctors had thus failed to become the habitués' advocates. This led to the passage of legislation that "overlooked the medical and physical needs of the sufferer."[44]

Leaders of the American Medical Association were distancing the profession from treating cases of drug addiction, and they did so with the support of many of their members. For several reasons, most doctors did not want to treat people who were addicted: the work was held in low esteem, nobody had identified an effective cure, and few asserted that addiction had a biological basis. Moreover, since few new cases of addiction resulted from medical malpractice, doctors no longer felt responsibility for having created "the problem of addiction."[45]

Rather than condemning government oversight of doctors' work, the AMA called on all levels of government to prevent doctors from providing addictive drugs to their patients. Some in the AMA supported the Harrison Act because they saw it as helping them to cure patients by closing off shady sources of drugs—the "illicit unprofessional peddler," in the words of Dr. Thomas Blair—that could delay or prevent an addicted person's recovery.[46] In addition, in an editorial in the AMA's journal soon after the decision in *United States* v. *Jin Fuey Moy* was issued, they asserted that as a matter of "public welfare," states should outlaw possession of habit-forming drugs. Possession of "opium, morphin, cocain and other forbidden drugs" they wrote, should be "presumptive evidence of possession for an unlawful purpose." They also maintained that it hurt a society if a doctor wrote a prescription "merely to satisfy the cravings of the victims of the drug habit." If the federal government could not act in a given case, they insisted, "state and municipal laws and ordinances can and should be applied." They expressed hope that the decision in *United States* v. *Jin Fuey Moy* would prompt such action.[47]

Also at that time, some physicians challenged maintenance advocates by suggesting that addiction could be cured quickly.[48] In 1920, the acting director of New York's Bureau of Public Health Education asserted that drug users could end their use and do so in less than a week. "Any form of cure can take an addict off his drug," Dr. S. Dana Hubbard insisted in a Department of Health publication. He added that it could be done "in 3 to 5 days, without discomfort to the patient."[49] In its study of the domestic drug problem, an AMA committee consulted with doctors and officials. According to its 1920 report, all had agreed it was important to "get the patient off the drug as soon as possible," and they saw such an approach as "better for the patient." The report implied that at most, the process of ending the person's use of the drug should take a week.[50]

Many doctors, meanwhile, advocated depriving habitués of access to their drugs by making the assertion—later proven false—that withdrawal symptoms were a psychological phenomenon, not a physical one. In remarks to New York City's Special Committee on Public Health in 1920, for example, Dr. Emil Pellini, a researcher at New York University and Bellevue Medical College, claimed that "withdrawal symptoms . . . have no physical basis." Many physicians shared this view. The person who recorded the session added, "All present agreed with the conclusions of Dr. Pellini." And when a committee of the AMA issued a report on the topic later that year, it echoed these assertions. Medical explanations of drug habituation sometimes changed as the population of users changed and as doctors' goals changed. As David Musto later observed, "It would appear that a desire to stop the dope doctors led prominent and able clinicians into believing that addiction withdrawal was functional"—that is, that it was psychological in nature, not physical.[51] Researchers, however, would later identify severe withdrawal symptoms as indicating a user's physical dependence on a drug.[52]

Increasingly, doctors explained addiction by focusing on the psychology of the user and suggesting that the person had criminal tendencies rather than acknowledging that the problem had a physical basis. Some asserted that people who were addicted had personality disorders and that the problem was therefore based in their minds, not their bodies.[53] Doctors also contended that these users threatened their communities, which bolstered support for responding with criminal charges rather than with medical treatment.[54] Alexander Lambert, president of the AMA, defended this stance. In 1920, he insisted that it was fair to conclude that a "heroin addict is of an inferior personality," unlike a morphine habitué. While doctors could treat morphine users, he added, he regarded heroin and cocaine users as a "social menace."[55]

Many, however, said that addiction was a disease and that people who were addicted would continue their use to avoid withdrawal. In 1919, a writer for *Youth's Companion* stated that the Harrison Act's goals could not be attained "without extreme cruelty to the victims of the drug habit." He allowed that the framers of the law had good intentions but insisted that they were "ignorant," as they considered addiction to be a "vice" when "it is distinctly a disease." A habitué was not taking opium "to give himself pleasure," the writer explained, "but to get surcease from pain."[56] In its 1919 report on the *Traffic in Narcotic Drugs*, the Department of the Treasury agreed that addiction was a disease. For that reason, the person needed either medical treatment or "the repeated administration of the drug of addiction to keep the body functioning normally." Without the drug, people who were addicted would experience "such painful disturbances" that they would go "to any extreme to procure more of the drug."[57]

Other doctors, meanwhile, challenged the allegation that drug dependency signified a moral lapse. Physicians J. B. Mattison and Charles Terry, for example, agreed that addiction was a disease and that habitués were "basically normal personalities addicted" through medical use, according to David Courtwright.[58] Around the time that the Harrison Act became law, Lucius P. Brown, Tennessee's Food and Drugs commissioner, insisted that a person who was addicted "should be studied and treated as a sick man and not as one always wilfully delinquent."[59] According to the Department of the Treasury, susceptibility to addiction was not limited to "any particular race, nationality, or class of people." Although some were more vulnerable than others, they added, anyone who took a narcotic repeatedly for more than a month would be "in grave danger of becoming an addict."[60]

Many doctors insisted that no effective treatment for addiction existed and that maintenance was therefore necessary. A committee appointed by the New York State Senate studied the drug problem in 1916 and 1917 and concluded that it was "impossible" for an addicted person to receive "competent treatment." Alleged cures were either dangerous or ineffective. "Many addicts have died under the methods of treatment existing today," they stated, and many of those who were supposedly cured in institutions resumed their drug use to end the "physical torture induced by improper withdrawal of their drug." They called for an investigation into suspect treatments and for more doctors to search for a cure. They believed that addicted people had an "absolute need" for their drugs and that the state should provide maintenance to "the confirmed addict" until a safe and effective treatment was available.[61]

There was, of course, a close connection between people's understanding of addiction and their attitudes toward maintenance policies. If addiction were merely a vice, then banning maintenance was "rational and, in the long run, humane," medical sociologist Catherine Charles has acknowledged. If, on the other hand, it was a disease, then outlawing maintenance was "at best premature and at worst a cruel injustice inflicted on a vulnerable addict population." David Musto agreed. In such a circumstance, "opiates could no more be withheld than digitalis from the chronic heart patient"—but in 1920, few regarded it as a disease.[62]

By outlawing drug maintenance, Congress and the Supreme Court—through their passage of the Harrison Act and interpretation of it—forced habitués either to end their drug use or to resort to illicit markets, and these markets grew as a result. People who were addicted found themselves unable to afford the inflated prices of the illicit market, and they turned to crime to sustain their habit.[63] As sociologist Erich Goode has explained, passage of the law gave rise to "a criminal class of addicts—*a criminal class that had not existed previously.*" In 1914, the "link between addiction and crime . . . was forged."[64] In a 1918 issue of *Outlook* magazine, writers Theodore H. Price and Richard Spillane declared, "There is a direct relationship between drug addiction and crime." Although future generations would see a clear connection between the two, this would have been new information to readers of *Outlook*. According to Price and Spillane, over half of American criminals were addicted, and almost all pickpockets were "dope fiends." They acknowledged, however, that the lack of legal access to drugs impelled criminal behavior. "When an addict craves a drug and cannot get it readily," they stated, "he will do almost anything to satisfy his desire."[65] Historian Richard Davenport-Hines also observed this, concluding, "It is not the supply of a drug that turns a user into a criminal but the illicitness of that supply."[66]

As users turned to crime to get money for drugs, a criminal network was willing to supply them. In its 1919 report, the Treasury Department stated that since passage of the Harrison Act, "the traffic by 'underground' channels has increased enormously." Most of the drugs were smuggled in from Mexico and Canada, though some came in along the coasts, from Europe and Asia.[67] Sales were lucrative. "It is said to be a slogan in the underworld," Price and Spillane reported, that "peddling dope" for six months "means independent wealth." The work attracted many "denizens of the underworld," who thus gave up "blowing safes, picking pockets, and other practices."[68] Although drug use decreased somewhat, the illegal market filled much of the void. According to a writer for *Outlook* soon after the Harrison Act went into effect, "many unlawful drug dealers and users are still able to obtain what they want."[69]

In 1921, journalist Frederick Bechdolt likened these unintended consequences of the Harrison Act to efforts to slay the many-headed Hydra of Greek mythology. With the Harrison Act, the government had cut off one of the heads of the drug problem. Then, however, "a dozen new heads sprang up" in its place, he lamented.[70]

*  *  *

Most middle-class morphine habitués had passed away by the early 1920s, leaving those with a recognized malady as the only habituated people who garnered public sympathy and could access drugs legally. The Harrison Act and the Supreme Court's interpretation of it "reflected and helped to produce a clear demographic division within the drug-using population," as Timothy Hickman has pointed out. There had been compassion for those who had become morphine users after seeking medical advice. Meanwhile, commentators were, at best, indifferent to the hardships of a later generation's heroin users, those who did not begin their use to treat a physical ailment. By 1920, as Hickman has pointed out, those whose use began for nonmedical reasons "came to be defined as *criminals* and were thus proper subjects of the penal system." Those with accepted medical circumstances, meanwhile, "were defined as innocent *patients*, something that was shown in part by their willingness to place themselves under the authority of professional medicine."[71]

Many who shaped drug policy focused on whether habitués had underlying ailments, but as they distinguished between the groups, they advanced the idea that only "respectable" people deserved help. In 1919, a committee of the Department of the Treasury concluded that addicted people "may be divided into two classes." One consisted "principally of addicts of the underworld," while almost all the others were "addicts in good social standing." Members of the former group tended to obtain heroin and cocaine from "associates"; most of the others received their drugs from doctors.[72] The following year, Dr. S. Dana Hubbard saw a similar division among habitual drug users. One group suffered from "a disease or ailment requiring the use of narcotic drugs," and the others "use narcotic drugs for the comfort these afford and solely by reason of an acquired habit."[73] This division was endorsed that same year by an AMA committee that described two types of habitués in a report based on information from "physicians and officials who have dealt with thousands of drug users." One group consisted of "legitimate medical cases," people suffering from an ailment that made narcotics necessary. The committee believed the term "addicts" only applied to the other group, those who first turned to narcotics "for the comfort they afford"—that is, marginalized people who used them for their restorative potential—and then kept using them.[74]

Some doctors ignored this division to excuse habitual drug use by white professionals regardless of the circumstances. Dr. Lawrence Kolb, who worked for the United States Public Health Service, sympathized with the many respected professional men who were morphine habitués, since they felt compelled to hide their usage and were ashamed of their dependency. They probably used drugs because they endured "unusual stresses," he suggested, and could be "quickly cured" once such stress had abated.[75] In his statement to Congress in 1923, Dr. William C. Fowler, who was the health officer for Washington, DC, would not blame any professional who had become addicted. They were "accidental addicts," he insisted. They included doctors, lawyers, and ministers— "very high-grade citizens," in his opinion. He believed the term "dope fiend" was appropriate only when referring to "underworld persons who were originally mentally and morally degenerates" and who began their use in order "to gratify certain sensual pleasure."[76] Kolb and Fowler supported basing responses to addiction on users' social status. They sympathized only with people with whom they could identify—other professional men. And Fowler proposed the use of different terms to denote the two groups of users, to make them appear more different from each other than they were.

Some saw members of the white middle class as more likely than others to be addicted, but rather than concluding that they deserved extra scrutiny or censure, they called for mercy, even when they relapsed. According to Maryland physician C. B. Pearson in 1918, "all classes of people are to be found in the ranks of morphine addiction." As he continued, however, he used language that referred to native-born citizens and that would have connoted that they were white: "the better class of the native American stock seem to be the most susceptible." He believed that "all right-thinking people" would want these users to receive "humane" treatment and to be restored to "complete health and happiness." Instead of blaming them for any lapses following treatment, Pearson saw them as victims of circumstance. A habitué's doctor should help him "in avoiding the dangers that threaten him during convalescence," he insisted. "We should not scold the addict for a relapse."[77] Dr. Charles Terry recognized this tendency to sympathize with more influential members of society. When he advocated drug maintenance, he played to this notion. In 1920, he suggested that many administrators did not support people who were addicted because they believed they were of poor character. It was important to know, he asserted, that "among the sufferers from this disease are numbered many of the highest intellectual types of men and women in the business and professional worlds."[78]

Some judges also favored leniency toward these users. In 1920, a San Francisco police court judge dismissed charges against a young couple who used morphine habitually. He explained that he did so because the "girl...came from a refined, high-class family" and he believed she might "have the 'spirit' to beat the game and break away from drugs." Perceiving her and her boyfriend as being in love, the judge advised them to "get married and try to quit the drugs." The reporter for the *San Francisco Examiner* presented the decision approvingly, characterizing the couple as "unfortunate victims of narcotic addiction." Meanwhile, as scholar Jim Baumohl points out, San Franciscans who were poor, or members of the working class, or Chinese American had "endured the frequent, fierce storms of local law enforcement long before the Harrison era."[79]

Some doctors connected economic marginalization with the likelihood of addiction, pointing out that many people who became addicted lacked access to high-quality medical care. In 1919, Dr. Thomas Blair, who headed Pennsylvania's Bureau of Drug Control, stated that people who endured "bad industrial and housing conditions" were more likely than others to become addicted to drugs. He saw this problem especially in coal-mining communities. He considered the absence of good medical and dental care, however, to be the most significant factor predisposing a person to addiction. Thousands of people, he explained, contracted illnesses that could be easily treated if they could see a doctor. Without that access, they became "chronic sufferers or even incurables" who then "drift into more or less permanent drug addiction." About half of the Pennsylvanians who struggled with addiction, he maintained, initially used drugs to treat a disease. Their subsequent "incapacity," he added, owed more to the addiction than to the original ailment. Few recognized this connection, but in much of the country, the "average worker and his family" did not have access to good medical care.[80]

* * *

Authorities would introduce new justifications for their starkly different approaches to treating people addicted to drugs. One theory maintained that only immoral people would derive pleasure from drug use. This gave the public another reason to accept a policy that would cause users to suffer. In 1925, Dr. Lawrence Kolb acknowledged that anyone could enjoy the release of pain on taking a pain reliever. But, he added, only "the emotionally unstable, the psychopath, or the neurotic" could feel euphoria—could experience a pleasure that raised the user "above his usual emotional plane." Definitions of "psychopath" varied. It could denote anyone with a mental illness, but it could also refer to a person who was anti-social and self-interested.[81] Kolb saw a correlation: those with the greatest "degree of psychopathy" would experience drug-induced joy most intensely. He deemed Thomas De Quincey the quintessential "psychopath," given his euphoria and his periods of depression. "Every psychopathic addict," Kolb asserted, "has an experience comparable to that recorded by De Quincey." Kolb was influential in the medical community—"the Osler of drug addiction" a colleague called him, referring to William Osler, one of the founders of Johns Hopkins Hospital. He did regard addiction as a mental illness and believed that those who were addicted deserved help.[82] He also, however, helped to popularize the notion that a gulf existed between two groups of habitués.

It appears, however, that the users were not seeking "pleasure"—a state of delight above the norm—so much as the drugs' restorative value: a way to endure life's troubles. Kolb quoted some of their explanations as to why drug use appealed to them:

> "It makes my troubles roll off my mind."
> "It is exhilarating and soothing."
> "You do not care for anything and you feel happy."
> "It makes you drowsy and feel normal."

While some acknowledged feeling exhilarated, they mainly indicated a wish to forget their problems and fit in. Kolb connected their drug use to their problems, but he offered no sympathy. He concluded that their addiction had a "neurotic basis," since their comments implied that they had "emotional conflicts or feelings of inadequacy, the relief from which is expressed as pleasure." These people, he stated, rarely enjoyed "mental peace and calm."[83]

* * *

As the century progressed, many white, middle-class Americans defended habitués within their circle while blaming the drug problem on people of color or foreigners. These tendencies shaped policy, as advocates of strict drug limitations found that they gained support for their goals when they blamed foreign nations for producing the drugs and "domestic ethnic minorities" for using them, as historian Douglas Clark Kinder has noted. Harry Anslinger, for example, who led the Federal Bureau of Narcotics from 1930 to 1962, recognized that playing to nativist sentiment was effective. He issued "hundreds" of false statements during his tenure, many of which played on xenophobic sentiments, in order to check criticism of the FBN's effectiveness, to garner funds for the Bureau, and to gain support for anti-drug legislation. In blaming outsiders, he ignored important parts of the story of American drug addiction: doctors' longtime practice of prescribing opiates excessively; Americans' enthusiasm for buying new and unregulated drugs, including proprietary treatments; the eagerness of mail-order houses and some druggists to sell them; and the absence of regulations, which allowed these transactions to take place. Advocates of drug laws, however, "refused to recognize that native-born citizens could misuse drugs without foreign instigation."[84]

Race, class, and "environment" continued to shape perceptions of drug users and, consequently, the responses to their behavior. In the 1950s, for example, legislators imposed mandatory sentences for drug-related charges. These sentences ensnared people of color, members of the working class, and the poor, but they were also applied to young, white, middle-class defendants. As a result, government officials revised or rescinded these measures. In 1956, for example, the federal government approved mandatory sentences of five years for a first offense of selling marijuana. This was changed in the late 1960s because many white, middle-class youth came before the court. Connecticut senator Thomas Dodd introduced legislation to remove the mandatory sentence, to protect defendants who were "not hardened criminals." He defined them as "college students and young people of middle and upper economic status." The modification had bipartisan support. And when white teenagers in the Dallas suburbs were arrested for marijuana use in 1973, new legislation reduced possession to a misdemeanor and provided a way for those arrested to avoid the mandatory sentence if they were found guilty of distributing it. The change in the law did not derive from the belief that it was inherently unfair or from the concerns of Latino or black families. A writer for *Texas Monthly* summed up the motivation behind the change in the law: "Too many of the wrong kids were being arrested."[85]

Also in 1973, New York state passed strict laws to reduce drug use. The purpose of the so-called Rockefeller Drug Laws, which were named for their main proponent, Governor Nelson Rockefeller, was to address New York City's extensive heroin problem.[86] Under the law, anyone convicted of the sale or possession of an illegal drug would face a mandatory prison sentence. The highest-level felonies resulted in sentences of at least fifteen years, with lifelong parole supervision on release.[87] Rockefeller maintained that the laws' severity would lead to drops in "illegal drug use and drug-related crime." The lack of judicial discretion in sentencing appeared to provide a dual advantage: potential criminals could choose to obey the law, since judges could not be lenient, and sentencing would theoretically be fair, since judicial bias would have no outlet.[88] The legislation had extensive public and political support.[89]

The laws, however, which were costly to enforce, did not diminish drug sales, and their implementation led to mass incarceration, primarily of people of color. Several years after the passage of the legislation, a committee concluded that these measures did not diminish the availability of drugs or reduce the crime rate.[90] Rockefeller had surmised that harsh penalties would discourage street dealing to such an extent that nobody would accept such work. He did not realize that potential profits would retain their appeal regardless of the risks and that this would especially be the case for dealers who endured "addiction-induced desperation," as historian Jessica Neptune has observed. The police focused primarily on nonwhite neighborhoods, which rendered moot the notion that consistent sentences for lawbreakers would result in impartial enforcement. The state's prison population doubled in the laws' first decade, and that population more than doubled again in the subsequent ten years.[91] Also in that first decade of the laws' existence, almost every other state followed New York's lead, attaching mandatory minimum sentences to anti-drug laws.[92]

Rockefeller presented the laws as protecting black communities by addressing drug addiction and drug-related crimes, but while these problems concerned black New Yorkers, most opposed his use of lengthy, mandatory sentences.[93] Delora Hercules, for example, was a principal in the Bronx who had seen students turn to drugs, and her husband had been robbed at gunpoint by men who he believed were addicted. She wanted criminals to be punished, but she opposed Rockefeller's plan. It would result in the "destruction of black and Puerto Rican people," she told a reporter soon after the governor introduced his plan. "I really feel it is a conspiracy, a way of destroying us."[94]

In subsequent decades, many white drug users and sellers remained able to elude legal consequences for their crimes. Beginning in 1986, for example, federal law mandated a prison sentence of at least five years for someone found guilty of possessing five grams of crack cocaine. About half of America's crack cocaine users were white, but African Americans constituted more than 85 percent of the defendants who were sentenced on these charges. Between 1988 and 1995, in fact, federal prosecutors in cities including Chicago and Los Angeles did not prosecute any white people on charges related to crack cocaine.[95] In the 1990s, sociologist Troy Duster identified why African American drug sellers were arrested to an extent that was out of proportion to their participation. There were many arrests of street-level sellers, many of them young black men whose sales were of low value, but there was far less attention to drug sellers in fraternity houses or "white bankers laundering huge sums of drug money."[96]

In the 2010s, there was growing support for a treatment-based response to drug addiction, in large part because so many who became addicted to opiates were white and middle class. Katharine Neill, a scholar of urban policy, connects these compassionate attitudes to the broader acceptance of marijuana use and to widespread sympathy for those who were addicted to opiates, since many people, for the first time, were acquainted with someone who was addicted. "Millions of Americans have or know someone who has taken prescription painkillers," she explains, and they were consequently inclined to champion treatment, rather than criminal charges, as the solution.[97] More important, many drug users had parents with sufficient clout to shape the official response. "Because the demographic of people affected are more white, more middle class, these are parents who are empowered," Michael Botticelli observed in 2015, while serving as the nation's drug czar. "They know how to call a legislator, they know how to get angry with their insurance company, they know how to advocate. They have been so instrumental in changing the conversation." Changes included a growing tendency to refer to people who were addicted as having a "substance abuse disorder," rather than using pejorative terms such as "addict" or "junkie." More substantively, they included the decisions of many police departments to direct heroin users to treatment rather than arresting them. Some people welcomed the change but lamented the fact that others who were addicted lacked powerful advocates and therefore faced much grimmer fates. Law professor Kimberlé Williams Crenshaw, for example, supported the compassionate response but points out that had there been similar support in earlier decades for African Americans who had become addicted, "the devastating impact of mass incarceration upon entire communities would never have happened."[98]

Many in the media continue to sympathize with white people who are addicted to drugs while perceiving and characterizing African Americans who are addicted as criminals and as people who lack support networks to encourage their recovery. As media analyst Michael Shaw has pointed out, when the media depicts white drug users, they tend to present color images of daytime scenes, often in homes, with an emphasis on bonds of family and community and the addicted person's resilience and recovery. Rather than blaming users for their crimes and dependency, journalists depict addiction as a disease—"a threat from outside." Meanwhile, images pertaining to African Americans' drug use are more likely to be taken at night "on seedy streets or dark alleys," in "starker black and white." Narratives focus on unfit mothers, children being placed in foster care, and other involvement from state agencies and the criminal justice system.[99] When writing about addiction in the black community, journalists could focus on the bonds of family or community or provide stories of users overcoming addiction and moving on, because these stories exist and could be shared. Rarely, however, are they reported.

* * *

Studying history can reveal a society's prejudices that, at one time undisguised, can persist and remain virulent, albeit in a muted form. Such beliefs can diminish over time. Sometimes, they resurge. They can be challenged and vocally rejected, but as long as they are at least whispered or promoted behind closed doors, they endure, shaping views and, by extension, policy. Analyzing those earlier voices, providing key context, and producing discomfort is a significant part of history's value and relevance.

Beginning in the Revolutionary era, Americans became increasingly familiar with the concepts of drug addiction and pleasure-seeking drug use, and their understanding was not necessarily value laden. Published writings about habitual or nonmedical use among Americans was sparse before the 1860s, and information from abroad filled the void. Americans read travelers' descriptions of pleasure-seeking drug consumption in parts of Africa and the Middle East and about the weakened condition of longtime users. They learned about concepts that would later be termed drug tolerance and withdrawal. Later, reports from South

America stated that cocaine use enhanced productivity by allaying hunger and promoting endurance. Responses to other reports indicated rigid views. Upon reading about English habituation, those who had believed that race, class, or nationality could insulate some people from addiction learned that this was not the case. Also, they read about widespread drug use in some lands and concluded that such use could render societies unable to advance in ways that they assumed should be universal. Due to the lack of appreciation for the risks, meanwhile, use of habit-forming drugs increased in the United States. They were sold without prescriptions to a curious public, and doctors prescribed them extensively. As the reality of addiction became clearer, many realized that most users could not end their use through willpower alone and that no effective treatments existed. Some doctors advocated maintenance programs for drug users and noted the importance of providing access to health care to diminish people's tendency to self-medicate.

Misperceptions and distortions deriving from prejudice clouded popular understanding. Two notions shaped the conventional wisdom: that drug use was acceptable only if it was necessary for medical or restorative purposes and that only members of the white middle class would likely need drugs for these reasons. This view justified extensive drug use by the white middle class and stigmatized others' use as indulgent. Many white people rejected the notion that African Americans could need drugs medicinally, suggesting instead that they feigned illness to avoid work or that their manual labor did not impose mental strain; consequently, they would have no need to use drugs for restorative purposes. Although international events sparked the move toward national legislation to control drug use, support for such laws was bolstered by the perception of many that typical users were young poor men who used drugs for their enjoyable effects rather than to treat a medical condition. This attitude accompanied comforting lies that addiction was merely a bad habit and that addicted people could end their use in a matter of days if they wanted to. Such ideas facilitated support for legislation that ended most habitués' legal access to drugs. Some also asserted that the impact of drug use on people was determined by their race and that only people of color would, as a result of their use, behave in a manner that could threaten the safety of those around them. This became another justification for withholding access.

The lies and exaggerations, however, tacitly acknowledged the common ground that existed among Americans, for those lies were necessary in order to persuade. Time and again when addressing drug abuse, people agreed as to what the response should be; disagreement arose only when someone persuasively misrepresented the circumstances. Those who endorsed letting drug users suffer, for example, rarely if ever suggested that habitués were blameless. Instead, they maintained that those users had criminal tendencies or that they chose not to be cured. As the prospect of treating drug users became increasingly unattractive to doctors, many of them embraced convenient but untrue notions that addiction was not a disease and that withdrawal symptoms had no physical basis.

Along racial lines, the contrast in the responses to drug use has been clear and consistent. In the 1980s and 1990s, many white people used crack cocaine with legal impunity, while black users were arrested disproportionately on possession charges. A century earlier, judges and department store managers repeatedly forgave the crimes of Annie Meyers, a well-to-do white woman who shoplifted to support her cocaine habit. Meanwhile, white people were exaggerating cocaine's propensity to cause African American users to become violent and were ignoring the violent behavior of some white users. And white Texans' concern that "too many of the wrong kids were being arrested" for marijuana use in the 1970s is akin to the dismay in San Francisco a century earlier, when the Board of Supervisors fretted that opium dens' white customers included not just people who were "vicious and depraved" but also "young men and women of respectable parentage."[100]

As the last example indicates, there has been an emphasis on protecting white, middle-class youth. In part, this perception derived from a widely held notion that these teenagers had uniquely bright futures and should therefore be insulated from the consequences of their actions. This view is on display in a 1952 episode of *Dragnet*, a TV police procedural that dramatized real cases from the files of the Los Angeles Police Department.[101] In the episode, Sergeant Joe Friday and his partner, Officer Frank Smith, are investigating a case of vandalism committed by a group of teenagers including Harry Everson, a white seventeen-year-old. At the scene of the crime, Harry had inadvertently dropped his marijuana supply. His family is well-to-do. When the detectives enter his family's two-story, colonial-style home—in a "better-than-average section of the city," as Friday notes—Smith says, "Sure a nice place, huh Joe?" to which Friday replies, "Yeah, beautiful furniture." They inform Harry's father that his son has been using marijuana. After Mr. Everson overcomes his disbelief, he states that the news hurts him more than it would hurt other parents:

EVERSON: I can't believe it. My own boy using marijuana. Can't tell you how I feel.
SMITH: Afraid there's going to be more folks feeling the same way before this is all cleaned up.
EVERSON: But it'd be different if Harry didn't have a chance. A good home, good training—always had the best I could give him.

Fortunately for Harry, the authorities are mainly concerned with the drug sellers. At the end of the episode, eight dealers are convicted and sent to San Quentin.[102]

By pointing out that Harry has "a chance," Everson implies that many youth do not—that their ambitions must be modest and, consequently, drug convictions that they might incur are of little concern, since they never had much to lose. By referring to Harry's "good home, good training," Everson implies that youth from affluent homes are the ones who have "a chance" and that drug convictions for them would be particularly tragic. The episode reflected a real if inflated concern with illegal drug use at the time among parents in California and elsewhere. As historian Matthew Lassiter has observed, Californians in the 1950s called for "lengthy mandatory-minimum sentences for dope 'pushers'" due to exaggerated allegations of teenagers' drug use. White teenagers, however, suffered few legal consequences, despite their involvement. Instead, they were depicted as "innocent white youth" and rarely got in trouble with the law. While the typical drug seller was an "older white teenage dealer or recreational marijuana user providing small quantities to friends and classmates," Lassiter adds, consequences were most dire for "minority youth and low-income neighborhoods."[103] The onset of the Rockefeller Drug Laws and subsequent mass incarceration created an even more stark disparity between the consequences for members of marginalized groups and white, middle-class users.

A study of drug policy through the lens of race reveals how easy it is to persuade people to embrace a theory that justifies their preferred decision and thereby soothes their consciences. Some people, many with political agendas, were all too willing to provide that justification—or, to borrow a metaphor that abolitionists used when referring to defenses of slavery, to provide the "opiate"—that would provide an artificial but soothing ease to an unsettled audience. Because the War on Drugs has focused extensively on people of color, abolitionists' use of the "opiate" metaphor to criticize the ingrained acceptance of anti-black slander still resonates. Now as then, people accept metaphorical "opiates" to allay their concerns about supporting immoral policies. In 1838, for example, a writer for the African American newspaper *Colored American*, based in New York, dismissed the suggestion that black people "Can't Take Care of Themselves." The writer added that nobody believed that notion, which was fabricated to erode support for abolition. The racist criticism was "a momentary opiate to the sting of conscience, and merely serves for the time being, as a shield against the arguments of the faithful."[104] Another writer for the publication insisted that "tyrants" sought out signs of immorality in the free black community to reinforce their proslavery stances. They were "waiting and praying for our deeper degradation, as an opiate for their consciences," he wrote, and to provide "an extenuation"—a partial excuse—"for their guilt."[105]

It is instructive to place these justifications alongside widely accepted pretexts for the disproportionate punishment of African Americans that has resulted from the War on Drugs. Data from 2015, for example, reveal that white adolescents in the United States sold drugs at approximately the same rate as black adolescents and were more likely than their black counterparts to use them.[106] The War on Drugs, meanwhile, "operates as a form of structural racism," according to sociologists Michael L. Rosino and Matthew W. Hughey, since its practices and policies have had "uniquely negative effects on families and communities of color and thus exacerbated racial inequality." Much of the public accepts the disproportionate arrests and incarcerations of African Americans by attributing the disparity to flaws in the black community rather than considering the impact of racist assumptions on the manner in which the law is applied. Rosino and Hughey analyzed coverage of the War on Drugs in American newspapers from 1983 to 2014, including articles, op-eds, and letters to the editor, and in the comments sections of relevant online news articles. They found widespread belief that the war's racially disparate results were "rational, natural, or just." Many people dismissed evidence that racism determined who was punished and who was not. Instead, they blamed black Americans and members of the Latinx community and asserted that the patterns of punishment resulted from an assumed "cultural pathology, inherent criminality, and racial inferiority" of the groups that were disproportionately punished.[107]

These false notions, these metaphorical opiates, help to perpetuate a system that ruins lives and, alongside its other devastating effects, that makes society less safe, not more so. To respond to addiction effectively, it is crucial to dispel these notions, to recognize addiction as a disease, to address it as a public health matter, and to address the underlying causes that have been the source of so much misery.

# NOTES

## Note on Terminology

1. *Oxford English Dictionary*, s.v. "habit" (n. 9e), updated March 2021, https://www-oed-com. proxy-tu.researchport.umd.edu/view/Entry/82978?rskey=ei9lyp&result=1#eid; *Oxford English Dictionary*, s.v. "addiction" (n. 1b), updated March 2021, https://www-oed-com. proxy-tu.researchport.umd.edu/view/Entry/2179?redirected From = addiction#eid.

## Introduction

1. "Hasheesh," *Frank Leslie's Popular Monthly* 8, no. 1 (January 1882), 110; *Oxford English Dictionary*, s.v. "Stimulant" (n. 2a), updated June 2020, https://www-oed-com.proxy-tu.resea rchport.umd.edu/view/Entry/190373?redirected From=Stimulant#eid.
2. [David W. Cheever], "Narcotics," *North American Review* (October 1862), 376.
3. Fitz Hugh Ludlow, "Hasheesh and Hasheesh Eaters," *Harper's New Monthly Magazine* (April 1858), 653; R. Gordon Wasson, *Soma: Divine Mushroom of Immortality* (New York: Harcourt Brace Jovanovich, 1968), 10, 153, 156; David T. Courtwright, *Forces of Habit: Drugs and the Making of the Modern World* (Cambridge, Mass.: Harvard University Press, 2001), 54; "Mission to the Sandwich Islands," *Missionary Herald* 17, no. 4 (April 1821), 118; Mariola Herbet and Ewa Jagiełło-Wójtowicz, "Datura Stramonium L.—Its Use over the Ages," *Acta Toxicologica* 14, 1/2 (2006), 6–8.
4. *The Writings of James Madison*, vol. 9, *1819–1836*, ed. Gaillard Hunt (New York: G. P. Putnam's Sons, 1910), 13–14. Emphasis in original.
5. *The Writings of James Madison*, 14.
6. [Cheever], "Narcotics," 386.
7. "Hasheesh and Its Smokers and Eaters," *Scientific American* 14 (October 23, 1858), 49.
8. Leslie E. Keeley, M.D., *The Morphine Eater: Or, From Bondage to Freedom* (Dwight, Ill.: C. L. Palmer, 1881), 195–96.
9. Alan Baumler, ed., *Modern China and Opium: A Reader* (Ann Arbor: University of Michigan Press, 2001), 28.
10. Quoted in "Use of Opium in this Country," *Medical and Surgical Reporter* 12, no. 27 (April 15, 1865), 438.
11. L. Barnes, M.D., "Opium—Morphine," *Ohio Medical and Surgical Reporter* (May 1868), 77.
12. Alcohol was the most widely consumed drug in America during the period under review, but other historians have thoroughly addressed its use and the impact of that use (e.g., W. J. Rorabaugh, *The Alcoholic Republic: An American Tradition* [New York: Oxford University Press, 1979]; William E. Unrau, *White Man's Wicked Water: The Alcohol Trade and Prohibition in Indian Country, 1802–1892* [Lawrence: University Press of Kansas, 1996]; Catherine Gilbert Murdock, *Domesticating Drink: Women, Men and Alcohol in America, 1870–1940*

[Baltimore: Johns Hopkins University Press, 1998]; Christine Sismondo, *America Walks into a Bar: A Spirited History of Taverns and Saloons, Speakeasies and Grog Shops* [New York: Oxford University Press, 2011]; and Matthew Warner Osborn, *Rum Maniacs: Alcoholic Insanity in the Early American Republic* [Chicago: University of Chicago Press, 2014]).

13. H. Wayne Morgan, *Drugs in America: A Social History, 1800–1980* (Syracuse, N. Y.: Syracuse University Press, 1981), ix–x.

14. David T. Courtwright, *Dark Paradise: A History of Opiate Addiction in America* (Cambridge, Mass.: Harvard University Press, 2001), 3–4.

15. Stephen R. Kandall, *Substance and Shadow: Women and Addiction in the United States* (Cambridge, Mass.: Harvard University Press, 1996), 7, 3, 8.

16. Diana L. Ahmad, *The Opium Debate and Chinese Exclusion Laws in the Nineteenth-Century American West* (Reno: University of Nevada Press, 2007), xi.

17. Timothy A. Hickman, *The Secret Leprosy of Modern Days: Narcotic Addiction and Cultural Crisis in the United States, 1870–1920* (Amherst: University of Massachusetts Press, 2007), 10. Emphasis in original.

18. David F. Musto, *The American Disease: Origins of Narcotic Control* (New York: Oxford University Press, 1999), 294.

19. "Opium Eater," *North-Carolina Free Press* [Halifax, N. C.], June 25, 1824, p. 4.

20. "Opium-Eating in New York," *Harper's Weekly* 1, no. 21 (May 23, 1857), 321–22.

21. Alonzo Calkins, *Opium and the Opium-Appetite* (Philadelphia: J. B. Lippincott, 1871), 40.

22. [George Parsons Lathrop], "The Sorcery of Madjoon," *Scribner's Monthly* 20 (July 1880), 421.

23. Courtwright, *Dark Paradise*, 41.

24. Morgan, *Drugs in America*, 38–40.

25. David T. Courtwright, *The Age of Addiction: How Bad Habits Became Big Business* (Cambridge, Mass.: Belknap Press of Harvard University Press, 2019), 7, 112.

26. E.g., Barbara Hahn, *Making Tobacco Bright: Creating an American Commodity, 1617–1937* (Baltimore: Johns Hopkins University Press, 2011); Frederick F. Siegel, *The Roots of Southern Distinctiveness: Tobacco and Society in Danville, Virginia, 1780–1865* (Chapel Hill: University of North Carolina Press, 1987); Allan Kulikoff, *Tobacco and Slaves: The Development of Southern Cultures in the Chesapeake, 1680–1800* (Chapel Hill: University of North Carolina Press, 1986); Drew A. Swanson, *Golden Weed: Tobacco and Environment in the Piedmont South* (New Haven, Conn.: Yale University Press, 2014); and Cassandra Tate, *Cigarette Wars: The Triumph of "The Little White Slaver"* (New York: Oxford University Press, 1999).

27. Benjamin R. Kracht, *Religious Revitalization among the Kiowas: The Ghost Dance, Peyote, and Christianity* (Lincoln: University of Nebraska Press, 2018), 70, 158–59; Martin Terry and Keeper Trout, "Regulation of Peyote (*Lophophora Williamsii*: Cactaceae) in the U.S.A.: A Historical Victory of Religion and Politics over Science and Medicine," *Journal of the Botanical Research Institute of Texas* 11, no. 1 (2017), 150–51.

28. Alan I. Leshner, "Addiction Is a Brain Disease, and It Matters," *Science* 278 (October 3, 1997), 45; Mark Kleiman et al., *Drugs and Drug Policy: What Everyone Needs to Know* (New York: Oxford University Press, 2011), 208–10, 212–13; *Oxford English Dictionary*, s.v. "endorphin" (n. 2), updated March 2021, https://www-oed-com.proxy-tu.researchport.umd.edu/view/Entry/61984?redirectedFrom=Endorphin#eid.

29. Leshner, "Addiction Is a Brain Disease," 45–46.

30. George M. Beard, "Certain Symptoms of Nervous Exhaustion," *Virginia Medical Monthly* 5, no. 3 (June 1878), 170–71; Anna Hayward Johnson, A. M., "Neurasthenia," *Philadelphia Medical Times* 11, no. 24 (August 27, 1881), 737; Brad Campbell, "The Making of 'American': Race and Nation in Neurasthenic Discourse," *History of Psychiatry* 18, no. 2 (June 2007), 161.

31. Diane Price Herndl, "The Invisible (Invalid) Woman: African-American Women, Illness, and Nineteenth-Century Narrative," *Women's Studies* 24, no. 6 (September 1995), 555–57.

32. Diane Price Herndl, *Invalid Women: Figuring Feminine Illness in American Fiction and Culture, 1840–1940* (Chapel Hill: University of North Carolina Press, 1993), 21, 23, 27–28.

33. Frederick Law Olmsted, *The Cotton Kingdom: A Traveller's Observations on Cotton and Slavery in the American Slave States* (New York: Mason Brothers, 1862), 118, 120–21.

34. Sven E. Wilson, "Prejudice and Policy: Racial Discrimination in the Union Army Disability Pension System, 1865–1906," *American Journal of Public Health* 100, no. S1 (April 2010), S63.

35. Michael K. Ostrowsky, *Self-Medication and Violent Behavior* (El Paso, Tex.: LFB Scholarly Publishing, 2009),96; "Rendered Insane by Cocaine," *Daily City News* [New Castle, Pa.], June 27, 1888, p. 1.

36. *Fifty-Seventh Annual Report of the Commissioner of Indian Affairs to the Secretary of the Interior* (Washington, D. C.: Government Printing Office, 1888), 95, 99.

37. [Hamilton Wright], "Opium Problem," Senate, 61st Congress, 2d session, Document No. 377 (ca. 1910), 50; Douglas J. Flowe, "'Tell the Whole White World': Crime, Violence, and Black Men in Early Migration New York City, 1890–1917" (PhD diss., University of Rochester, 2014), 119–22.

38. E.g., "Crazed by a Weed, Man Murders," *El Paso* [Tex.] *Herald*, January 2, 1913, p. 2; Bob Chessey, "El Paso's 1915 Marihuana Ordinance: Myth and Reality," *Password* 58, no. 1 (2014), 34–35.

39. Annie C. Meyers, *Eight Years in Cocaine Hell* (Chicago: St. Luke Society, 1902), 11; Michael M. Cohen, "Jim Crow's Drug War: Race, Coca Cola, and the Southern Origins of Drug Prohibition," *Southern Cultures* 12, no. 3 (2006), 70.

40. Thomas A. Horrocks, "'The Poor Man's Riches, The Rich Man's Bliss': Regimen, Reform, and the *Journal of Health*, 1829–1833," *Proceedings of the American Philosophical Society* 139, no. 2 (June 1995), 121, 127, 134.

41. E.g., Mrs. Ellet, *The Queens of American Society* (New York: Charles Scribner, 1867), 457–58.

42. Gilbert G. Weigle, "Cupid Guides Addicts' Way to New Life," *San Francisco Examiner,* October 19, 1920, p. 5; Meyers, *Eight Years in Cocaine Hell,* 25–26.

43. David T. Courtwright, "The Female Opiate Addict in Nineteenth-Century America," *Essay in Arts and Sciences* 10 (March 1982), 166–67.

44. Joseph F. Spillane, *Cocaine: From Medical Marvel to Modern Menace in the United States, 1884–1920* (Baltimore: Johns Hopkins University Press, 2002), 119–21; e.g., C. B. Pearson, M.D., "The Treatment of Morphinism," *Medical Times* (August 1914), 245; Charles B. Towns, *Habits That Handicap; The Menace of Opium, Alcohol, and Tobacco, and the Remedy* (New York: Century Co., 1916), 244.

45. Martin Booth, *Cannabis: A History* (New York: St. Martin's Press, 2003), 162; Harrison Narcotic Act, 38 Stat. 785 (1914).

46. Catherine A. Charles, "Doctors and Addicts: A Case Study of Demedicalization" (PhD diss., Columbia University, 1979), 100, 136–37, 129, 123; Marcus Aurin, "Chasing the Dragon: The Cultural Metamorphosis of Opium in the United States, 1825–1935," *Medical Anthropology Quarterly* 14, no. 3 (September 2000), 436.

47. Hickman, *Secret Leprosy of Modern Days*, 130, 10.

48. "Solving the Narcotic Problem," *Druggists Circular* 67, no. 4 (April 1923), 141; Spillane, *Cocaine,* 103.

49. Matthew D. Lassiter, "Impossible Criminals: The Suburban Imperatives of America's War on Drugs," *Journal of American History* 102, no. 1 (June 2015), 127, 129, 133, 135–36; "Rates of Drug Use and Sales, by Race; Rates of Drug Related Criminal Justice Measures, by Race," Hamilton Project, Brookings Institution, last modified October 21, 2016, https://www.hamiltonproject.org/charts/rates_of_drug_use_and_sales_by_race_rates_of_drug_related_criminal_justice.

50. *Oxford English Dictionary,* s.v. "opiate" (n. 1a), updated June 2021, https://www-oed-com.proxy-tu.researchport.umd.edu/view/Entry/131849?rskey=ET3ZoX&result=1&isAdvanced=false#eid; *Oxford English Dictionary,* s.v. "opioid" (n. A), updated June 2020, https://www-oed-com.proxy-tu.researchport.umd.edu/view/Entry/131913?redirectedFrom=opioid&.

51. H. H. Kane, M.D., "The Chinese Opium-Pipe as a Therapeutic Agent," *Medical Record* 20, no. 19 (November 5, 1881), 515; Diana Lynn Ahmad, "'Caves of Oblivion': Opium Dens and Exclusion Laws, 1850–1882" (PhD diss., University of Missouri-Columbia, 1997), 72; "Opium Smoking as a Therapeutic Means," *Journal of the American Medical Association* (July 26, 1884), 100.

52. H. Kalant, "Opium Revisited: A Brief Review of Its Nature, Composition, Non-medical Use and Relative Risks," *Addiction* 92, no. 3 (1997), 270.

53. Robert Morrison, "De Quincey's Addiction," *Romanticism* 17, no. 3 (2011), 273; Colin Dickey, "The Addicted Life of Thomas De Quincey," *Lapham's Quarterly* 6, no. 1 (Winter 2013); Laura Miller, "The Romantics and the Opium-Eater," Slate.com, last modified November 7, 2016, http://www.slate.com/articles/arts/books/2016/11/biography_of_thomas_de_quincey_guilty_thing_by_frances_wilson_reviewed.html.

54. W. B. O'Shaughnessy, "On the Preparations of the Indian Hemp, or Gunjah (*Cannabis Indica*)," *Provincial Medical Journal and Retrospect of the Medical Sciences* 123 (February 4, 1843), 364–68; [Fitz Hugh Ludlow], *The Hasheesh Eater: Being Passages from the Life of a Pythagorean* (New York: Harper & Brothers, 1857), 15–18.

55. Spillane, *Cocaine*, 8, 14; "The New Anæsthetic Chloral," *Scientific American* 22, no. 24 (June 11, 1870), 377.

56. William Willard, "The First Amendment, Anglo-Conformity and American Indian Religious Freedom," *Wicazo Sa Review* 7, no. 1 (Spring 1991), 29–30; D. W. Prentiss and Francis P. Morgan, "Mescal Buttons," *Transactions of the Association of American Physicians* 11 (Philadelphia, 1896), 306–7.

57. *Life and Letters of Dolly Madison*, ed. Allen C. Clark (Washington, D. C.: W. F. Roberts, 1914), 80–81.

58. Courtwright, *Dark Paradise*, 67; Mrs. E. V. Robbins, "Chinese Slave Girls: A Bit of History," *Overland Monthly* 1, no. 1 (January 1908), 100.

59. Henry G. Cole, *Confessions of an American Opium Eater: From Bondage to Freedom* (Boston: James H. Earle, 1895), 106; William L. White, "Addiction as a Disease: Birth of a Concept," *Counselor* 1 (2000), 49.

60. Dale H. Gieringer, "The Forgotten Origins of Cannabis Prohibition in California," *Contemporary Drug Problems* 26 (Summer 1999), 251–55, 258.

61. Cohen, "Jim Crow's Drug War," 66, 70, 73; NIDA, "Coca-Cola's Scandalous Past," National Institute on Drug Abuse, accessed January 3, 2022, last modified March 1, 2012, https://teens.drugabuse.gov/blog/post/coca-colas-scandalous-past.

62. *Opium Eating: An Autobiographical Sketch by an Habituate* (Philadelphia: Claxton, Remsen and Haffelfinger, 1876), 113.

63. "Order No. 1254—Prohibiting Opium Smoking Dens," *San Francisco Examiner*, November 24, 1875, p. 2; Ahmad, *The Opium Debate and Chinese Exclusion Laws*, 82; Musto, *American Disease*, 59–60.

64. Courtwright, *Dark Paradise*, 2, 33.

65. *Yearbook of the United States Department of Agriculture, 1908* (Washington, D. C.: Government Printing Office, 1909), 775.

66. Courtwright, *Dark Paradise*, 2, 50–51, 53, 110; Anne L. Foster, "Prohibition as Superiority: Policing Opium in South-East Asia, 1898–1925," *International History Review* 22, no. 2 (2000), 256.

67. Edward Huntington Williams, "The Drug-Habit Menace in the South," *Medical Record* (February 7, 1914), 247.

68. Our Special Correspondent, "Happy Days in Hollywood," *Vanity Fair* (May 1922), 73.

69. Lassiter, "Impossible Criminals," 127, 129–30, 132; Matthew Lassiter, "Pushers, Victims, and the Lost Innocence of White Suburbia: California's War on Narcotics during the 1950s," *Journal of Urban History* 41, no. 5 (2015), 790, 798, 796; Benjamin T. Smith and Wil G. Pansters, "US Moral Panics, Mexican Politics, and the Borderlands Origins of the War on Drugs, 1950–62," *Journal of Contemporary History* 55, no. 2 (2020), 369.

70. Bill Bryan, "14 Are Facing Charges Tied to Trafficking of Heroin Here," *St. Louis Post-Dispatch*, September 27, 2001, p. 16; Julie Netherland and Helena B. Hansen, "The War on Drugs That Wasn't: Wasted Whiteness, 'Dirty Doctors,' and Race in Media Coverage of Prescription Opioid Misuse," *Culture, Medicine and Psychiatry: An International Journal of Cross-Cultural Health Research* 40, no. 4 (December 2016), 671, 673, 669; Caryn Sullivan, "Parents—Lock Up Your Prescription Drugs," *TwinCitiesPioneerPress.com*, May 26, 2011.

## Chapter 1

1. [David W. Cheever], "Narcotics," *North American Review* 95, no. 197 (October 1862), 399.
2. Anne L. Foster, "Prohibition as Superiority: Policing Opium in South-East Asia, 1898–1925," *International History Review* 22, no. 2 (June 2000), 256.
3. [Cheever], "Narcotics," 409.
4. *Baltimore: Past and Present* (Baltimore: Richardson & Bennett, 1871), 89; Lance Lee Humphries, "Robert Gilmor, Jr. (1774–1848): Baltimore Collector and American Art Patron" (PhD diss., University of Virginia, 1998), I: 318, 75–76.
5. "The Diary of Robert Gilmor," *Maryland Historical Magazine* 17, no. 3 (September 1922), 232, 252–53.
6. Humphries, "Robert Gilmor, Jr.," 87; "Diary of Robert Gilmor," 234.
7. Richard Dorsey Papers, MS 1764, H. Furlong Baldwin Library, Maryland Center for History and Culture.
8. U.S. Congress, *American State Papers. Documents, Legislative and Executive, of the Congress of the United States*, Second Series, vol. 6 (Washington: Gales & Seaton, 1859), 418–19.
9. "The State vs. James Wilson," *Baltimore Sun*, February 14, 1840, p. 2; "City Court—February Term," *Baltimore Sun*, February 13, 1841, p. 1.
10. "Slavery Convention," *Baltimore Sun*, December 6, 1841, p. 2.
11. James S. Lewis, Philadelphia, to Richard Dorsey, June 26 (or 20), 1809, Dorsey Papers, Maryland Center for History and Culture.
12. J. Swaine to Richard Dorsey, July 6, 1809, Collection LCP.in.HSP134 Rush Family Papers, vol. 16, p. 114, Library Company of Philadelphia on deposit at Historical Society of Pennsylvania.
13. W. Hammond to Richard Dorsey, December 25, 1809, Dorsey Papers, Maryland Center for History and Culture.
14. David T. Courtwright, *Dark Paradise: A History of Opiate Addiction in America* (Cambridge, Mass.: Harvard University Press, 2001), 26.
15. David Johnson, *John Randolph of Roanoke* (Baton Rouge: Louisiana State University Press, 2012), 247n29, 8, 4.
16. Southgate to King, July 19, 1800, vol. 33: Letterbook, American Letters of Introduction to Rufus King, 1796–1802, Rufus King Papers, 1766–1899 (Bulk 1783–1826), MS 1660, New-York Historical Society.
17. David T. Courtwright, "The Female Opiate Addict in Nineteenth-Century America," *Essay in Arts and Sciences* 10 (March 1982), 164.
18. Emma Hitt Nichols, "Understanding Addiction: Dopamine and Brain Function," *MD Conference Express* 14, no. 8 (June 2014), 6–7; Mark A. R. Kleiman, Jonathan P. Caulkins, and Angela Hawken, *Drugs and Drug Policy: What Everyone Needs to Know* (New York: Oxford University Press, 2011), 207.
19. Benjamin Breen, *The Age of Intoxication: Origins of the Global Drug Trade* (Philadelphia: University of Pennsylvania Press, 2019), 125.
20. H. Wayne Morgan, *Drugs in America: A Social History, 1800–1980* (Syracuse, N. Y.: Syracuse University Press, 1981), 2.
21. "Advertisements," *South-Carolina Gazette*, August 22, 1743; *The Druggist's Manual, Being a Price Current of Drugs, Medicines, Paints, Dye-Stuffs, Glass, Patent Medicines, &c. . . .* (Philadelphia: Solomon W. Conrad, 1826), 28; Robley Dunglison, M.D., *Medical Lexicon: A New Dictionary of Medical Science . . .* (Philadelphia: Lea & Blanchard, 1842), 691.
22. John Theobald, M.D., *Every Man His Own Physician* (London: W. Griffin, and Boston: Cox and Berry, 1767), 35.
23. "To the Printers of the Pennsylvania Gazette," *Pennsylvania Gazette*, August 31, 1769, p. 1.
24. John Tennent, *Every Man His Own Doctor: OR, The Poor Planter's Physician* (Williamsburg and Annapolis: William Parks, 1734), 55, 56. Emphasis in original.
25. Day Book, 1800–1801, John Harrison Records, Amb.4258, Historical Society of Pennsylvania.
26. E. D. G. Prime, *Around the World: Sketches of Travel Through Many Lands and over Many Seas* (New York: Harper & Brothers, 1874), 241.
27. "Something Besides Tobacco," *Beadle's Monthly* 2 (August 1866), 135; Hast Handy, *An Inaugural Dissertation on Opium . . .* (Philadelphia: T. Lang, 1791), 6–7; John Awsiter, M.D.,

*An Essay on the Effects of Opium* (London: Printed for G. Kearsly, 1767), 7; Daniel M. Perrine, *The Chemistry of Mind-Altering Drugs: History, Pharmacology, and Cultural Context* (Washington, D. C.: American Chemical Society, 1996), 45; The Reverend Isaac Pierson, "Opium in China," *Missionary Herald* 73, no. 3 (March 1877), 76; Antony Wild, *The East India Company: Trade and Conquest from 1600* (New York: Lyons Press, 2000), 173.

28. "Persian Opium," *American Journal of Pharmacy* (September 1880), 464; J. Carson, M.D., "Note upon India Opium," *American Journal of Pharmacy* (July 1849), 197; "Another Dose of Physic," *Friends' Review* 12, no. 50 (August 20, 1859), 796; George W. Carpenter, *Observations and Experiments on the Pharmaceutical Preparations and Constituent Principles of Opium* (Philadelphia: s.n. 1827), 4; David H. Finnie, *Pioneers East: The Early American Experience in the Middle East* (Cambridge, Mass.: Harvard University Press, 1967), 20.

29. "North Carolina," *Baltimore Weekly Magazine* (December 31, 1800), 164.

30. David Ramsay, *The History of South-Carolina, from Its First Settlement in 1670, to the Year 1808* (Charleston: David Longworth, 1809), II: 347.

31. "Domestic Opium," *New England Journal of Medicine and Surgery* 1, no. 3 (July 1812), 315.

32. Milton Anthony, "Observations on the Cultivation of the Poppy and the Formation of Opium," *Philadelphia Medical Museum*, n.s. 1, no. 3 (1810), 142.

33. "On Making Opium," *Archives of Useful Knowledge* 2, no. 2 (October 1811), 169–70, 175, 177.

34. Joyce E. Chaplin, "Creating a Cotton South in Georgia and South Carolina, 1760–1815," *Journal of Southern History* 57, no. 2 (May 1991), 194.

35. Dr. Alexander Jones, "Observations Relative to the Culture of the Poppy," *Southern Agriculturist* 4, no. 4 (April 1831), 188–89.

36. Dr. Alexander Jones, "On the Culture of the Persian Poppy," *Southern Agriculturist* 3, no. 11 (November 1830), 571.

37. E.g., "Something Besides Tobacco," *Beadle's Monthly* 2 (August 1866), 137; D. W. Tyndall, "Opium," *Prairie Farmer* 20, no. 12 (September 21, 1867), 179.

38. C. F. Holder, "The Opium Industry in America," *Scientific American* 78, no. 10 (March 5, 1898), 147.

39. M. I. Wilbert, "Some Early Botanical and Herb Gardens," *American Journal of Pharmacy* 80 (September 1908), 426.

40. Morgan, *Drugs in America*, 2.

41. E.g., "Editorial Miscellany," *De Bow's Review* 28, no. 4 (October 1860), 494; E. B. Haskins, "Clinical Observations in Private Practice," *Western Journal of Medicine and Surgery* 7 (January 1851), 8.

42. Diane Price Herndl, "The Invisible (Invalid) Woman: African-American Women, Illness, and Nineteenth-Century Narrative," *Women's Studies* 24, no. 6 (September 1995), 555–57.

43. *The American Farmer's New and Universal Hand-book* (Philadelphia: Cowperthwait, Desilver, & Butler, 1854), 275–76; G. W. Briggs, M.D., "Hog Plague," *American Farmer* 6, no. 5 (May 1877), 168; J. Carver, "Veterinary Pharmacopœia," *Farrier's Magazine* (June 1, 1818), 99; H. J. G., "New Remedy for the Bots," *Southern Planter* 9, no. 1 (January 1849), 4.

44. Ronald Hamowy, "Introduction: Illicit Drugs and Government Control," in *Dealing with Drugs: Consequences of Government Control*, ed. Ronald Hamowy (Lexington, Mass.: D. C. Heath, 1987), 10–11.

45. Paul C. Nagel, *The Lees of Virginia: Seven Generations of an American Family* (New York: Oxford University Press, 1990), 149–51.

46. John Burns, *Popular Directions for the Treatment of the Diseases of Women and Children* (New-York: Thomas A. Ronalds, 1811), 181–82.

47. Cathy N. Davidson, *Revolution and the Word: The Rise of the Novel in America* (Oxford: Oxford University Press, 1987), 289.

48. "Forms of Disease in which Opiates Are Indicated," *Half-Yearly Abstract of the Medical Sciences* 1 (January–June 1845), 88–92. Emphases in original.

49. Abigail Adams, *The Quotable Abigail Adams*, ed. John P. Kaminski (Cambridge, Mass.: Belknap Press of Harvard University Press, 2009), xxxv.

50. Dr. John Jones, *The Mysteries of Opium Reveal'd* (London: Printed for Richard Smith, 1701), 42. Emphasis in original.

51. Robert A. East, *John Quincy Adams: The Critical Years: 1785–1794* (New York: Bookman, 1962), 94–95, 100–104; William G. Ross, "The Legal Career of John Quincy Adams," *Akron Law Review* 23, no. 3 (Spring 1990), 420–21; George Paulson, "Illnesses of the Brain in John Quincy Adams," *Journal of the History of the Neurosciences* 13, no. 4 (December 2004), 341–43; *Life in a New England Town: 1787, 1788: Diary of John Quincy Adams* (Boston: Little, Brown, 1903), 68.

52. Samuel K. Jennings, *The Married Lady's Companion, or, Poor Man's Friend* (Richmond: T. Nicolson, 1804), 20.

53. Catherine Clinton, *Plantation Mistress: Woman's World in the Old South* (New York: Pantheon, 1982), 172.

54. Benjamin Rush, M.D., *Medical Inquiries and Observations, upon the Diseases of the Mind* (Philadelphia: Kimber & Richardson, 1812), 319–20.

55. Sally G. McMillen, *Motherhood in the Old South: Pregnancy, Childbirth, and Infant Rearing* (Baton Rouge: Louisiana State University Press, 1990), 176.

56. Elizabeth Powel letter to Bushrod Washington, June 22, 1785, Series 3b, Box 4, Folder 3, Powel Family Papers, 1681–1938, Collection 1582, Historical Society of Pennsylvania.

57. "Life of the Late Dr. John Jones," *American Medical and Philosophical Register* 3 (January 1813), 333.

58. Franklin to Jane Mecom, March 24, 1790, in *The Writings of Benjamin Franklin*, vol. 10, *1789–1790*, ed. Albert Henry Smyth (New York: Macmillan, 1907), 92.

59. Joseph J. Ellis, *Founding Brothers: The Revolutionary Generation* (New York: Vintage Books, 2000), 26.

60. *Quotable Abigail Adams*, xxxv; David McCullough, *John Adams* (New York: Simon and Schuster, 2001), 613.

61. Rush, *Medical Inquiries and Observations*, 329.

62. Gerald N. Grob, *Mental Institutions in America: Social Policy to 1875* (London: Routledge, 2009), 167–68.

63. William H. Simmons, *An Essay on Some of the Effects of Contusions of the Head* (Philadelphia: Archibald Bartram, 1806), 17–18.

64. "Cases of Insanity," *American Journal of Insanity* 3 (January 1847), 193–94.

65. D. Y. DeLyser and W. J. Kasper, "Hopped Beer: The Case for Cultivation," *Economic Botany* 48, no. 2 (April–June 1994), 166–70; Wakeman Bryarly, *An Inaugural Essay, on the Lupulus Communis, or Gærtner; or the Common Hop* (Philadelphia: John H. Oswald, 1805), 29.

66. Richard Saunders, *Poor Richard improved: Being an Almanack and Ephemeris of the Motions of the Sun and Moon . . .* (Philadelphia: D. Hall and W. Sellers, 1767). Emphasis in original.

67. J. Worth Estes, *Hall Jackson and the Purple Foxglove: Medical Practice and Research in Revolutionary America, 1760–1820* (Hanover, N. H.: University Press of New England, 1979), 6.

68. J. B., "Oil of Turpentine in Burns," *New-England Journal of Medicine and Surgery* 1, no. 2 (April 1812), 195.

69. *The Continental Almanac, For the Year of our Lord, 1780* (Philadelphia: Francis Bailey, [1779]).

70. Morgan, *Drugs in America*, 6.

71. John Westley, *Primitive Physick . . .* (Philadelphia: Andrew Steuart, 1764), xvii–xviii. Emphases in original.

72. *Biographies of Successful Philadelphia Merchants* (Philadelphia: James K. Simon, 1864), 124–27; George W. Carpenter [of Philadelphia], "Observations and Experiments on Opium," *American Journal of Science* 13, no. 1 (January 1828), 17.

73. C. Ellis, "Patent Medicines," *American Journal of Pharmacy* 5, no. 1 (April 1839), 70–71.

74. Franklin Scott, *Experiments and Observations on the Means of Counteracting the Deleterious Effects of Opium . . .* (Philadelphia: H. Maxwell, 1803), 7.

75. James Cocke, "Rules for the Recovery of the Apparently Dead," *Baltimore Medical and Physical Recorder* (1809), 9.

76. "Effects of Opium Eating," *Boston Medical and Surgical Journal* 6, no. 8 (April 4, 1832), 130–31.

77. Thomas Calhoun Nelson, "An Inaugural Dissertation on the Effects of Emetics in Mercurial Salivation," *Transylvania Journal of Medicine and the Associate Sciences* 3, no. 2 (May 1830), 243–44.

78. A. B. Shipman, M.D., "Case of Poisoning with Opium," *American Journal of the Medical Sciences* (August 1840), 508.

79. Franklin B. Hough, *A History of Lewis County, in the State of New York* ... (Albany: Munsell and Rowland, 1860), 211n4.

80. "Charlestown," *South-Carolina Gazette*, July 8, 1732.

81. "To the Printers of the Pennsylvania Gazette ...," p. 1.

82. "Literary, Philosophic, &c.," *Pittsburgh Recorder* 3 (September 7, 1824), 188.

83. Sarah Waln Recipe Book, Am.1743 (1800), 14–15, Historical Society of Pennsylvania.

84. "Novel Case," *Monthly Traveller* 7, no. 6 (June 1836), 205–6; James Conquest Cress, "Case of Poisoning by Opium, Successfully Treated by Cold Affusions," *Philadelphia Journal of the Medical and Physical Sciences* 8, no. 16 (1824), 398–400.

85. Morgan, *Drugs in America*, 6.

86. "From the *New England Weekly Journal*, May 12," *Pennsylvania Gazette*, June 25, 1741. Emphases in original.

87. Dr. Barent P. Staats, "A Case of Poisoning by Opium Successfully Treated by Cold Affusions," *New-York Medical and Physical Journal* 3, no. 4 (October–December 1824), 473.

88. David B. Slack, "Opium in Cholera, Dysentery and Diarrhœa," *Boston Medical and Surgical Journal* 3 (September 28, 1830), 532.

89. "Opium Eater," *North-Carolina Free Press* [Halifax, N. C.], June 25, 1824, p. 4; Jones, *Mysteries of Opium Reveal'd*, 19; John Burns, *Popular Directions for the Treatment of the Diseases of Women and Children* (New-York: Thomas A. Ronalds, 1811), vi; Richard Holmes, *Coleridge: Darker Reflections, 1804–1834* (New York: Pantheon Books, 1998), 355n. Emphases in original.

90. *Saturday Evening Post* 9 (September 11, 1830), 2.

91. "Medical Jurisprudence," *American Medical Recorder* 1, no. 3 (July 1818), 386; *Trial and Execution of Abraham Kesler* ... (Albany, 1818).

92. Douglas V. Shaw, "Infanticide in New Jersey: A Nineteenth-Century Case Study," *New Jersey History* 115, no. 1/2 (Spring/Summer 1997), 3; Katie M. Hemphill, "'Driven to the Commission of This Crime': Women and Infanticide in Baltimore, 1835–1860," *Journal of the Early Republic* 32, no. 3 (Fall 2012), 446.

93. *The Liberator*, June 18, 1852, p. 3.

94. *The Liberator*, March 16, 1849, p. 3.

95. W. J. Rorabaugh, *The Alcoholic Republic: An American Tradition* (New York: Oxford University Press, 1979), 126–27, 131; Ric N. Caric, "The Man with the Poker Enters the Room: Delerium Tremens and Popular Culture in Philadelphia, 1828–1850," *Pennsylvania History* 74, no. 4 (Autumn 2007), 454–55.

96. Rorabaugh, *Alcoholic Republic*, 29–30, 7.

97. Peter C. Mancall, "'I Was Addicted to Drinking Rum': Four Centuries of Alcohol Consumption in Indian Country," in Sarah W. Tracy and Caroline Jean Acker, eds., *Altering American Consciousness: The History of Alcohol and Drug Use in the United States, 1800–2000* (Amherst, Mass.: University of Massachusetts Press, 2004), 95–96.

98. Benjamin Rush, M.D., *An Inquiry into the Effects of Ardent Spirits upon the Human Body and Mind* (Philadelphia: Thomas Dobson, 1805), 10, 6; Scott C. Martin, "'He is an Excellent Doctor if Called when Sober': Temperance, Physicians and the American Middle Class, 1800–1860," *Social History of Alcohol and Drugs* 24, no. 1 (Winter 2010), 22.

99. Rush, *Inquiry into the Effects of Ardent Spirits*, 9, 8, 11, 14, 10; Subhash C. Pandey, Adip Roy, Huaibo Zhang, and Tiejun Xu, "Partial Deletion of the cAMP Response Element-Binding Protein Gene Promotes Alcohol-Drinking Behaviors," *Journal of Neuroscience* 24, no. 21 (May 26, 2004), 5022–30.

100. Thomas Trotter, M.D., *An Essay, Medical, Philosophical, and Chemical, on Drunkenness, and Its Effects on the Human Body* (London: Longman Hurst, Rees, and Orme, 1804), 8.

101. Harry Gene Levine, "The Discovery of Addiction: Changing Conceptions of Habitual Drunkenness in America," *Journal of Studies on Alcohol* 39, no. 1 (1978), 152.

102. Matthew Warner Osborn, "A Detestable Shrine: Alcohol Abuse in Antebellum Philadelphia," *Journal of the Early Republic* 29, no. 1 (Spring 2009), 103–4, 110, 123–25.

103. Katherine A. Chavigny, "Reforming Drunkards in Nineteenth-Century America: Religion, Medicine, Therapy," in Tracy and Acker, eds., *Altering American Consciousness*, 110–13.

104. Benjamin Rush, M.D., *Medical Inquiries and Observations* (Philadelphia: J. Conrad & Co., 1805), 391.

105. Tho. Chadbourne, M.D., "Cases of Uterine Polypi," *Boston Medical and Surgical Journal* 21, no. 18 (December 11, 1839), 291.

106. "Philadelphia Hospital," *American Medical Intelligencer* 3, no. 16 (November 15, 1839), 249.

107. Alexander Hamilton, M.D., *A Treatise on the Management of Female Complaints, and of Children in Early Infancy* (New-York: Samuel Campbell, 1792), 236.

108. Mara L. Keire, "Dope Fiends and Degenerates: The Gendering of Addiction in the Early Twentieth Century," *Journal of Social History* 31, no. 4 (Summer 1998), 811.

109. Nancy Isenberg, *Fallen Founder: The Life of Aaron Burr* (New York: Penguin, 2007), 72–73.

110. Diane Price Herndl, *Invalid Women: Figuring Feminine Illness in American Fiction and Culture, 1840–1940* (Chapel Hill: University of North Carolina Press, 1993), 1, 23–24.

111. Thomas W. Ruble, M.D., *American Medical Guide for the Use of Families* (Richmond, Ky.: E. Harris, 1810), 34.

112. Thomas Cooper, Esq. M.D., *Tracts on Medical Jurisprudence* (Philadelphia: James Webster, 1819), 137.

113. Elizabeth Drinker, *The Diary of Elizabeth Drinker: The Life Cycle of an Eighteenth-Century Woman*, ed. and abridged by Elaine Forman Crane (Boston: Northeastern University Press, 1994), 135.

114. Letter dated July 2, 1824, Dr. James Carmichael Papers, 1816–1832 and n.d., Accession #11373, Special Collections Department, University of Virginia Library.

115. "Miscellaneous Intelligence: Effects of Opium Eating," *Western Journal of the Medical and Physical Sciences* 5, no. 4 (January–March 1832), 629–30.

116. Jones, *Mysteries of Opium Reveal'd*, 32. Emphases in original.

117. J. C. Rousseau, M.D., "Sketches on Venereal Complaints," *American Medical Recorder* 3, no. 2 (April 1820), 180.

118. John Lofland, *The Poetical and Prose Writings of Dr. John Lofland, the Milford Bard, Consisting of Sketches in Poetry and Prose* (Baltimore: John Murphy & Co., 1853), 14.

119. Alonzo Calkins, M.D., *Opium and the Opium-Appetite* (Philadelphia, J. B. Lippincott & Co., 1871), 98.

120. Johnson, *John Randolph of Roanoke*, 4; Dumas Malone, ed., *Dictionary of American Biography* (New York: Charles Scribner's Sons, 1935), 15: 364–65; Richard Heath Dabney, *John Randolph: A Character Sketch* (Chicago: University Association, 1898), 87.

121. James Thomas Flexner, *States Dyckman: American Loyalist* (Boston: Little, Brown, 1980), 119–25, 140–41.

122. *The Porter Family. Proceedings at the Reunion of the Descendants of John Porter, of Danvers, Held at Danvers, Mass., July 17th, 1895* (Danvers, [Mass.]: Eben Putnam, 1897), 50.

123. Eliza Southgate Bowne, *A Girl's Life Eighty Years Ago: Selections from the Letters of Eliza Southgate Bowne* (New York: Charles Scribner's Sons, 1887), 26, 69.

124. Ronald Hoffman and Sally D. Mason, *Princes of Ireland, Planters of Maryland: A Carroll Saga, 1500–1782* (Chapel Hill: University of North Carolina Press, 2000), 372.

125. Ronald Hoffman, Sally D. Mason, and Eleanor S. Darcy, eds., *Dear Papa, Dear Charley: The Peregrinations of a Revolutionary Aristocrat . . .* (Chapel Hill: University of North Carolina Press, 2001), 97.

126. Hoffman and Mason, *Princes of Ireland, Planters of Maryland*, 372, 382.

127. Richard Dorsey to Dorsey, January 18, 1836, Dorsey Papers, Maryland Center for History and Culture.

128. Jones, *Mysteries of Opium Reveal'd*, 51, 84; Louise Foxcroft, *The Making of Addiction: The 'Use and Abuse' of Opium in Nineteenth-Century Britain* (Burlington, Vt.: Ashgate, 2007), 171. Emphases in original.

129. "Biographical Memoir of Dr. Samuel Bard," *American Medical Recorder* 4, no. 4 (October 1821), 620.

130. Charles Francis Adams, ed., *Letters of John Adams, Addressed to His Wife* (Boston: Charles C. Little and James Brown, 1841), II: 173.

131. Virginia Berridge and Griffith Edwards, *Opium and the People: Opiate Use in Nineteenth-Century England* (New Haven, Conn.: Yale University Press, 1987), xxi.

132. John Leigh, M.D., *An Experimental Inquiry into the Properties of Opium, and Its Effects on Living Subjects* (Edinburgh: Printed for Charles Elliot, 1786), 113–17.

133. Scott, *Experiments and Observations*, 18.

134. Rush, *Medical Inquiries and Observations* (1805), IV: 382.

135. "Heermann's Case of Anomalous Disease," *New-York Medical Magazine* 1 (January 1814), 130; Lewis Heermann, *Directions for the Medicine Chest* (New-Orleans: John Mowry, & Co., 1811), 26.

136. Tracy and Acker, eds., *Altering American Consciousness*, 6.

137. John Hodgkinson, *A Narrative of His Connection with the Old American Company . . .* (New-York: J. Oram, 1797), 6, 7, 10, 11, 12; George O. Seilhamer, *History of the American Theatre: New Foundations* (Philadelphia: Globe Printing House, 1891), 115; Henry Collins Brown, ed., *Valentine's Manual of the City of New York for 1916–7* (New York: Valentine Company, 1916), 233. Emphasis in original.

138. Stephen Olin, *The Life and Letters of Stephen Olin, D.D., LL.D.* (New York: Harper & Brothers, 1853), I: 131–32; Rev. George G. Smith, A.M., *The Life and Letters of James Osgood Andrew* (Nashville, Tenn.: Southern Methodist Publishing House, 1882), 310.

139. George Cheyne, *The English Malady* (London: G. Strahan, 1733), i, ii; Serena R. Zabin, *Dangerous Economies: Status and Commerce in Imperial New York* (Philadelphia: University of Pennsylvania Press, 2009), 81. Emphases in original.

140. Thomas Trotter, M.D., *A View of the Nervous Temperament . . .* (London: Longman, Hurst, Rees, and Orme, 1807), 238, 242, 237; Peter Melville Logan, *Nerves and Narratives: A Cultural History of Hysteria in Nineteenth-Century British Prose* (Berkeley: University of California Press, 1997), 16.

141. Ramsay, *History of South-Carolina*, II: 392–93.

142. S., "Reid on Nervous Affections," *Portico* 4, nos. 1 and 2 (July/August 1817), 18. Emphasis in original.

143. "Taking Laudanum," *Journal of Health* 1 (February 10, 1830), 161–63.

144. Thomas A. Horrocks, "'The Poor Man's Riches, The Rich Man's Bliss': Regimen, Reform, and the *Journal of Health*, 1829–1833," *Proceedings of the American Philosophical Society* 139, no. 2 (June 1995), 119, 125–26; Frank Luther Mott, *A History of American Magazines, 1741–1850* (Cambridge, Mass.: Harvard University Press, 1966), 440.

145. "Review: Trotter's View of the Nervous Temperament," *New-York Medical and Philosophical Journal and Review* 1 (June 1809), 243.

146. Robert E. Lee, ed., *The Revolutionary War Memoirs of General Henry Lee* (New York: Da Capo Press, 1998), 69.

147. "Taking Laudanum," 163.

148. Lisa Norling, *Captain Ahab Had a Wife: New England Women and the Whalefishery, 1720–1870* (Chapel Hill: University of North Carolina Press, 2000), 283–84n3; Tupper is identified in "Boston, June 28, 1788," *New-Haven Gazette, and the Connecticut Magazine* 3, no. 30 (July 31, 1788), 2; J. Hector St. John de Crèvecoeur, *Letters from an American Farmer and Sketches of Eighteenth-Century America* (New York: Penguin Books, 1981; orig. pub. 1782), 160.

149. Crèvecoeur, *Letters*, 160.

150. Nathaniel Philbrick, "The Nantucket Sequence in Crèvecoeur's *Letters from an American Farmer*," *New England Quarterly* 64, no. 3 (September 1991), 420, mentioned in Norling, *Captain Ahab Had a Wife*, 296–97n86; Courtwright, "The Female Opiate Addict," 164.

151. James J. Kirschke, *Gouverneur Morris: Author, Statesman, and Man of the World* (New York: St. Martin's Press, 2005), 261.

152. Gouverneur Morris, *The Diary and Letters of Gouverneur Morris*, ed. Anne Cary Morris (New York: Da Capo Press, 1970), II: 548.

153. John Adams, *Statesman and Friend: Correspondence of John Adams with Benjamin Waterhouse, 1784–1822*, ed. Worthington Chauncey Ford (Boston: Little, Brown, 1927), 157–58.

154. Courtwright, *Dark Paradise*, 45.
155. "Taking Laudanum," 161–63.
156. Horace Greeley, *Recollections of a Busy Life* (New York: J. B. Ford & Co., 1868), 103.
157. Edward Hitchcock, *An Essay on Alcoholic & Narcotic Substances, as Articles of Common Use. Addressed Particularly to Students* (Amherst, [Mass.]: J. S. & C. Adams, 1830), 1, 7.
158. "Cure of an Opium-Eater," *New-York Mirror* 12, no. 23 (December 6, 1834), 177–78.
159. "Taking Laudanum," 161–63.
160. Rush, *Medical Inquiries and Observations* (1805), I: 365.
161. Howard Padwa, *Social Poison: The Culture and Politics of Opiate Control in Britain and France, 1821–1926* (Baltimore: Johns Hopkins University Press, 2012), 15.
162. "Curious Facts: Opium," *New-York Mirror, and Ladies' Literary Gazette* 3, no. 41 (May 6, 1826), 322–23.
163. Edward Hitchcock, *An Essay on Temperance* (Amherst: J. S. & C. Adams, 1830), 8.
164. Morgan, *Drugs in America*, 4.
165. John Reid, M.D., *Essays on Hypochondriacal and Other Nervous Affections* (Philadelphia: M. Carey & Son, 1817), 65.
166. "Miscellaneous Intelligence: Effects of Opium Eating," 628.
167. "Opium Eating," *Boston Medical and Surgical Journal* 9, no. 4 (September 4, 1833), 66.
168. C. L. Seeger, M.D., "Opium Eating," *Boston Medical and Surgical Journal* 9, no. 8 (October 2, 1833), 118–20. Seeger's great-great-grandson was folk singer Pete Seeger (Studs Terkel, *And They All Sang: Adventures of an Eclectic Disc Jockey* [New York: New Press, 2006], 213–14).
169. Seeger, "Opium Eating," 117, 120.
170. "Opium Eating," 67.
171. "Opium Eating," 66.

## Chapter 2

1. [David W. Cheever], "Narcotics," *North American Review* 95, no. 197 (October 1862), 375, 409.
2. "Opium-Eating in New York," *Harper's Weekly* 1, no. 21 (May 23, 1857), 321–22.
3. "Opium-Eating in New York," 321–22.
4. Rudolf Schmitz, "Friedrich Wilhelm Sertürner and the Discovery of Morphine," *Pharmacy in History* 27 (1985), 69n10, 61; David T. Courtwright, *Dark Paradise: A History of Opiate Addiction in America* (Cambridge, Mass.: Harvard University Press, 2001), 45.
5. H. Wayne Morgan, *Drugs in America: A Social History, 1800–1980* (Syracuse, N.Y.: Syracuse University Press, 1981), 23; David T. Courtwright, *Forces of Habit: Drugs and the Making of the Modern World* (Cambridge, Mass.: Harvard University Press, 2001), 37.
6. Sarah W. Tracy and Caroline Jean Acker, eds., *Altering American Consciousness: The History of Alcohol and Drug Use in the United States, 1800–2000* (Amherst: University of Massachusetts Press, 2004), 4–5.
7. David F. Musto, *The American Disease: Origins of Narcotic Control* (New York: Oxford University Press, 1999), 2.
8. "Use of Opium in the United States," *American Journal of Pharmacy* 37 (September 1865), 393. The article was widely reprinted.
9. Courtwright, *Dark Paradise*, 20.
10. Alonzo Calkins, M.D., *Opium and the Opium-Appetite* (Philadelphia: J. B. Lippincott and Co., 1871), 41.
11. "Confessions of a Medicine-Chest," *Merry's Museum* 11, no. 1 (January 1846), 21.
12. Sharon Lowe, "Behind the Soothing Mist: Women and Opiate Use in the Mining West, 1860–1900" (PhD diss., Union Institute and University, 2006), 283.
13. Edward R. Squibb, "Materia Medica and Pharmacy," *American Medical Times*, September 29, 1860, p. 230.
14. Courtwright, *Dark Paradise*, 45; Marcus Aurin, "Chasing the Dragon: The Cultural Metamorphosis of Opium in the United States, 1825–1935," *Medical Anthropology Quarterly* 14, no. 3 (September 2000), 418.

15. Charles E. Rosenberg, *The Cholera Years: The United States in 1832, 1849, and 1866* (Chicago: University of Chicago Press, 1987), 22.

16. Jno. Stainback Wilson, M.D., "Health Department," *Godey's Lady's Book and Magazine,* March 1861, 272; Dr. Charles P. Uhle, "Health Department," *Godey's Lady's Book and Magazine,* June 1870, 574.

17. Mrs. Mary S. Gove, *Lectures to Ladies on Anatomy and Physiology* (Boston: Saxton and Peirce, 1842), 45.

18. Prof. Geo. W. Winterburn, Ph.D., M.D., "A Seductive Drug," *American Medical Journal* 12, no. 3 (March 1884), 116–17.

19. William A. Alcott, "On the Study of Physiology as a Branch of General Education," *American Annals of Education and Instruction* 3, no. 9 (September 1833), 395n.

20. "Opium—The Poor Child's Nurse," *Harper's Weekly,* January 29, 1859, 80.

21. "The Laudanum Bottle, or 'I've Killed it!,'" *Parley's Magazine,* January 1844, 357.

22. Catherine Gilbert Murdock, *Domesticating Drink: Women, Men, and Alcohol in America, 1870–1940* (Baltimore: Johns Hopkins University Press, 1998), 4.

23. Jno. Stainback Wilson, M.D., "Health Department," *Godey's Lady's Book and Magazine,* November 1858, 467.

24. Allan Nevins and Milton Halsey Thomas, eds., *The Diary of George Templeton Strong: Young Man in New York, 1835–1849* (New York: MacMillan, 1952), 203. Emphasis in original.

25. "Opium Eating in England," *Water-Cure Journal, and Herald of Reforms* 8 (August 1849), 56.

26. *Public Laws of the State of Maine, from 1853 to 1857 Inclusive* (Augusta: Fuller and Fuller, 1856), 166; Murdock, *Domesticating Drink*, 12.

27. Quoted in "Appetite for Stimulants—Policy of Prohibition," *National Era* [Washington, D. C.], April 19, 1855.

28. Clarence Cook, "More About the Permanent Free Picture Gallery," *Independent* 7 (August 23, 1855), 265.

29. *Transactions of the Medical Society of the State of Pennsylvania, at its Twentieth Annual Session, Held at Erie, June, 1869* (Philadelphia: Collins, 1869), II: 316.

30. "Intemperance in Maine," *Boston Post,* February 10, 1879, p. 1.

31. *Oxford English Dictionary*, s.v. "ether" (n. 5a), updated March 2014, https://www-oed-com.proxy-tu.researchport.umd.edu/view/Entry/64728?rskey=AjevD6&result=2&is Advanced = false#eid; *Oxford English Dictionary*, s.v. "chloroform," updated 1989, https://www-oed-com.proxy-tu.researchport.umd.edu/view/Entry/32055?rskey=IJ7niQ &result = 1&isAdvanced = false#eid.

32. Richard Davenport-Hines, *The Pursuit of Oblivion: A Global History of Narcotics* (New York: W. W. Norton, 2002), 119–20.

33. David T. Courtwright, "Opiate Addiction as a Consequence of the Civil War," *Civil War History* 24 (1978), 107–8.

34. Jonathan Lewy, "The Army Disease: Drug Addiction and the Civil War," *War in History* 21, no. 1 (January 2014), 105, 103; Byron Stinson, "The Army Disease," *American History Illustrated* 6, no. 5 (August 1971), 10.

35. Lukasz Kamieński, *Shooting Up: A Short History of Drugs and War* (Oxford: Oxford University Press, 2016), 71.

36. Courtwright, "Opiate Addiction as a Consequence of the Civil War," 109, 103.

37. *Opium Eating: An Autobiographical Sketch by an Habituate* (Philadelphia: Claxton, Remsen and Haffelfinger, 1876), 59.

38. "Medical and Surgical Society of Baltimore: Opium Poisoning," *Medical and Surgical Reporter* 37, no. 4 (July 28, 1877), 68–69.

39. Jonathan S. Jones, "Then and Now: How Civil War-Era Doctors Responded to Their Own Opiate Epidemic," *Civil War Monitor,* November 3, 2017; email correspondence with Jonathan Jones, October 17, 2019.

40. Lewy, "The Army Disease," 112.

41. Jonathan S. Jones, "Opium Slavery: Civil War Veterans and Opiate Addiction," *Journal of the Civil War Era* 10, no. 2 (June 2020), 202–3.

42. T. D. Crothers, M.D., *Morphinism and Narcomanias from Other Drugs* (Philadelphia: W. B. Saunders, 1902), 75–76.

43. American Association for the Study and Cure of Inebriety, *The Disease of Inebriety from Alcohol, Opium and Other Narcotic Drugs* ... (New York: E. B. Treat, 1893), 323.

44. James D. Richardson, ed., *A Compilation of the Messages and Papers of the Presidents, 1789–1897* (Washington, D. C.: Government Printing Office, 1898), VIII: 699.

45. "One of Cleveland's Vetoes," *Indianapolis Journal*, August 13, 1888, p. 5.

46. Jones, "Opium Slavery," 196, 193, 201.

47. Jones, "Opium Slavery," 189–90, 199, 186, 193.

48. *Louisa May Alcott: Her Life, Letters, and Journals*, ed. Ednah D. Cheney (Boston: Roberts Brothers, 1889), 230.

49. Horace Day, *The Opium Habit, with Suggestions as to the Remedy* (New York: Harper and Brothers, 1868), 7.

50. "Opium and Its Consumers," *New York Tribune*, July 10, 1877, p. 2.

51. Leslie E. Keeley, *Opium: Its Use, Abuse and Cure; or, From Bondage to Freedom* (Dwight, Ill.: Leslie E. Keeley Co., 1892), 18.

52. David T. Courtwright, "The Hidden Epidemic: Opiate Addiction and Cocaine Use in the South, 1860–1920," *Journal of Southern History* 49, no. 1 (February 1983), 65.

53. Mark A. Quinones, "Drug Abuse During the Civil War (1861–1865)," *Substance Use and Misuse* 10, no. 6 (1975), 1019.

54. Courtwright, "Opiate Addiction as a Consequence of the Civil War," 102.

55. Quinones, "Drug Abuse During the Civil War," 1009; Lewy, "The Army Disease," 104–5; Courtwright, *Dark Paradise*, 46–47.

56. Morgan, *Drugs in America*, 24.

57. Stephen R. Kandall, *Substance and Shadow: Women and Addiction in the United States* (Cambridge, Mass.: Harvard University Press, 1999), 8.

58. Ann Douglas Wood, "'The Fashionable Diseases': Women's Complaints and Their Treatment in Nineteenth-Century America," *Journal of Interdisciplinary History* 4, no. 1 (Summer 1973), 27.

59. Diane Price Herndl, *Invalid Women: Figuring Feminine Illness in American Fiction and Culture, 1840–1940* (Chapel Hill: University of North Carolina Press, 1993), 1, 27, 23, 21.

60. Mara L. Keire, "Dope Fiends and Degenerates: The Gendering of Addiction in the Early Twentieth Century," *Journal of Social History* 31, no. 4 (Summer 1998), 809.

61. Scott C. Martin, *Devil of the Domestic Sphere: Temperance, Gender, and Middle-Class Ideology, 1800–1860* (DeKalb: Northern Illinois University Press, 2008), 37.

62. Frederick Hollick, M.D., *The Matron's Manual of Midwifery* (New-York: T. W. Strong, 1849), v. Emphases in original.

63. Abba Goold Woolson, *Woman in American Society* (Boston: Roberts Brothers, 1873), 136. Emphasis in original.

64. Wood, "'The Fashionable Diseases,'" 26.

65. Herndl, *Invalid Women*, 24.

66. Wood, "'The Fashionable Diseases,'" 27.

67. Carroll Smith-Rosenberg, *Disorderly Conduct: Visions of Gender in Victorian America* (New York: Oxford University Press, 1985), 208.

68. Herndl, *Invalid Women*, 28, 30, xiii, 39.

69. "Opium Eating," *New-York Observer* 33, no. 15 (April 12, 1855), 117.

70. Smith-Rosenberg, *Disorderly Conduct*, 200, 202, 208.

71. Quoted in Sally G. McMillen, *Motherhood in the Old South: Pregnancy, Childbirth, and Infant Rearing* (Baton Rouge: Louisiana State University Press, 1990), 176.

72. Dr. E. W. Shipman, "The Promiscuous Use of Opium in Vermont," *Transactions of the Vermont State Medical Society, for the Year 1890* (Burlington, Vt.: The Society, 1890), 75.

73. Katherine McVane Armstrong, "Thy Will Lord, Not Mine: Parents, Grief, and Child Death in the Antebellum South" (PhD diss., Emory University, 2011), 146–47.

74. "Opium," *Times-Picayune* [New Orleans, La.], April 4, 1840, p. 2.

75. Summarized in "Improper Use of Laudanum," *Scientific American* 10, no. 41 (June 23, 1855), 325.

76. Calkins, *Opium and the Opium-Appetite*, 139.

77. "Opium-Eaters and the Opium Trade," *Flag of Our Union* 12, no. 22 (May 23, 1857), 164.

78. "Drunkenness," *Hall's Journal of Health* 9, no. 3 (March 1862), 66.
79. J. B. Mattison, M.D., "Opium Addiction Among Medical Men," *Medical Record* 23, no. 23 (June 9, 1883), 621.
80. Thos. S. Blair, M.D., "Making the Narcotic Laws Help the Doctor and Not Hinder Him in His Work," *American Medicine* 26 (July 1920), 375.
81. Barry Milligan, "Morphine-Addicted Doctors, the English Opium-Eater, and Embattled Medical Authority," *Victorian Literature and Culture* 33, no. 2 (September 2005), 541.
82. Kristina Aikens, "A Pharmacy of Her Own: Victorian Women and the Figure of the Opiate" (PhD diss., Tufts University, 2008), 32; Joseph Michael Gabriel, "Gods and Monsters: Drugs, Addiction, and the Origins of Narcotic Control in the Nineteenth-Century Urban North" (PhD diss., Rutgers University, 2006), 242–43.
83. *The Writings of Henry David Thoreau: Journal*, vol. 2, *1850–September 15, 1851*, ed. Bradford Torrey (Boston: Houghton Mifflin, 1906), 194.
84. Margaret Fuller Ossoli, *At Home and Abroad; Or, Things and Thoughts in America and Europe*, ed. Arthur B. Fuller (Boston: Brown, Taggard and Chase, 1860), 202–3.
85. "Dangers of Using Ether and Chloroform—Extraordinary Revelations of Dentists—Sympathy for Dr. Beale," *Lancaster Ledger* [S. C.], January 17, 1855, p. 2.
86. James V. Ricci, M.D., *The Development of Gynæcological Surgery and Instruments* (San Francisco: Norman Publishing, 1990), 286.
87. "The Thing 'Ladies' Get Tight On," *Cincinnati Enquirer*, July 27, 1869, p. 4.
88. Calkins, *Opium and the Opium-Appetite*, 291.
89. R. P. Talley, "The Hypodermatic Use of Bimuriate of Quinine and Urea in the Practice of Medicine," *Medical and Surgical Reporter* 56, no. 19 (May 7, 1887), 577.
90. Gabriel, "Gods and Monsters," 257.
91. "The Chloroform Habit as Described by One of Its Victims," *Detroit Lancet* 8, no. 6 (December 1884), 251–54.
92. Morgan, *Drugs in America*, 13.
93. Nathan Allen, "Abuse of Opiates," *Friends' Intelligencer* 27, no. 51 (February 18, 1871), 813.
94. "New-York City," *New-York Daily Times*, April 14, 1852.
95. Amelia Fitzgerald Poe, Baltimore, to George Woodberry, August 28, 1884. George Edward Woodberry papers concerning Edgar Allan Poe, 1829–1928. MS Am 790.5 (46) Houghton Library, Harvard University.
96. Amelia Poe to George Woodberry, September 13, 1884. Woodberry Papers, Harvard University.
97. A Patient, "Original Communications: Opium and Alcohol," *New York Medical Times* 3, no. 2 (November 1853), 40.
98. Keeley, *Opium*, 50.
99. Day, *The Opium Habit*, 15.
100. *Opium Eating: An Autobiographical Sketch*, 66–67.
101. Thomas Dormandy, *Opium: A History* (New Haven, Conn.: Yale University Press, 2012), 182.
102. Quoted in Calkins, *Opium and the Opium-Appetite*, 389.
103. "Inquest," *Brooklyn Daily Eagle*, February 5, 1855.
104. Morgan, *Drugs in America*, 69.
105. William W. Smithers, *The Life of John Lofland, "The Milford Bard"* (Philadelphia: Wallace M. Leonard, 1894), 74–75, 92, 94–95, 122. Emphasis in original.
106. *Opium Eating: An Autobiographical Sketch*, 116–17.
107. "Eating Opium," *Baltimore Sun*, February 1, 1841, p. 1.
108. James McCune Smith, M.D., "On the Influence of Opium upon the Catamenial Functions," *New York Journal of Medicine* 2 (January 1844), 57; W. H. Van Buren, M.D., "Amputation of the Thigh, and Subsequent Amputation at the Hip-Joint, Followed by Perfect Recovery," *New-York Journal of Medicine* 7 (July 1851), 50, 52–56.
109. Susan Zieger, *Inventing the Addict: Drugs, Race, and Sexuality in Nineteenth-Century British and American Literature* (Amherst: University of Massachusetts Press, 2008), 98.
110. Leslie E. Keeley, *The Morphine Eater: Or, From Bondage to Freedom* (Dwight, Ill.: C. L. Palmer and Co., 1881), 36.

111. Henry G. Cole, *Confessions of an American Opium Eater* (Boston: James H. Earle, 1895), 136.

112. L. Barnes, M.D., *Opium* (Cleveland: Beckwith and Co., 1868), 5.

113. L. Barn[e]s, M.D., "The Late Rev. G. W. Brush," *Delaware* [Ohio] *Gazette* (January 31, 1868), 2; L. Barnes, M.D., "Opium—Morphine," *Ohio Medical and Surgical Reporter* 2, no. 3 (May 1868), 68, 71, 72.

114. Moses Clark White, *Dissertation on the Abuses of Opium*, M.D. Thesis, Yale University, 1854, Cushing-Hay Library.

115. Julian Hawthorne, *Nathaniel Hawthorne and His Wife: A Biography* (Boston: James R. Osgood and Company, 1885), I: 483.

116. Journal 9, p. 205. Charles Edward French diaries, 1851–1904, P-787, 6 reels (microfilm), Massachusetts Historical Society.

117. Sylvanus Cobb Jr. to Robert, October 30, 1867, Sylvanus Cobb, Letters, 1827–1867, Clifton Waller Barrett Library, Accession #7507, 7507-a, Special Collections Department, University of Virginia Library.

118. Samuel Chipman, *Report of an Examination of Poor-Houses, Jails, &c. in the State of New-York* (Albany: Hoffman and White, 1834), 63; John Hayward, *New-England and New-York Law-Register, for the Year 1835* (Boston: John Hayward, 1834), 242. Emphasis in original.

119. *New-York Times*, February 10, 1860, p. 1.

120. [D. W. Nolan], "The Opium Habit," *Catholic World* 33, no. 198 (September 1881), 827.

121. Abby K. Foster, "A Female Impostor," *Liberator* [Boston, Mass.], August 5, 1853.

122. Wm. A. Brown, "An Interesting Case of Malingering," *Ohio Medical and Surgical Journal* 12 (March 1860), 285–90.

123. "Relations Between the Clerical and Medical Professions: The Christian Examiner and the Hydropathic Delusion," *Boston Medical and Surgical Journal* 38, no. 26 (July 26, 1848), 517n.

124. A. B. Shipman, "Accidents from Taking Strychnine," *Boston Medical and Surgical Journal* 41, no. 6 (September 12, 1849), 114.

125. "Opium Eaters," *Adams Sentinel* [Gettysburg, Pa.], October 10, 1842, p. 1.

126. "Disorderly Men and Women—A Hasheesh Eater," *New-York Times*, October 28, 1866; "Law Reports: A Depraved Appetite," *New-York Times*, October 31, 1866.

127. "Psychology of Opium and Hasheesh: Opium," *Dial* 1, no. 9 (September 1860), 557.

128. "The Necessity of Caution in Prescribing Opiates," *Medical and Surgical Reporter* 33 (November 13, 1875), 397.

129. Sylvanus Cobb Jr. to Robert, October 30, 1867, Sylvanus Cobb, Letters, 1827–1867, University of Virginia Library.

130. Gerald Bordman and Thomas S. Hischak, *Oxford Companion to American Theatre* (New York: Oxford University Press, 2004), 135; Madeleine B. Stern, *Louisa May Alcott: A Biography* (Lebanon, N. H.: Northeastern University Press, 1996), 141.

131. George Combe, *A System of Phrenology* (Edinburgh: MacLachlan and Stewart, 1836), I: 44; Nathan Allen, M.D., *An Essay on the Opium Trade* (Boston: John P. Jewett and Co., 1850), 30.

132. "The Chemistry of Common Life," *Ladies' Repository* (May 1855), 292.

133. Calkins, *Opium and the Opium-Appetite*, 85. Emphasis in original.

134. Diane Price Herndl, "The Invisible (Invalid) Woman: African-American Women, Illness, and Nineteenth-Century Narrative," *Women's Studies* 24, no. 6 (September 1995), 555–57.

135. Jim Downs, *Sick from Freedom: African-American Illness and Suffering During the Civil War and Reconstruction* (New York: Oxford University Press, 2012), 9, 34–35.

136. In his extensive study of opiate addiction among Civil War veterans, Jonathan Jones found no African American habitués. He believes that this is largely because black soldiers "lacked equitable access to physicians" [Jones, "Opium Slavery," 205–6n5].

137. Courtwright, *Dark Paradise*, 49.

138. J. D. Roberts, M.D., "Opium Habit in the Negro," *North Carolina Medical Journal* 16, no. 4 (October 1885), 207.

139. J. Young, M.D., "Medical and Obstetrical Cases," *American Journal of the Medical Sciences* (April 1852), 426–27.

140. "Local Matters," *Daily Morning Post* [Pittsburgh, Pa.], May 20, 1850, p. 2.

141. J. S. Scofield, M.D., "Opium Eating," *New-York Daily Times*, November 4, 1852.

## Chapter 3

1. [David W. Cheever], "Narcotics," *North American Review* 95, no. 197 (October 1862), 403.
2. [Cheever], "Narcotics," 404, 379–80. Emphasis in original.
3. M. C. Cooke, *The Seven Sisters of Sleep* (London: James Blackwood, 1860), 163, 195. Emphasis mine.
4. [Cheever], "Narcotics," 408.
5. George Wheelock Grover, M. D., *Shadows Lifted or Sunshine Restored in the Horizon of Human Lives* (Chicago: Stromberg, Allen and Co., 1894), 82–83; "Miscellaneous: Hasheesh Candy," *New York Daily Herald*, September 5, 1862, p. 6; "Hasheesh Candy," *Baltimore Sun*, December 12, 1863, 2.
6. "Hasheesh and Its Smokers and Eaters," *Scientific American* 14 (October 23, 1858), 49.
7. Grover, *Shadows Lifted or Sunshine Restored*, 82–84.
8. Barney Warf, "High Points: An Historical Geography of Cannabis," *Geographical Review* 104, no. 4 (October 2014), 418–22, 424, 425; John Edward Philips, "African Smoking and Pipes," *Journal of African History* 24, no. 4 (1983), 312–13; Brian M. du Toit, "Man and Cannabis in Africa: A Study of Diffusion," *African Economic History* 1 (Spring 1976), 17–20, 28; David T. Courtwright, *Forces of Habit: Drugs and the Making of the Modern World* (Cambridge, Mass.: Harvard University Press, 2001), 40.
9. Martin Booth, *Cannabis: A History* (New York: St. Martin's Press, 2003), 39.
10. Stephen Snelders, Charles Kaplan, and Toine Pieters, "On Cannabis, Chloral Hydrate, and Career Cycles of Psychotropic Drugs in Medicine," *Bulletin of the History of Medicine* 80, no. 1 (Spring 2006), 98–99.
11. Ernest L. Abel, *Marihuana: The First Twelve Thousand Years* (New York: Plenum Press, 1980), 121.
12. Daniele Piomelli and Ethan B. Russo, "The *Cannabis sativa* Versus *Cannabis indica* Debate: An Interview with Ethan Russo, MD," *Cannabis and Cannabinoid Research* 1, no. 1 (January 1, 2016), 44–46. DOI: 10.1089/can.2015.29003.ebr.
13. Warf, "High Points," 416.
14. Cooke, *The Seven Sisters of Sleep*, 217.
15. [Cheever], "Narcotics," 403; George M. Beard, M. D., *Stimulants and Narcotics; Medically, Philosophically, and Morally Considered* (New York: G. P. Putnam and Sons, 1871), 20.
16. M. L. Thomas, "Something Besides Tobacco," *Beadle's Monthly* 2 (August 1866), 139–40.
17. Booth, *Cannabis*, 26.
18. Courtwright, *Forces of Habit*, 39.
19. Booth, *Cannabis*, 26, 52–53.
20. Booth, *Cannabis*, 7, 10; Warf, "High Points," 416.
21. Thomas Trotter, M.D., *An Essay, Medical, Philosophical, and Chemical, on Drunkenness, and Its Effects on the Human Body* (London: T. N. Longman, 1804), 10, 35. Emphasis in original.
22. "Intoxicating Effects of Wild Hemp," *Roanoke* [North Carolina] *Advocate*, August 23, 1832, p. 4.
23. E.g., "The Poisons We Indulge In," *Lancaster* [Pa.] *Examiner*, March 21, 1855, p. 1.
24. Joseph Michael Gabriel, "Gods and Monsters: Drugs, Addiction, and the Origins of Narcotic Control in the Nineteenth-Century Urban North" (PhD diss., Rutgers University, 2006), 171–72; W. B. O'Shaughnessy, "On the Preparations of the Indian Hemp, or Gunjah, (*Cannabis Indica*)," *Provincial Medical Journal and Retrospect of the Medical Sciences* 123 (February 4, 1843), 363n, 364–68.
25. Snelders et al., "On Cannabis, Chloral Hydrate," 101–2.
26. E. H. Squibb, M. D., "Brief Comments on the Materia Medica, Pharmacy, and Therapeutics of the Year Ending October 1, 1891, Alphabetically Arranged," *Transactions of the New York State Medical Association, for the Year 1891* 8 (New York City: The Association, 1892), 516. Emphasis in original.
27. "India: Part First—Ancient India," *Christian Review* 24, no. 97 (July 1859), 466.
28. "Hasheesh and Its Smokers and Eaters," 49.
29. "Hasheesh," *Frank Leslie's Popular Monthly* 13, no. 1 (January 1882), 110.
30. Booth, *Cannabis*, 45.

31. [Cheever], "Narcotics," 403.

32. Booth, *Cannabis*, 5, 37–38, 40.

33. G. Melvin Herndon, "Hemp in Colonial Virginia," *Agricultural History* 37 (April 1963), 91–92.

34. Eugene D. Genovese, *Roll, Jordan, Roll: The World the Slaves Made* (New York: Vintage, 1976), 641.

35. Thomas Jefferson to George Fleming, December 29, 1815, in *The Writings of Thomas Jefferson*, ed. H. A. Washington (Washington, D. C.: Taylor and Maury, 1854), VI: 506.

36. Courtwright, *Forces of Habit*, 41.

37. Chris S. Duvall, *The African Roots of Marijuana* (Durham, N. C.: Duke University Press, 2019), 148.

38. David A. Guba Jr., "Antoine Isaac Silvestre de Sacy and the Myth of the Hachichins: Orientalizing Hashish in Nineteenth-century France," *Social History of Alcohol and Drugs* 30 (2016), 51.

39. Mirt Komel, "Re-orientalizing the Assassins in Western Historical-fiction Literature: Orientalism and Self-Orientalism in Bartol's *Alamut*, Tarr's *Alamut*, Boschert's *Assassins of Alamut* and Oden's *Lion of Cairo*," *European Journal of Cultural Studies* 17, no. 5 (2014), 529.

40. Farhad Daftary, *Historical Dictionary of the Ismailis* (Lanham, Md.: Scarecrow Press, 2012), li–lii; Farhad Daftary, *The Assassin Legends: Myths of the Isma'ilis* (London: I. B. Tauris, 1994), 3.

41. Daryoush Mohammad Poor, "Secular/Religious Myths of Violence: The Case of Nizārī Ismailis of the Alamūt Period," *Studia Islamica* 114, no. 1 (2019), 51, 60, 61, 50.

42. Daftary, *The Assassin Legends*, 6, 2.

43. Guba, "Antoine Isaac Silvestre de Sacy," 50–51, 58–59.

44. Guba, "Antoine Isaac Silvestre de Sacy," 59.

45. Komel, "Re-orientalizing the Assassins in Western Historical-fiction Literature," 529.

46. Lukasz Kamieński, *Shooting Up: A Short History of Drugs and War* (Oxford: Oxford University Press, 2016), 37, 38; Guba, "Antoine Isaac Silvestre de Sacy," 50–52, 56, 57, 59–61.

47. "Von Hammer's *History of the Assassins*," *Foreign Quarterly Review* 1 (November 1827), 461. Emphasis in original. The review was reprinted, under the same title, in two Philadelphia publications: *Port–Folio* 2 (1827), 361–71, and *Museum of Foreign Literature, Science, and Art* 13 (May 1828), 1–11. The *Southern Literary Messenger* also presented Hammer's explanation in "Pinakidia," 2, no. 9 (August 1836), 575.

48. Bayard Taylor, *The Lands of the Saracen; or, Pictures of Palestine, Asia Minor, Sicily, and Spain* (New York: G. P. Putnam and Co., 1855), 133.

49. "Narcotics," *Friend* 36 (December 6, 1862), 110.

50. Juan Cole, *Napoleon's Egypt: Invading the Middle East* (New York: Palgrave Macmillan, 2008), 13, 110, 130; Kamieński, *Shooting Up*, 51.

51. David Alan Guba Jr., "Empire of Illusion: The Rise and Fall of Hashish in Nineteenth-century France" (PhD diss., Temple University, 2018); Booth, *Cannabis*, 77; Kamieński, *Shooting Up*, 51–54.

52. Michael Löwy and Robert Sayre, *Romanticism Against the Tide of Modernity*, trans. Catherine Porter (Durham, N. C.: Duke University Press, 2001), 9, 26.

53. Booth, *Cannabis*, 81–84.

54. "Editors' Book Table," *Godey's Magazine and Lady's Book* (December 1849), 465.

55. Alexandre Dumas, *The Count of Monte-Cristo* (London: George Routledge and Sons, 1888), II: 64–69.

56. "The Hashish: Singular Effects of an Oriental Drug," *Vermont Watchman & State Journal*, May 31, 1849, p. 1.

57. [Bayard Taylor], "The Vision of Hasheesh," *Putnam's Monthly* 3, no. 16 (April 1854), 403–4, emphasis in original; Susan Zieger, *Inventing the Addict: Drugs, Race, and Sexuality in Nineteenth-Century British and American Literature* (Amherst: University of Massachusetts Press, 2008), 34.

58. Taylor, *Lands of the Saracen*, 133, 138, 141–42.

59. Taylor, *Lands of the Saracen*, 142, 144–47.

60. James Todd Uhlman, "Gas-Light Journeys: Bayard Taylor and the Cultural Work of the American Travel Lecturer in the Nineteenth Century," *American Nineteenth Century History* 13, no. 3 (September 2012), 377, 383.

61. Susan Nance, *How the Arabian Nights Inspired the American Dream, 1790–1935* (Chapel Hill: University of North Carolina Press, 2009), 77; Uhlman, "Gas-Light Journeys," 386.

62. Uhlman, "Gas-Light Journeys," 385–87.

63. Zieger, *Inventing the Addict*, 17.

64. [Fitz Hugh Ludlow], *The Hasheesh Eater: Being Passages from the Life of a Pythagorean* (New York: Harper and Brothers, 1857), 15–18.

65. James F. Johnston, *The Chemistry of Common Life* (New York: D. Appleton and Company, 1863), 95.

66. [Ludlow], *Hasheesh Eater*, 30–31.

67. Quoted in [Cheever], "Narcotics," 405–6.

68. Taylor, *Lands of the Saracen*, 143, 138.

69. [Ludlow], *Hasheesh Eater*, 37–38, 132–33.

70. [Ludlow], *Hasheesh Eater*, 108.

71. [Fitz Hugh Ludlow], "Hasheesh and Hasheesh Eaters," *Harper's New Monthly Magazine* 16, no. 95 (April 1858), 653.

72. [Ludlow], *Hasheesh Eater*, 328, 349–51.

73. [Ludlow], *Hasheesh Eater*, xiii–xiv, 214, 92, 86, 260, 262, 273–74, 270.

74. [Ludlow], *Hasheesh Eater*, 47, 227–32. Emphasis in original.

75. Gabriel, "Gods and Monsters," 205.

76. [Ludlow], *Hasheesh Eater*, 280.

77. "Literary Notices," *Russell's Magazine* 2, no. 4 (January 1858), 382.

78. "Notices of Recent Publications," *Christian Examiner and Religious Miscellany* 23, no. 2 (March 1855), 304–5.

79. Leonard Warren, *Adele Marion Fielde: Feminist, Social Activist, Scientist* (London: Routledge, 2002), 32–33, 36–37, 40–41.

80. A. M. Fielde, "An Experience in Hasheesh-Smoking," *Therapeutic Gazette* 4, no. 7 (July 16, 1888), 449–51.

81. "Mental Science: Psychic Effects of Hasheesh," *Science* 12, no. 297 (October 12, 1888), 175; "Psychic Effects of Hasheesh," *Medical and Surgical Reporter* 59, no. 19 (November 10, 1888), 604; "The Dreams of a Hasheesh Smoker," *Cincinnati Medical Journal* 4, no. 1 (January 1889), 30–31.

82. Mary C. Hungerford, "An Overdose of Hasheesh," *Popular Science Monthly* 24 (February 1884), 509–14.

83. Letter 102 [undated; March 1862?]. Homans Family Correspondence, 1850–1938, bulk (1862–1864). MssCol 1427, Box 1. Manuscripts and Archives Division, New York Public Library, Astor, Lenox and Tilden Foundations.

84. Homans Family Correspondence, April 2, 1862, #103.

85. Homans Family Correspondence, January 9, 1864 #171.

86. L. M. A., "Perilous Play," *Frank Leslie's Chimney Corner* 8, no. 194 (February 13, 1869), 180–91.

87. Mrs. Ellet, *The Queens of American Society* (New York: Charles Scribner and Company, 1867), 457–58.

88. William Roscoe Thayer, *The Life and Letters of John Hay* (Boston: Houghton Mifflin Company, 1915), I: 47, 50; Tyler Dennett, *John Hay: From Poetry to Politics* (New York: Dodd, Mead, 1933), 22; John Taliaferro, *All the Great Prizes: The Life of John Hay, from Lincoln to Roosevelt* (New York: Simon and Schuster, 2013), 1, 8.

89. "Mr. Binns's Curious Experiences," *Baltimore Sun*, March 6, 1884, p. 4.

90. "Mr. Binns Tries Hasheesh," *New-York Times*, March 7, 1884.

91. "Delightful Drug," *St. Louis Post-Dispatch* (December 25, 1892), p. 7.

## Chapter 4

1. [David W. Cheever], "Narcotics," *North American Review* 95, no. 197 (October 1862), 377.

2. [Cheever], "Narcotics," 384–86; Diana Lynn Ahmad, "'Caves of Oblivion': Opium Dens and Exclusion Laws, 1850–1882" (PhD diss., University of Missouri-Columbia, 1997), 72.

3. E.g., Norman E. Zinberg, *Drug, Set, and Setting: The Basis for Controlled Intoxicant Use* (New Haven, Conn.: Yale University Press, 1984).

4. Hast Handy, *An Inaugural Dissertation on Opium . . .* (Philadelphia: T. Lang, 1791), 5, 11, 7–8, 13–14.

5. Joseph Michael Gabriel, "Gods and Monsters: Drugs, Addiction, and the Origins of Narcotic Control in the Nineteenth-Century Urban North" (PhD diss., Rutgers University, 2006), 164; Richard Davenport-Hines, *The Pursuit of Oblivion: A Global History of Narcotics* (New York: W. W. Norton, 2002), 25.

6. John Leigh, M.D., *An Experimental Inquiry into the Properties of Opium, and Its Effects on Living Subjects* (Edinburgh: Printed for Charles Elliot, 1786), 22, 26, 129.

7. Franklin Scott, *Experiments and Observations on the Means of Counteracting the Deleterious Effects of Opium* (Philadelphia: H. Maxwell, 1803), 20.

8. Benjamin Rush, *Medical Inquiries and Observations* (1805), I: 452–53.

9. "Opium," *Boston Medical and Surgical Journal* 16, no. 1 (February 8, 1837), 7; "Reports of Societies: Eating Opium," *New-York Mirror* 17, no. 40 (March 28, 1840), 317; "Eating Opium," *New York Evangelist* 11, no. 15 (April 11, 1840), 60.

10. Ernest L. Abel, *Marijuana: The First Twelve Thousand Years* (New York: Plenum Press, 1980), 110.

11. Margaret Goldsmith, *The Trail of Opium: The Eleventh Plague* (London: Robert Hale, 1939), 31; Martin Booth, *Opium: A History* (New York: St. Martin's Press, 1996), 25; Leigh, *Experimental Inquiry into the Properties of Opium*, 13, 14, 17, 18.

12. Alonzo Calkins, M.D., *Opium and the Opium-Appetite* (Philadelphia, J. B. Lippincott and Co., 1871), 21–22.

13. Albert G. Hess, "Deviance Theory and the History of Opiates," *International Journal of the Addictions* 6, no. 4 (December 1971), 589.

14. Samuel Crumpe, M.D., *An Inquiry into the Nature and Properties of Opium* (London: G. G. and J. Robinson, 1793), 48.

15. Hess, "Deviance Theory and the History of Opiates," 586–88; Virginia Berridge and Griffith Edwards, *Opium and the People: Opiate Use in Nineteenth-Century England* (New Haven, Conn.: Yale University Press, 1987), xxii; AB Damania, "The Origin, History, and Commerce of the Opium Poppy (*Papaver somniferum*) in Asia and the United States," *Asian Agri-History* 15, no. 2 (2011), 109–10; John D. Loeser, "Opiophobia and Opiophilia," in Marcia L. Meldrum, ed., *Opioids and Pain Relief: A Historical Perspective* (Seattle: IASP Press, 2003), 2.

16. Barney Warf, "High Points: An Historical Geography of Cannabis," *Geographical Review* 104, no. 4 (October 2014), 418–20, 424; David Alan Guba Jr., "Empire of Illusion: The Rise and Fall of Hashish in Nineteenth-Century France" (PhD diss., Temple University, 2018), 7; Brian M. du Toit, "Man and Cannabis in Africa: A Study of Diffusion," *African Economic History* 1 (Spring 1976), 17; David T. Courtwright, *Forces of Habit: Drugs and the Making of the Modern World* (Cambridge, Mass.: Harvard University Press, 2001), 40.

17. Gabriel G. Nahas, "Hashish in Islam 9th to 18th century," *Bulletin of the New York Academy of Medicine* 58, no. 9 (December 1982), 819–21; Franz Rosenthal, *The Herb: Hashish Versus Medieval Muslim Society* (Leiden: E. J. Brill, 1971), 160.

18. Courtwright, *Forces of Habit*, 64.

19. Booth, *Opium*, 21.

20. Francisco Guerra, "Sex and Drugs in the 16th Century," *British Journal of Addiction to Alcohol & Other Drugs* 69, no. 3 (September 1974), 285.

21. Steven B. Karch, M.D., *A Brief History of Cocaine* (Boca Raton, Fla.: CRC Press, 1998), 16–17.

22. Leo Africanus, *A Geographical Historie of Africa*, trans. John Pory (London, 1600), 249. The fact that "Lhasis" is hashish is noted in Leo Africanus, *The History and Description of Africa, and of the Notable Things Therein Contained*, trans. John Pory, ed. Robert Brown (London: Hakluyt Society, 1896), III: 755n46; I: xiv.

23. Martin Booth, *Cannabis: A History* (New York: Picador, 2003), 74; Guerra, "Sex and Drugs in the 16th Century," 274–76.

24. Quoted in Glenn Sonnedecker, "Emergence of the Concept of Opiate Addiction," *Journal mondial de pharmacie* 3 (1962), 279.

25. Samuel Purchas, *Purchas His Pilgrimage, or Relations of the World and the Religions Observed in All Ages . . .* (London: William Stansby, 1614), V: 508.

26. Matthew Dimmock, "Faith, Form and Faction: Samuel Purchas's Purchas His Pilgrimage (1613)," *Renaissance Studies* 28, no. 2 (2014), 264.

27. Quoted in Guerra, "Sex and Drugs in the 16th Century," 282.

28. Nahas, "Hashish in Islam 9th to 18th century," 821; Guba, "Empire of Illusion," 10.

29. Asli Çirakman, "From Tyranny to Despotism: The Enlightenment's Unenlightened View of the Turks," *International Journal of Middle East Studies* 33 (2001), 60; Davenport-Hines, *Pursuit of Oblivion*, 60.

30. "Travels," *Analytical Review* 15, no. 1 (January 1793), 35. Emphasis in original.

31. John Awsiter, M.D., *An Essay on the Effects of Opium. Considered as a Poison* (London: Printed for G. Kearsly, 1767), 3. Emphases in original.

32. Scott, *Experiments and Observations*, 20.

33. Davenport-Hines, *Pursuit of Oblivion*, 27.

34. Quoted in W. Golden Mortimer, M.D., *Peru: History of Coca, "The Divine Plant" of the Incas* (New York: J. H. Vail, 1901), 155.

35. Purchas, *Purchas His Pilgrimage*, II: 1541. Emphases in original.

36. [Erasmus Darwin], *The Botanic Garden. A Poem, in Two Parts* (New-York: T. and J. Swords, 1807), II: 57n.

37. Dr. John Jones, *The Mysteries of Opium Reveal'd* (London: Printed for Richard Smith, 1701), 215. Emphases in original.

38. "State of Medicine in Turkey," *Eclectic Journal of Medicine* 2, no. 5 (March 1838), 181.

39. [Cheever], "Narcotics," 374.

40. Peter Kolben, *The Present State of the Cape of Good-Hope* (London: W. Innys, 1731), 168; Eron Ackerman, "Ruling Pleasures and Growing Pains: Drugs and Colonial Expansion in Southern Africa, 1652–1850," 30, Alcohol and Drugs History Society, last modified July 12, 2013, https://alcoholanddrugshistorysociety.org. Emphasis in original.

41. David Gordon, "From Rituals of Rapture to Dependence: The Political Economy of Khoikhoi Narcotic Consumption, c. 1487–1870," *South African Historical Journal* 35 (November 1996), 63, 73–76, 80–81, 80n79; Booth, *Cannabis*, 55.

42. "Proofs that the People of the Southern Climes Have a Much Stronger Propensity to Heating and Intoxicating Liquors and Drugs than Those of the Northern," *Literary Magazine, and American Register* 2, no. 7 (April 1804), 74, 79.

43. Courtwright, *Forces of Habit*, 33.

44. Charles Caldwell, M.D., *Medical & Physical Memoirs . . .* (Philadelphia: Thomas and William Bradford, 1801), 204–5.

45. Jean-Baptiste Tavernier, *The Six Voyages of John Baptista Tavernier, Baron of Aubonne . . .* (London: Robert Littlebury and Moses Pitt, 1677), I: 242. Emphasis in original.

46. Richard Mead, *A Mechanical Account of Poisons in Several Essays* (London: J. R. for Ralph South, 1702), 138–39. Emphases in original.

47. Goldsmith, *Trail of Opium*, 31; Booth, *Opium*, 25.

48. Tavernier, *Six Voyages of John Baptista Tavernier*, I: 242; *Oxford English Dictionary*, s.v. "stupid" (n. 2a), updated June 2019, https://www-oed-com.proxy-tu.researchport.umd.edu/view/Entry/192218?redirectedFrom=stupid#eid.

49. Quoted in Gabriel, "Gods and Monsters," 164.

50. "The Cruelty of Avarice—The Opium Smokers of China," *National Magazine*, April 1855, 314–20.

51. Alex. Russell, M.D., *The Natural History of Aleppo, and Parts Adjacent* (London: A. Millar, 1756), 84.

52. "State of Medicine in Turkey," *New York Medical and Physical Journal* (January 1830), 402.

53. "Proofs that the People of the Southern Climes," 77.

54. "Horrors of Opium Eating," *Water-Cure Journal* 1, no. 3 (January 1, 1846), 39.

55. Quoted in Guerra, "Sex and Drugs in the 16th Century," 283–84.

56. Purchas, *Purchas His Pilgrimage*, V: 508.

57. Jones, *Mysteries of Opium Reveal'd*, 32. Emphases in original.

58. William Hunter, *Travels in the Year 1792 Through France, Turkey, and Hungary, to Vienna* (London: printed by J. Davis, for B. and J. White, 1796), 365.

59. Scott, *Experiments and Observations*, 41.

60. Davenport-Hines, *Pursuit of Oblivion*, 59; "From the Memoirs of Baron de Tott, on the Turks and Tartars," *New-Haven Gazette, and the Connecticut Magazine*, October 2, 1788, 39.

61. "Memoirs of the Baron de Tott . . . ," *Pennsylvania Packet*, December 4, 1788, 4.

62. Crumpe, *Inquiry into the Nature and Properties of Opium*, 51–53; George W. Carpenter, "Observations and Experiments on Opium," *American Journal of Science* 13, no. 1 (January 1828), 30n.

63. "Turkish Opium Takers," *American Phrenological Journal* (1848), 197–98.

64. Daniel Wilson, *An Inaugural Dissertation on the Morbid Effects of Opium Upon the Human Body* (Philadelphia: Solomon W. Conrad, 1803), 28–30, 30n.

65. Hans Derks, *History of the Opium Problem: The Assault on the East, ca. 1600–1950* (Leiden: Brill, 2012), 26.

66. Booth, *Opium*, 74. Emphasis in original.

67. Gunnar F. Kwakye et al., "*Atropa belladonna* Neurotoxicity: Implications to Neurological Disorders," *Food and Chemical Toxicology* 116 (2018), 347.

68. William Cadogan, *A Dissertation on the Gout . . .* (London: J. Dodsley, 1771), 88n.

69. James Mease, *An Inaugural Dissertation on the Disease Produced by the Bite of a Mad Dog or Other Rabid Animal* (Philadelphia: Thomas Dobson, 1792), 49.

70. Quoted in Booth, *Opium*, 25.

71. Jones, *Mysteries of Opium Reveal'd*, 21. Emphases in original.

72. Thomas Percival, M.D., *Father's Instructions . . .* (Philadelphia: Printed for Thomas Dobson, 1788), 193n.

73. Valentine Seaman, *An Inaugural Dissertation on Opium* (Philadelphia: Johnston and Justice, 1792), 11.

74. Guerra, "Sex and Drugs in the 16th Century," 269–70.

75. Courtwright, *Forces of Habit*, 102–3.

76. Jones, *Mysteries of Opium Reveal'd*, 24. Emphases in original.

77. Guerra, "Sex and Drugs in the 16th Century," 284.

78. Calkins, *Opium and the Opium-Appetite*, 30.

79. Sonnedecker, "Emergence of the Concept of Opiate Addiction," 280; Booth, *Opium*, 25.

80. Hunter, *Travels in the Year 1792*, 364–65.

81. Dumas Malone, ed., *Dictionary of American Biography* (New York: Charles Scribner's Sons, 1936), XIX: 530; "Review," *Philadelphia Medical and Physical Journal* 1, no. 3 (1805), 177.

82. [Cheever], "Narcotics," 393.

83. "Opium-Eating," *Boston Medical and Surgical Journal* 18, no. 8 (March 28, 1838), 129. It also appeared in G.H.V., "Opium and the Opium Trade," *American Quarterly Register and Magazine* 1, no. 1 (May 1848), 167, and Joel Shew, M.D., "Dangers of Drugs—Opium," *Water-Cure Journal* 20, no. 3 (September 1855), 50–52.

84. "Curious Historical and Descriptive Particulars Respecting the Inhabitants of the Kingdom of Canary on the Coast of Malabar," *Massachusetts Magazine: or, Monthly Museum* 8, no. 6 (June 1796), 316, 319.

85. Nathan Allen, M.D., *An Essay on the Opium Trade* (Boston: John P. Jewett and Co., 1850), 43–44.

86. Calkins, *Opium and the Opium-Appetite*, 113.

87. "To the Publisher of the Weekly Magazine," *New-Haven Gazette, and the Connecticut Magazine* 3, no. 23 (June 12, 1788), 3.

88. "Of the Oriental Learning and Philosophy," *Port Folio* (February 7, 1807), 94.

89. "Reports of Societies: Eating Opium," 317.

90. Mary Louise Pratt, *Imperial Eyes: Travel Writing and Transculturation* (London: Routledge, 1992), 44.

91. Chris S. Duvall, *The African Roots of Marijuana* (Durham, N. C.: Duke University Press, 2019), 18–19.

92. Russel Viljoen, "Aboriginal Khoikhoi Servants and Their Masters in Colonial Swellendam, South Africa, 1745–1795," *Agricultural History* 75, no. 1 (Winter 2001), 43.

93. Anthony Benezet, *A Short Account of the Part of Africa, Inhabited by the Negroes* (Philadelphia: W. Dunlap, 1762), 16–19.

94. Jayeeta Sharma, "'Lazy' Natives, Coolie Labour, and the Assam Tea Industry," *Modern Asian Studies* 43, no. 6 (2009), 1295–96.

95. Syed Hussein Alatas, *The Myth of the Lazy Native* (London: Frank Cass, 1977), 2.

96. J. M. Coetzee, *White Writing: On the Culture of Letters in South Africa* (New Haven, Conn.: Yale University Press, 1988), 16, 23.

97. Derks, *History of the Opium Problem*, xiii.

98. Sharma, "'Lazy' Natives, Coolie Labour," 1297.

99. Alatas, *Myth of the Lazy Native*, 8.

100. David Spurr, *The Rhetoric of Empire: Colonial Discourse in Journalism, Travel Writing, and Imperial Administration* (Durham, N. C.: Duke University Press, 1993), 15, 22.

101. Hissei Imai, Yusuke Ogawa, Kiyohito Okumiya, and Kozo Matsubayashi, "Amok: A Mirror of Time and People. A Historical Review of Literature," *History of Psychiatry* 30, no. 1 (March 2019), 49.

102. John Hawkesworth, ed., *A New Voyage Round the World, in the Years 1768, 1769, 1770, and 1771* (New-York: James Rivington, 1774), I: 218, 220–22.

103. Benjamin Rush, M.D., *Medical Inquiries and Observations, Upon the Diseases of the Mind* (Philadelphia: Kimber and Richardson, 1812), 177.

104. "Cafe and Divan at Algiers," *Flag of Our Union* 12, no. 15 (April 11, 1857), 116. Emphasis in original.

105. "Hasheesh and Its Smokers and Eaters," *Scientific American* 14, no. 7 (October 23, 1858), 49.

106. Jedidiah Morse, *The American Universal Geography* . . . (Boston: J. T. Buckingham, 1805), I: 391–92.

107. R. Brookes, *Brookes's General Gazetteer Improved, or, A New and Compendious Geographical Dictionary* . . . (Philadelphia: Jacob Johnson, and Co., 1806), "Turkey" entry.

108. J. Aikin, M.D., *Geographical Delineations, or, A Compendious View of the Natural and Political State of All Parts of the Globe* (Philadelphia: F. Nichols, 1807), 156.

109. Louis Lewin, M.D., *Phantastica* (Rochester, Vt.: Park Street Press, 1998), 32.

110. The Rev. R. Walsh, LL.D., *A Residence at Constantinople* (London: Frederick Westley and A. H. Davis, 1836), I: 255.

111. Hatice Aynur and Jan Schmidt, "A Debate Between Opium, Berş, Hashish, Boza, Wine and Coffee; The Use and Perception of Pleasurable Substances Among Ottomans," *Journal of Turkish Studies* 31, no. 1 (2007), 61, 63, 67.

112. Alex. Russell, M.D., *The Natural History of Aleppo, and Parts Adjacent* (London: A. Millar, 1756), 83. Emphasis in original.

113. Crumpe, *An Inquiry into the Nature and Properties of Opium*, 48.

114. "Foreign News: Constantinople," *Susquehanna Democrat* [Wilkes-Barre, Pa.], May 14, 1824, p. 2; "Opium Eaters," *Spirit of the English Magazines* 1, no. 5 (June 1, 1824), 205.

115. "The Turks," *Long-Island Star*, May 7, 1829.

116. Quoted in Booth, *Opium*, 25.

117. James Windle, "How the East Influenced Drug Prohibition," *International History Review* 35, no. 5 (2013), 1189–91.

118. Ronald D. Renard, "The Making of a Problem: Narcotics in Mainland Southeast Asia," in Don McCaskill and Ken Kampe, eds., *Development or Domestication? Indigenous Peoples of Southeast Asia* (Chiang Mai, Thailand: Silkworm Books, 1997), 319.

119. Quoted in Gabriel, "Gods and Monsters," 164.

120. John Barrow, *Travels in China* . . . (London: A. Strahan, 1804), 152–53.

121. N. P. Willis, *Pencillings by the Way* (London: John Macrone, 1835), II: 264.

122. Stephen Olin, *Greece, and the Golden Horn* (New York: J. C. Derby, 1854), 228.

123. James R. Rush, "Opium in Java: A Sinister Friend," *Journal of Asian Studies* 44, no. 3 (May 1985), 558.

124. R. R. Madden, Esq., *Travels in Turkey, Egypt, Nubia, and Palestine, in 1824, 1825, 1826, and 1827* (London: Henry Colburn, 1829), I: 12–13, 24–25; Dr. J. Oscar Noyes, "Intemperance in Europe and the East," *Ohio Medical and Surgical Journal* 9, no. 3 (January 1, 1857), 246. Emphases in original.

125. Madden, *Travels in Turkey, Egypt, Nubia, and Palestine*, I: 25–27.
126. "Opium Eaters," *Boston Medical and Surgical Journal* 2, no. 32 (September 22, 1829), 503; "Opium-Eaters and Snuff-Chewers," *Journal of Health* 1, no. 19 (June 9, 1830), 297–99; Shew, "Dangers of Drugs—Opium," 50–52; "Miscellany: Opium Eaters," *Weekly Gleaner* [Winston-Salem, N. C.], September 29, 1829, p. 1; [Cheever], "Narcotics," 388.
127. "Opium," *Boston Medical and Surgical Journal* 16, no. 7 (March 22, 1837), 101.
128. Davenport-Hines, *Pursuit of Oblivion*, 21–22.

## Chapter 5

1. [David W. Cheever], "Narcotics," *North American Review* 95, no. 197 (October 1862), 387, 400.
2. [Cheever], "Narcotics," 393–94.
3. Susan Zieger, *Inventing the Addict: Drugs, Race, and Sexuality in Nineteenth-Century British and American Literature* (Amherst: University of Massachusetts Press, 2008), 19.
4. *Saturday Magazine*, 2, nos. 2–21 (January 5–May 25, 1822).
5. Thomas De Quincey, *Confessions of an English Opium-Eater and Suspiria de Profundis* (Boston: Ticknor, Reed, and Fields, 1850), 52–53, x–xii.
6. De Quincey, *Confessions*, ix, 112, 3.
7. Richard Davenport-Hines, *The Pursuit of Oblivion: A Global History of Narcotics* (New York: W. W. Norton, 2002), 69–70.
8. Horace Day, *The Opium Habit, with Suggestions as to the Remedy* (New York: Harper and Brothers, 1868), 77.
9. Alonzo Calkins, M.D., *Opium and the Opium-Appetite* (Philadelphia, J. B. Lippincott and Co., 1871), 70.
10. De Quincey, *Confessions*, 50–53, 3, 66, 59, 53.
11. De Quincey, *Confessions*, 93–95, 91, 89, 96–97, 104–5, 98, 111. Emphasis in original.
12. Davenport-Hines, *Pursuit of Oblivion*, 69, 70.
13. Colin Dickey, "The Addicted Life of Thomas De Quincey," *Lapham's Quarterly* 6, no. 1 (Winter 2013).
14. "Notices of New Works, and Literary Intelligence," *Southern Literary Messenger* 7 (November 1841), 814.
15. Eric Schaefer, *"Bold! Daring! Shocking! True!": A History of Exploitation Films, 1919–1959* (Durham, N. C.: Duke University Press, 1999), 220; Tatum O'Neal, *A Paper Life* (New York: Harper Entertainment, 2004); Mackenzie Phillips, *High on Arrival* (New York: Gallery Books, 2009).
16. "Notices of New Works: Confessions of an Opium Eater," *Southern Literary Messenger* (December 1850), 764.
17. David F. Musto, *The American Disease: Origins of Narcotic Control* (New York: Oxford University Press, 1999), 69.
18. Robert Morrison, "De Quincey's Addiction," *Romanticism* 17, no. 3 (2011), 270, 272–73.
19. C. F., "Willard Phillips," *Dictionary of American Biography*, ed. Dumas Malone (New York: Charles Scribner's Sons, 1934), XIV: 547.
20. [Willard Phillips], "Confessions of an English Opium-Eater," *North American Review* 18 (January 1824), 90–98. Phillips's authorship of the review is established in Julius H. Ward, "The North American Review," *North American Review* 201, no. 710 (January 1915), 127.
21. "Confessions of an English Opium-eater," *United States Literary Gazette* (May 15, 1824), 38–40.
22. "Opiologia; or Confessions of an English Opium-Eater," *American Medical Recorder* 5 (July 1822), 553, 543.
23. Rev. Walter Colton, U.S.N., *Visit to Constantinople and Athens* (New-York: Leavitt, Lord and Co., 1836), 80, 84.
24. "Thomas De Quincey," *Yale Literary Magazine* 16, no. 6 (April 1851), 226.
25. Jane Addams, *Twenty Years at Hull-House with Autobiographical Notes* (New York: Macmillan, 1911), 46.

26. Dr. C. H. Hughes, "The Opium Psycho-Neurosis—Chronic Meconism or Papaverism," *Alienist and Neurologist* 5 (1884), 137.

27. Virginia Berridge and Griffith Edwards, *Opium and the People: Opiate Use in Nineteenth-Century England* (New Haven, Conn.: Yale University Press, 1987), 53.

28. Richard Mead, *A Mechanical Account of Poisons in Several Essays* (London: Ralph Smith, 1708), 137–54.

29. John Awsiter, *An Essay on the Effects of Opium. Considered as a Poison* (London: G. Kearsly, 1763), 5. Emphasis in original.

30. George Young, M.D., *A Treatise on Opium, Founded Upon Practical Observations* (London: Printed for A. Millar, 1753), iii–vi.

31. "The Opium Eater," *New-England Magazine* (March 1833), 217–29. Whittier acknowledged his authorship in John B. Pickard, "John Greenleaf Whittier and Mary Emerson Smith," *American Literature* 38 (January 1967), 497.

32. William Blair, "An Opium-Eater in America," *Knickerbocker* 20, no. 1 (July 1842), 47–57.

33. William W. Smithers, *The Life of John Lofland, "The Milford Bard"* (Philadelphia: Wallace M. Leonard, 1894), 122.

34. Jill Jonnes, *Hep-Cats, Narcs, and Pipe Dreams: A History of America's Romance with Illegal Drugs* (Baltimore: Johns Hopkins University Press, 1999), 212.

35. "Literary Notices: The Hasheesh-Eater," *Knickerbocker* 51 (February 1858), 197–98.

36. "Slaves to Opium: Increase of the Vice in California," *Zion's Herald* 58, no. 29 (July 21, 1881), 227.

37. William Rosser Cobbe, *Doctor Judas: A Portrayal of the Opium Habit* (Chicago: S. C. Griggs and Company, 1895), 12.

38. "Confessions of an English Opium-Eater," *Christian Examiner* (November 1841), 274.

39. Peter Melville Logan, *Nerves and Narratives: A Cultural History of Hysteria in Nineteenth-Century British Prose* (Berkeley: University of California Press, 1997), 89.

40. Berridge and Edwards, *Opium and the People*, 53.

41. "Opium," *Inter Ocean* [Chicago, Ill.], August 17, 1874, p. 4.

42. H. T. Tuckerman, "Something About Wine," *Knickerbocker* 52 (August 1858), 151–52.

43. De Quincey, *Confessions*, 4, 2.

44. The Rev. J. Townley Crane, "Drugs as an Indulgence," *Methodist Quarterly Review* 10 (October 1858), 564.

45. "Psychology of Opium and Hasheesh: Opium," *Dial* (September 1860), 564.

46. "Thomas de Quincey," *Saturday Evening Post* 57 (July 28, 1877), 4.

47. Martin Booth, *Opium* (New York: St. Martin's Griffin, 1996), 36.

48. Quoted in Althea Hayter, *Opium and the Romantic Imagination* (Berkeley: University of California Press, 1968), 215–16; Elisabeth Schneider, *Coleridge, Opium and Kubla Khan* (Chicago: University of Chicago Press, 1953), 23; Samuel Taylor Coleridge, "Kubla Khan, or a Vision in a Dream," lines 1–4.

49. Berridge and Edwards, *Opium and the People*, 50.

50. Hayter, *Opium and the Romantic Imagination*, 297.

51. Julia Ward Howe, *Words for the Hour* (Boston: Ticknor and Fields, 1857), 145, 146.

52. Hayter, *Opium and the Romantic Imagination*, 297.

53. "Psychology of Opium and Hasheesh: Opium," 557.

54. De Quincey, *Confessions*, 60, 61–62.

55. "The Chemistry of Common Life," *Ladies' Repository*, May 1855, 292.

56. [Cheever], "Narcotics," 386, 396.

57. Chandra Ford and Nina T. Harawa, "A New Conceptualization of Ethnicity for Social Epidemiologic and Health Equity Research," *Social Science & Medicine* 71, no. 2 (July 2010), 251–58.

58. Norman E. Zinberg, *Drug, Set, and Setting: The Basis for Controlled Intoxicant Use* (New Haven, Conn.: Yale University Press, c.1984).

59. Morrison, "De Quincey's Addiction," 274.

60. "Thomas de Quincey," *Yale Literary Magazine*, 225.

61. K., "Literary Notices," *Universalist Quarterly*, 322.

62. "Mr. Cottle and His Friends," *Harper's New Monthly Magazine* 8, no. 43 (December 1853), 74–75.
63. E.g., "Thomas de Quincey and His Works," *Graham's Magazine* 45, no. 3 (September 1854), 272–84; "Thomas De Quincey and His Works," *Eclectic Magazine of Foreign Literature, Science, and Art* (July 1854), 289.
64. Mrs. Ellen M. Mitchell, "Thomas De Quincey," *Arthur's Illustrated Home Magazine* 45, no. 4 (April 1877), 185.
65. Paul Youngquist, "Rehabilitating Coleridge: Poetry, Philosophy, Excess," *ELH* 66 (Winter 1999), 885, 903, 887.
66. "Editor's Table," *Southern Literary Messenger* 30, no. 1 (January 1860), 77.
67. "Thomas de Quincey," *Saturday Evening Post* 57 (July 28, 1877), 4.
68. "Literary Notices," *National Era*, April 7, 1853.
69. "Editor's Table," 77.
70. S. Ryan Johansson, "Medics, Monarchs and Mortality, 1600–1800: Origins of the Knowledge-Driven Health Transition in Europe," University of Oxford, Discussion Papers in Economic and Social History 85 (October 2010), 1.
71. "Reminiscences of Coleridge," *North American Review* 65 (October 1847), 402, 440; David Masson, *De Quincey* (New York: Harper and Brothers, 1882), 133.
72. "On the Influence of Opium-eating on Health and Longevity," *American Journal of the Medical Sciences* 10 (May 1832), 252–54; G. G. Sigmond, "Influence of Opium Eating on Health and Longevity," *American Journal of the Medical Sciences* (February 1838), 523; Davenport-Hines, *Pursuit of Oblivion*, 66–68; J. W. Dickson, W. H. Dunbar, et al., *The Scottish Jurist* (Edinburgh: Michael Anderson, 1832), IV: 386; R. P., "Christison on Poisons," *Transylvania Journal of Medicine and the Associate Sciences* 8 (1836), 549.
73. "On the influence of Opium-eating on Health and Longevity," 252–54; Sigmond, "Influence of Opium Eating on Health and Longevity," 523; Davenport-Hines, *Pursuit of Oblivion*, 66–68, 567; Dickson et al., *Scottish Jurist*, IV: 386.
74. R. H. Semple, Esq., "Lecture on Vegetable Poisons," *Pharmaceutical Journal* 2, no. 7 (January 1, 1843), 438.
75. De Quincey, *Confessions*, 54, 55, xii.
76. De Quincey, *Confessions*, 56.
77. Howard Padwa, *Social Poison: The Culture and Politics of Opiate Control in Britain and France, 1821–1926* (Baltimore: Johns Hopkins University Press, 2012), 26.
78. "Taking Laudanum," *Journal of Health* 1 (February 10, 1830), 161–62.
79. Calkins, *Opium and the Opium-Appetite*, 281. Emphasis in original.
80. Richard Holmes, *Coleridge: Early Visions, 1772–1804* (New York: Pantheon Books, 1989), 111, 127; James Dykes Campbell, *Samuel Taylor Coleridge: A Narrative of the Events of His Life* (London: Macmillan and Co., 1896), 123.
81. Youngquist, "Rehabilitating Coleridge," 888–89.
82. Louise Foxcroft, *The Making of Addiction: The 'Use and Abuse' of Opium in Nineteenth-Century Britain* (Routledge, 2007), 30–31; Youngquist, "Rehabilitating Coleridge," 890; Holmes, *Coleridge: Early Visions, 1772–1804*, 111, 127, 337; Campbell, *Samuel Taylor Coleridge*, 123; Robert Morrison, "Opium-Eaters and Magazine Wars: De Quincey and Coleridge in 1821," *Victorian Periodicals Review* 30 (Spring 1997), 28.
83. Earl Leslie Griggs and Seymour Teulon Porter, "Samuel Taylor Coleridge and Opium," *Huntington Library Quarterly* 17, no. 4 (August 1954), 368, 364, 365.
84. M. C. Cooke, *The Seven Sisters of Sleep: Popular History of the Seven Prevailing Narcotics of the World* (London: James Blackwood, 1860), 147–48.
85. Youngquist, "Rehabilitating Coleridge," 903.
86. "Mr. Cottle and His Friends," 74–75; "Literary: Samuel Taylor Coleridge," *New-York Daily Times* (June 4, 1853), 2.
87. Quoted in Youngquist, "Rehabilitating Coleridge," 905, and Molly Lefebure, *Samuel Taylor Coleridge: A Bondage of Opium* (Stein and Day, 1974), 40. Emphasis in original.
88. "Mr. Cottle and His Friends," 73.
89. "Reminiscences of Coleridge," 401. Emphasis in original.
90. "Review of New Books," *Graham's Magazine* 31, no. 5 (November 1847), 274–75.

91. "Mr. Cottle and His Friends," 74–75.
92. "Coleridge," *Princeton Review* 20, no. 2 (April 1848), 155–56.
93. Lefebure, *Samuel Taylor Coleridge: A Bondage of Opium*, 49.
94. "Life and Writings of Coleridge," *American Review* (November 1849), 534.
95. De Quincey, *Confessions*, 3, 1.
96. Tobias Smollett, *The Miscellaneous Works of Tobias Smollett, M. D.* (Edinburgh: Mundell, Doig and Stevenson, 1806), III: 358.
97. De Quincey, *Confessions*, 61.
98. Davenport-Hines, *Pursuit of Oblivion*, 68.
99. De Quincey, *Confessions*, 72, 75.
100. Berridge and Edwards, *Opium and the People*, 52–53.
101. K., "Literary Notices: The Complete Works of Samuel Taylor Coleridge," *Universalist Quarterly and General Review* 10 (July 1853), 322.
102. "Thomas De Quincey," *Harper's New Monthly Magazine*, July 1850, 149.
103. De Quincey, *Confessions*, 74–75, 88, 89.
104. Morrison, "De Quincey's Addiction," 271.
105. "Cure of an Opium-Eater," *New-York Mirror* 12 (December 6, 1834), 178.
106. Kristina Aikens, "A Pharmacy of Her Own: Victorian Women and the Figure of the Opiate" (PhD diss., Tufts University, 2008), 8; Berridge and Edwards, *Opium and the People*, 35–36, 44, 144–45.
107. Sally G. McMillen, *Motherhood in the Old South: Pregnancy, Childbirth, and Infant Rearing* (Baton Rouge: Louisiana State University Press, 1990), 176.
108. Keith Humphreys, "Thomas de Quincey, Confessions of an English Opium Eater," *Addiction* 99, no. 9 (September 2004), 1221–22.

## Chapter 6

1. [David W. Cheever], "Narcotics," *North American Review* 95, no. 197 (October 1862), 393.
2. [Cheever], "Narcotics," 395–96.
3. Keith McMahon, *The Fall of the God of Money: Opium Smoking in Nineteenth-Century China* (Lanham, Md.: Rowman and Littlefield, 2002), 33, 35.
4. Jerry Wylie and Richard E. Fike, "Chinese Opium Smoking Techniques and Paraphernalia," in Priscilla Wegars, ed., *Hidden Heritage: Historical Archaeology of the Overseas Chinese* (Amityville, N. Y.: Baywood, c. 1993), 259.
5. Mrs. Henrietta Shuck, *Scenes in China: or, Sketches of the Country, Religion, and Customs, of the Chinese* (Philadelphia: American Baptist Publication Society, 1852), 148–51. Emphases in original.
6. Stephen A. Siegel, "Francis Wharton's Orthodoxy: God, Historical Jurisprudence, and Classical Legal Thought," *American Journal of Legal History* 46, no. 4 (October 2004), 423; Francis Wharton, "China and the Chinese Peace," *Hunt's Merchants' Magazine* (March 1843), 206.
7. H. H. Kane, M.D., "American Opium-Smokers," *Harper's Weekly* (September 24, 1881), 646; H. H. Kane, M.D., *Opium-Smoking in America and China* (New York: G. P. Putnam's Sons, 1882), 15.
8. Stewart Culin, "Opium Smoking by the Chinese in Philadelphia," *American Journal of Pharmacy* (October 1891), 498.
9. Leslie E. Keeley, *The Morphine Eater: Or, From Bondage to Freedom* (Dwight, Ill.: C. L. Palmer and Co., 1881), 175.
10. Diana Lynn Ahmad, "'Caves of Oblivion': Opium Dens and Exclusion Laws, 1850–1882" (PhD diss., University of Missouri-Columbia, 1997), 72.
11. Kane, "American Opium-Smokers," 646; "Society Proceedings," *Medical Gazette* (January 21, 1882), 28; Kane, *Opium-Smoking in America and China*, 90; Culin, "Opium Smoking by the Chinese in Philadelphia," 501.
12. "The Chinese Opium Pipe as a Therapeutic Agent," *Quarterly Epitome of American Practical Medicine and Surgery . . .* 9 (March 1882), 5; H. Kalant, "Opium Revisited: A Brief Review of Its Nature, Composition, Non-Medical Use and Relative Risks," *Addiction* 92, no. 3 (1997),

270–72; Keith McMahon, "Opium Smoking and Modern Subjectivity," *Postcolonial Studies* 8, no. 2 (May 2005), 166.

13. Carl Trocki, *Opium, Empire and the Global Political Economy: A Study of the Asian Opium Trade 1750–1950* (London: Routledge, 1999), 37.

14. R. K. Newman, "Opium Smoking in Late Imperial China: A Reconsideration," *Modern Asian Studies* 29, no. 4 (October 1995), 786, 781.

15. Frank Dikötter, Lars Laamann, and Zhou Xun, "Narcotic Culture: A Social History of Drug Consumption in China," *British Journal of Criminology* 42, no. 2 (Spring 2002), 324.

16. Kalant, "Opium Revisited," 272.

17. Richard Davenport-Hines, *The Pursuit of Oblivion: A Global History of Narcotics* (New York: W. W. Norton, 2002), 45–46.

18. James Windle, "How the East Influenced Drug Prohibition," *International History Review* 35, no. 5 (2013), 1191.

19. A. C. Sahu, "Genesis and Growth of Indo-Chinese Opium Monopoly under East India Company," *Journal of Indian History* 57, no. 1 (April 1979), 163; Davenport-Hines, *Pursuit of Oblivion*, 48; Lukasz Kamieński, *Shooting Up: A Short History of Drugs and War* (Oxford: Oxford University Press, 2016), 60.

20. Windle, "How the East Influenced Drug Prohibition," 1191.

21. Peter Ward Fay, *The Opium War, 1840–1842: Barbarians in the Celestial Empire in the Early Part of the Nineteenth Century and the War by Which They Forced Her Gates Ajar* (Chapel Hill: University of North Carolina Press, 1998), 17, 55; Diana S. Kim, *Empires of Vice: The Rise of Opium Prohibition Across Southeast Asia* (Princeton, N. J.: Princeton University Press, 2020), 31–32; Kamieński, *Shooting Up*, 60.

22. Davenport-Hines, *Pursuit of Oblivion*, 48.

23. Martin Booth, *Opium* (New York: St. Martin's Griffin, 1996), 111–12.

24. Michael Greenberg, *British Trade and the Opening of China 1800–42* (Cambridge: Cambridge University Press, 1969), 104. Emphasis in original.

25. Thomas N. Layton, *The Voyage of the "Frolic": New England Merchants and the Opium Trade* (Stanford, Calif.: Stanford University Press, 1997), 29; "Monthly Commercial Chronicle," *Hunt's Merchants' Magazine* 12 (January 1845), 74; Windle, "How the East Influenced Drug Prohibition," 1191.

26. Greenberg, *British Trade and the Opening of China*, 50.

27. Ibrahim Ihsan Poroy, "Expansion of Opium Production in Turkey and the State Monopoly of 1828–1839," *International Journal of Middle East Studies* 13, no. 2 (May 1981), 191.

28. E. W. Stoughton, "The Opium Trade—England and China," *Hunt's Merchants' Magazine* 2 (May 1840), 402.

29. Virginia Berridge, *Demons: Our Changing Attitudes to Alcohol, Tobacco and Drugs* (Oxford: Oxford University Press, 2013), 122; McMahon, *Fall of the God of Money*, 12, 98.

30. Frank Dikötter, Lars Laamann, and Zhou Xun, *Narcotic Culture: A History of Drugs in China* (Chicago: University of Chicago Press, 2004), 44–45.

31. Kane, *Opium-Smoking in America and China*, 117. Emphases in original.

32. Charles C. Stelle, "American Trade in Opium to China, Prior to 1820," *Pacific Historical Review* (December 1940), 425.

33. John K. Fairbank, "America and China: The Mid-Nineteenth Century," in Ernest R. May and James C. Thomson Jr., eds., *American-East Asian Relations: A Survey* (Cambridge, Mass.: Harvard University Press, 1972), 24.

34. Stelle, "American Trade in Opium to China, Prior to 1820," 442.

35. I explore domestic reactions to Americans' role in the opium trade in E. K. Gray, "The Trade-Off: Chinese Opium Traders and Antebellum Reform in the United States, 1815–1860," in James H. Mills and Patricia Barton, eds., *Drugs and Empires: Essays in Modern Imperialism and Intoxication, c. 1500–c. 1930* (Basingstoke, UK: Palgrave Macmillan, 2007), 220–42.

36. *The Journals of Major Samuel Shaw* (Boston: Wm. Crosby and H. P. Nichols, 1847), 238, 265.

37. Quoted in Jonathan Goldstein, *Philadelphia and the China Trade, 1682–1846: Commercial, Cultural, and Attitudinal Effects* (University Park: Pennsylvania State University Press, 1978), 52.

38. Perkins and Co. letter, Canton, August 7, 1819. Thomas Handasyd Perkins Papers, P-334, 17 reels, Massachusetts Historical Society. Emphasis in original.

39. Jacques M. Downs, "American Merchants and the China Opium Trade, 1800–1840," *Business History Review* 42, no. 4 (Winter 1968), 428–29.

40. Quoted in Jonathan Goldstein, "A Clash of Civilizations in the Pearl River Delta: Stephen Girard's Trade with China, 1787–1824," in Paul A. Van Dyke, ed., *Americans and Macao: Trade, Smuggling, and Diplomacy on the South China Coast* (Hong Kong: Hong Kong University Press, 2012), 22.

41. Fay, *The Opium War*, 45.

42. Geoffrey C. Ward and Frederic Delano Grant Jr., "'A Fair, Honorable, and Legitimate Trade,'" *American Heritage* 37, no. 5 (August–September 1986), 54.

43. *Letters from China: The Canton-Boston Correspondence of Robert Bennet Forbes, 1838–1840*, ed. Phyllis Forbes Kerr (Mystic, Conn.: Mystic Seaport Museum, c. 1996), 101.

44. Jacques M. Downs, "Fair Game: Exploitive Role-Myths and the American Opium Trade," *Pacific Historical Review* 41, no. 2 (May 1972), 133–34, 143.

45. Layton, *Voyage of the "Frolic,"* 30.

46. Jacques M. Downs, *The Golden Ghetto: The American Commercial Community at Canton and the Shaping of American China Policy, 1784–1844* (Bethlehem, Pa: Lehigh University Press, 1997), 134.

47. Zhen Zou, "'Smoke Gets in Your Eyes': American Writers on the Opium Issue in China, 1840–1860" (PhD diss., Purdue University, 2006), 175, 178–79.

48. Steffen Rimner, *Opium's Long Shadow: From Asian Revolt to Global Drug Control* (Cambridge, Mass.: Harvard University Press, 2018), 26.

49. Fay, *The Opium War*, 195.

50. Mao Haijian, *The Qing Empire and the Opium War* (Cambridge: Cambridge University Press, 2018), 105.

51. Trocki, *Opium, Empire and the Global Political Economy*, 97–100; Michael C. Lazich, "American Missionaries and the Opium Trade in Nineteenth-Century China," *Journal of World History* 17, no. 2 (June 2006), 211–14.

52. Windle, "How the East Influenced Drug Prohibition," 1191–92.

53. Wm. B. Diver, "Facts Concerning the Opium Trade," *Christian Observer* 21, no. 10 (March 11, 1842), 38.

54. P. E. Caquet, "Notions of Addiction in the Time of the First Opium War," *Historical Journal* 58, no. 4 (2015), 1019.

55. Robert B. Forbes, *Personal Reminiscences* (Boston: Little, Brown, 1882), 144.

56. Ward and Grant, "'A Fair, Honorable, and Legitimate Trade,'" 55–56.

57. Henry Blaney, *Journal of Voyages to China and Return* (Boston: Privately printed, 1913), 57.

58. H. L., "Evils of Opium in South-Eastern Asia," *Episcopal Recorder* 12, no. 24 (September 13, 1834), 97.

59. John Upton Terrell, *Furs by Astor* (New York: William Morrow, 1963), 292; Carl Seaburg and Stanley Paterson, *Merchant Prince of Boston: Colonel T. H. Perkins, 1764–1854* (Cambridge, Mass.: Harvard University Press, 1971), 372; 26th Congress, 1st sess., Doc. No. 40.

60. Ward and Grant, "'A Fair, Honorable, and Legitimate Trade,'" 52; Fay, *The Opium War*, 84; Robert Charles, "Olyphant and Opium: A Canton Merchant Who 'Just Said "No,"'" *International Bulletin of Missionary Research* 16, no. 2 (April 1, 1992), 67.

61. Richard Harvey Brown, "The Opium Trade and Opium Policies in India, China, Britain, and the United States: Historical Comparisons and Theoretical Interpretations," *Asian Journal of Social Science* 30 (2002), 629.

62. Stelle, "American Trade in Opium to China, Prior to 1820," 436.

63. "Commerce and the Opium Trade at Hong Kong," *Hunt's Merchants' Magazine* 16, no. 1 (January 1847), 122.

64. "Miscellany: Opium Smuggling," *American Journal of Pharmacy* 14 (January 1848), 76–78.

65. Geo. Francis Train, *An American Merchant in Europe, Asia, and Australia . . .* (New York: G. P. Putnam and Co., 1857), 161, 162.

66. [William S. W. Ruschenberger], "Notes and Commentaries, on a Voyage to China: Chapter XXV," *Southern Literary Messenger* 19 (November 1853), 687.

67. E.g., Elizabeth Kelly Gray, "'Whisper to Him the Word "India"': Trans-Atlantic Critics and American Slavery, 1830–1860," *Journal of the Early Republic* 27, no. 3 (Fall 2008): 379–406.

68. "Other Societies," *Baptist Missionary Magazine* 21, no. 2 (February 1841), 52.

69. Zou, "'Smoke Gets in Your Eyes,'" 91.

70. "England and China," *United States Magazine and Democratic Review* 7, no. 30 (June 1840), 516.

71. Reprinted in "Late and Important from China," *Tioga Eagle* [Wellsboro, Pa.] (March 25, 1840), 3.

72. "A Day's Death Record," *New-York Times*, January 8, 1882, p. 7; Stoughton, "The Opium Trade—England and China," 406, 391.

73. "England and China," *Boston Recorder* 25, no. 28 (July 10, 1840), 110.

74. "The Opium War, and Its Justice," *Christian Examiner*, May 1841, 228–29.

75. Henry M. Field, D. D., *From Egypt to Japan* (New York: Scribner, Armstrong and Co., 1877), 390.

76. W., "The Destruction of Opium in Canton," *Monthly Miscellany* 2, no. 1 (January 1840), 37.

77. Nathan Allen, *An Essay on the Opium Trade* (Boston, 1850), 51.

78. A Chinese Missionary, "The Opium Trade in the East," *National Magazine*, January 1855, 41.

79. A Chinese Missionary, "The Opium Trade in the East," *National Magazine*, May 1855, 434–35, 438.

80. Howard Malcom, *Travels in South-Eastern Asia* (Boston: Gould, Kendall, and Lincoln, 1839), II: 160; Allen, *Essay on the Opium Trade*, 61.

81. N. A., "Slavery and the Opium Trade," *New-York Observer* 31, no. 12 (March 24, 1853), 93. Emphasis in original.

82. *Speeches of John C. Calhoun* (New-York: Harper and Brothers, 1843), 389.

83. Alastair Su, "'The Cause of Human Freedom': John Quincy Adams and the Problem of Opium in the Age of Emancipation," *Journal of the Early Republic* 40, no. 3 (Fall 2020), 467.

84. "New-Haven, June 21," *New-Haven Gazette and the Connecticut Magazine*, June 21, 1787, 142.

85. "England and China," *United States Magazine*, 528.

86. B. E., "Chinese Materia Medica," *Journal of the Philadelphia College of Pharmacy* 1, no. 2 (July 1829), 150, 151.

87. "China," *Advocate of Peace* 3, no. 4 (December 1839), 81; Harry F. Lee and David D. Zhang, "A Tale of Two Population Crises in Recent Chinese History," *Climatic Change* 116 (2013), 285–308, https://doi.org/10.1007/s10584-012-0490-9.

88. "The Opium War, and Its Justice," 227.

89. "Opium Smoking in China," *Boston Medical and Surgical Journal* 26, no. 16 (May 25, 1842), 247; Lisa Sturm-Lind, *Actors of Globalization: New York Merchants in Global Trade, 1784–1812* (Leiden: Brill, 2018), 64.

90. "Habitual Use of Opium," *American Journal of the Medical Sciences* 20 (October 1850), 499.

91. "The Opium Trade," *Evangelist* 32, no. 35 (August 28, 1862), 1.

92. "Notes and Notices," *Godey's Lady's Book* 82, no. 489 (March 1871), 288.

93. "The Opium Trade," *Gleason's Pictorial* 5 (October 22, 1853), 272.

94. [Cheever], "Narcotics," 395.

95. McMahon, *Fall of the God of Money*, 106, 197.

96. McMahon, *Fall of the God of Money*, 207, 204, 197, 198.

97. McMahon, *Fall of the God of Money*, 205–7, 198.

98. McMahon, *Fall of the God of Money*, 212–13.

99. McMahon, *Fall of the God of Money*, 109, 200–201, 209, 204.

100. Francis Wharton, "East India, and the Opium Trade," *Hunt's Merchants' Magazine* 4, no. 1 (January 1841), 9.

101. Stoughton, "The Opium Trade—England and China," 389.

102. "Speech of Mr. Miller, of N. Jersey, on the Expediency of Recognizing the Independence of Liberia," *Frederick Douglass' Paper* [Rochester, N. Y.], March 25, 1853, p. 1.

103. Allen, *Essay on the Opium Trade*, 49.

104. Dr. Ely, "China in One Thousand Eight Hundred and Fifty-Three," *De Bow's Review* 14, no. 4 (April 1853), 360.

105. David Courtwright, *Dark Paradise: A History of Opiate Addiction in America* (Cambridge, Mass.: Harvard University Press, 2001), 65.

106. Stuart Creighton Miller, *The Unwelcome Immigrant: The American Image of the Chinese, 1785–1882* (Berkeley: University of California Press, 1969), 148, 11.

107. Hyungju Hur, "Staging Modern Statehood: World Exhibitions and the Rhetoric of Publishing in Late Qing China, 1851–1910" (PhD diss., University of Illinois, 2012), 100.

## Chapter 7

1. [David W. Cheever], "Narcotics," *North American Review* 95, no. 197 (October 1862), 375, 384.

2. David T. Courtwright, *Dark Paradise: A History of Opiate Addiction in America* (Cambridge, Mass.: Harvard University Press, 2001), 20.

3. Diana L. Ahmad, *The Opium Debate and Chinese Exclusion Laws in the Nineteenth-Century American West* (Reno: University of Nevada Press, 2007), 32.

4. Barbara Berglund, "Chinatown's Tourist Terrain: Representation and Racialization in Nineteenth-Century San Francisco," *American Studies* 46, no. 2 (Summer 2005), 9–10.

5. Samuel Williams, *The City of the Golden Gate: A Description of San Francisco in 1875* (San Francisco: Book Club of California, 1921), 39–41.

6. "The City of the Golden Gate," *Scribner's Monthly* 10, no. 3 (July 1875), 281–84; "The City of the Golden Gate," *Holton* [Kan.] *Recorder and Express,* July 8, 1875, p. 3; Berglund, "Chinatown's Tourist Terrain," 6.

7. Diana L. Ahmad, "To Preserve Moral Virtue: Opium Smoking in Nevada and the Pressure for Chinese Exclusion," *Nevada Historical Society Quarterly* 41, no. 3 (September 1998), 141–43; Martin Booth, *Opium* (New York: St. Martin's Griffin, 1996), 175; Hsin-Yun Ou, "Chinese Ethnicity and the American Heroic Artisan in Henry Grimm's *The Chinese Must Go* (1879)," *Comparative Drama* 44, no. 1 (2010), 68.

8. Lisa Lowe, *The Intimacies of Four Continents* (Durham, N. C.: Duke University Press, 2015), 98.

9. Ronald Takaki, *Iron Cages: Race and Culture in 19th-Century America* (Oxford: Oxford University Press, 2000), 216.

10. Sucheng Chan, "The Exclusion of Chinese Women, 1870–1943," in Sucheng Chan, ed., *Entry Denied: Exclusion and the Chinese Community in America, 1882–1943* (Philadelphia: Temple University Press, 1994), 94–95.

11. Lenore Metrick-Chen, *Collecting Objects/Excluding People: Chinese Subjects and American Visual Culture, 1830–1900* (Albany: State University of New York Press, 2012), 25.

12. Stephen E. Ambrose, *Nothing Like It in the World: The Men Who Built the Transcontinental Railroad, 1863–1869* (New York: Simon and Schuster, 2000), 149.

13. Edwin L. Sabin, *Building the Pacific Railway* (Philadelphia: J. B. Lippincott, 1919), 111.

14. Sharon Lowe, "Behind the Soothing Mist: Women and Opiate Use in the Mining West, 1860–1900" (PhD diss., Union Institute and University, 2006), 40.

15. Aaron H. Palmer, *Memoir, Geographical, Political, and Commercial, on the Present state, productive resources, and capabilities for commerce, of Siberia, Manchuria, and the Asiatic islands of the Northern Pacific ocean; and on the importance of opening commercial intercourse with those countries, &c.* Senate, 30th Congress, 1st Session, Miscellaneous No. 80 ([Washington, D. C.]: 1848), 60.

16. Ou, "Chinese Ethnicity and the American Heroic Artisan," 78.

17. [Thomas J. Vivian], "John Chinaman in San Francisco," *Scribner's Monthly* 12, no. 6 (October 1876), 872.

18. Stuart Creighton Miller, *The Unwelcome Immigrant: The American Image of the Chinese, 1785–1882* (Berkeley: University of California Press, 1969), 197–98.

19. Ou, "Chinese Ethnicity and the American Heroic Artisan," 70, 64–65.

20. Wong Chin Foo, "The Chinese in New York," *Cosmopolitan* 5, no. 4 (June 1888), 309; "How Opium Is Smoked," *Christian Recorder* 13, no. 41 (October 14, 1875), 7.

21. Thomas Byrnes, *Professional Criminals of America* (New York: Cassell and Company, 1886), 383, preface.

22. David T. Courtwright, *Forces of Habit: Drugs and the Making of the Modern World* (Cambridge, Mass.: Harvard University Press, 2001), 35.

23. Booth, *Opium*, 177.

24. Williams, *The City of the Golden Gate*, 36.

25. George H. Fitch, "A Night in Chinatown," *Cosmopolitan* 2, no. 6 (February 1887), 358.

26. "Opium Smokers," *Saturday Evening Post* 55, no. 9 (September 25, 1875), 7.

27. John L. Fagan, "The Chinese Cannery Workers of Warrendale, Oregon, 1876–1930," in Priscilla Wegars, ed., *Hidden Heritage: Historical Archaeology of the Overseas Chinese* (Amityville, N. Y.: Baywood, c. 1993), 226.

28. Mrs. E. V. Robbins, "Chinese Slave Girls: A Bit of History," *Overland Monthly* 1, no. 1 (January 1908), 100.

29. Loren B. Chan, "The Chinese in Nevada: An Historical Survey, 1856–1970," in Arif Dirlik, ed., *Chinese on the American Frontier* (Lanham, Md.: Rowman and Littlefield, 2001), 107.

30. Ahmad, *The Opium Debate and Chinese Exclusion Laws*, 1.

31. Quoted in Lowe, "Behind the Soothing Mist," 47.

32. Ambrose, *Nothing Like It in the World*, 150.

33. Diana Lynn Ahmad, "'Caves of Oblivion': Opium Dens and Exclusion Laws, 1850–1882" (PhD diss., University of Missouri-Columbia, 1997), 44–45.

34. [Stephen Crane], "Opium's Varied Dreams," [New York] *Sun*, May 17, 1896.

35. Lowe, "Behind the Soothing Mist," 255.

36. Courtwright, *Dark Paradise*, 67.

37. Grace Greenwood, "The Chinese in San Francisco," *Youth's Companion* 46, no. 30 (July 24, 1873), 236.

38. Mrs. Frank Leslie, *California: A Pleasure Trip from Gotham to the Golden Gate* (New York: G. W. Carleton, 1877), 159.

39. "The Chinese Opium Pipe as a Therapeutic Agent," *Quarterly Epitome of American Practical Medicine and Surgery . . .* 9 (March 1882), 5; H. Kalant, "Opium Revisited: A Brief Review of Its Nature, Composition, Non-Medical Use and Relative Risks," *Addiction* 92, no. 3 (1997), 272; Carl Trocki, *Opium, Empire and the Global Political Economy: A Study of the Asian Opium Trade 1750–1950* (London: Routledge, 1999), 37.

40. H. H. Kane, "American Opium-Smokers," *Harper's Weekly* (September 24, 1881), 646; "The Chinamen," *Massachusetts Ploughman* 45 (August 14, 1886), 3.

41. Lee Meriwether, "The 'Labor Question' on the Pacific Coast," *Harper's Weekly* (October 13, 1888), 778–79.

42. Mark Twain, *Roughing It* (New York: Penguin Books, 1985), 395.

43. "How Opium Is Smoked," *Saturday Evening Post* 55, no. 10 (October 2, 1875), 7.

44. Frederick J. Masters, "The Opium Traffic in California," *Chautauquan* 24, no. 1 (October 1896), 54.

45. "The Chinamen," 3; "Opium Eating in Chicago," *St. Louis Post-Dispatch* (September 17, 1880), 2; Helen H. Jun, "Black Orientalism: Nineteenth-Century Narratives of Race and U.S. Citizenship," *American Quarterly* 58, no. 4 (December 2006), 1052; Arnold Shankman, "Black on Yellow: Afro-Americans View Chinese-Americans, 1850–1935," *Phylon* 39, no. 1 (Spring 1978), 10.

46. Allen S. Williams, *The Demon of the Orient, and His Satellite Fiends of the Joints* (New York: The Author, 1883), 16–18. Emphasis in original.

47. "Demoniacal Dens," *River Press* [Fort Benton, Mont.], January 19, 1881, p. 8.

48. H. H. Kane, M. D., *Opium-Smoking in America and China* (New York: G. P. Putnam's Sons, 1882), 54–56.

49. David T. Courtwright, "Opiate Addiction in the American West, 1850–1920," *Journal of the West* 21, no. 3 (July 1982), 26.

50. Huping Ling, "'Hop Alley': Myth and Reality of the St. Louis Chinatown, 1860s–1930s," *Journal of Urban History* 28, no. 2 (January 2002), 186.

51. Kane, *Opium-Smoking in America and China*, 5; Timothy J. Gilfoyle, *A Pickpocket's Tale: The Underworld of Nineteenth-Century New York* (New York: W. W. Norton, 2006), 83.

52. Ahmad, *The Opium Debate and Chinese Exclusion Laws*, 31.

53. "Chinese in New-York: How They Live, and Where," *New-York Times* (December 26, 1873), 3.

54. Wong, "The Chinese in New York," 311.
55. Rev. O. [Otis] Gibson, A. M., *The Chinese in America* (Cincinnati: Hitchcock and Walden, 1877), 42.
56. Allan Forman, "Celestial Gotham," *Arena* 7, no. 41 (April 1893), 626–27.
57. Helen F. Clark, "The Chinese of New York; Contrasted with Their Foreign Neighbors," *Century Magazine* 53, no. 1 (November 1896), 110.
58. "The Silver Lining to an Opium Cloud," *Puck* 17, no. 440 (August 12, 1885), 370.
59. Quoted in James B. Jones Jr., "Selected Aspects of Drug Abuse in Nineteenth- and Early Twentieth-Century Tennessee History, ca. 1830–1920," *West Tennessee Historical Society Papers* 48 (1994), 7.
60. Huping, " 'Hop Alley,' " 200.
61. [Vivian], "John Chinaman in San Francisco," 870.
62. Augustine E. Costello, *Our Police Protectors: History of the New York Police* (New York, 1885), 523.
63. Wong, "The Chinese in New York," 311.
64. Charles H. Brown, "Correspondence. The Opium Habit," *Medical News* 78, no. 11 (March 16, 1901), 433–34; Richard Davenport-Hines, *The Pursuit of Oblivion: A Global History of Narcotics* (New York: W. W. Norton, 2002), 124.
65. Gregory Yee Mark, "Political, Economic and Racial Influences on America's First Drug Laws" (PhD diss., University of California, Berkeley, 1978), 108–9; Masters, "The Opium Traffic in California," 55; Williams, *The Demon of the Orient*, 38.
66. Gilfoyle, *A Pickpocket's Tale*, 87.
67. Courtwright, *Dark Paradise*, 67–68.
68. H. H. Kane, M.D., "The Chinese Opium-Pipe as a Therapeutic Agent," *Medical Record* 20, no. 19 (November 5, 1881), 515; "Opium Smoking as a Therapeutic Means," *Journal of the American Medical Association* (July 26, 1884), 100.
69. Henry G. Cole, *Confessions of an American Opium Eater: From Bondage to Freedom* (Boston: James H. Earle, 1895), 106.
70. William Rosser Cobbe, *Doctor Judas: A Portrayal of the Opium Habit* (Chicago: S. C. Griggs and Company, 1895), 124–25.
71. Timothy A. Hickman, "Drugs and Race in American Culture: Orientalism in the Turn-of-the-Century Discourse of Narcotic Addiction," *American Studies* 41, no. 1 (Spring 2000), 81.
72. Stephen Crane, "Dope Smokers," *Atlanta Constitution*, May 17, 1896, p. 26.
73. Diana L. Ahmad, "Opium Smoking, Anti-Chinese Attitudes, and the American Medical Community, 1850–1890," *American Nineteenth Century History* 1, no. 2 (Summer 2000), 55.
74. Ahmad, *Opium Debate and Chinese Exclusion Laws*, 14.
75. "Topics in the Sagebrush," *New-York Times*, February 21, 1881, p. 1.
76. "Opium 'Joints' in the Black Hills," *Chambers's Journal* 5, no. 250 (October 13, 1888), 654–55.
77. Williams, *Demon of the Orient*, 67.
78. Gilfoyle, *Pickpocket's Tale*, 143.
79. Kane, *Opium-Smoking in America and China*, 70.
80. Williams, *Demon of the Orient*, 60.
81. Will. Brooks, "A Fragment of China," *Californian* 6, no. 31 (July 1882), 9–10.
82. Horace Greeley, *An Overland Journey, from New York to San Francisco, in the Summer of 1859* (New York: C. M. Saxton, Barker and Co., 1860), 288–89.
83. Louis J. Beck, *New York's Chinatown* (New York: Bohemia Publishing Company, 1898), 168.
84. Williams, *Demon of the Orient*, 49.
85. "Ex-Inspector Byrnes Ill," *New York Times*, February 1, 1910, p. 7; Byrnes, *Professional Criminals of America*, 387.
86. Kane, *Opium-Smoking in America and China*, 71–72.
87. Kane, "American Opium-Smokers" (September 24, 1881), 646.
88. W. I. Lincoln Adams, "Flash Light Photography," *Outing* 17, no. 3 (December 1890), 177.
89. W. I. Lincoln Adams, "Flash Light Photography," *Outing* 17, no. 4 (January 1891), 262.
90. Lee Meriwether, "The Labor Question on the Pacific Coast," *Harper's Weekly* (October 13, 1888), 778, quoted in Berglund, "Chinatown's Tourist Terrain," 33–34n19.

91. A Member of the Party, "The Opium Den Pictures—How They Were Taken," *Californian Illustrated Magazine* 1, no. 6 (May 1892), 627–30.
92. [Hamilton Wright], "Opium Problem," Senate, 61st Congress, 2d session, Document No. 377 (ca. 1910), 37.
93. Kane, "American Opium-Smokers" (September 24, 1881), 646–47; H. H. Kane, "American Opium-Smokers," *Harper's Weekly* 25, no. 1294 (October 8, 1881), 682–84.
94. Jacob August Riis, *How the Other Half Lives: Studies Among the Tenements of New York* (New York: Charles Scribner's Sons, 1890), 92.
95. [Vivian], "John Chinaman in San Francisco," 868; Ella Sterling Cummins, *The Story of the Files: A Review of Californian Writers and Literature* (San Francisco: Co-operative Printing Co., 1893), 208.
96. Berglund, "Chinatown's Tourist Terrain," 5–6; Sabine Haenni, "Filming 'Chinatown': Fake Visions, Bodily Transformations," in Peter X. Feng, ed., *Screening Asian Americans* (New Brunswick, N. J.: Rutgers University Press, 2002), 22.
97. Fitch, "A Night in Chinatown," 351, 355, 349.
98. Berglund, "Chinatown's Tourist Terrain," 27.
99. J. Philip Gruen, *Manifest Destinations: Cities and Tourists in the Nineteenth-Century American West* (Norman: University of Oklahoma Press, 2014), 187–88.
100. Rev. O. T. Gifford, "China-Town, San Francisco," *Lebanon* [Pa.] *Daily News*, February 21, 1883, p. 1.
101. Quoted in Joseph Michael Gabriel, "Gods and Monsters: Drugs, Addiction, and the Origins of Narcotic Control in the Nineteenth-Century Urban North" (PhD diss., Rutgers University, 2006), 436.
102. Ahmad, "'Caves of Oblivion,'" iii; Courtwright, *Dark Paradise*, 62–63.
103. [Crane], "Opium's Varied Dreams," 27.
104. Costello, *Our Police Protectors*, 524.
105. Stewart Culin, "Opium Smoking by the Chinese in Philadelphia," *American Journal of Pharmacy* (October 1891), 497–98.
106. "Local Paragraphs," *Memphis Daily Appeal*, May 24, 1879, p. 4; "Local Paragraphs," *Memphis Daily Appeal*, June 17, 1879, p. 4; "Opium Smoking," *Memphis Daily Appeal*, June 28, 1879, p. 4.
107. "The Chinese Curse," *San Francisco Chronicle*, February 9, 1894, p. 10.
108. George W. Walling, *Recollections of a New York Chief of Police* (New York: Caxton Book Concern, 1887), 420.
109. Summarized in "Opium Smoking in Nevada," *New-York Times*, July 29, 1877, p. 10.
110. "A Growing Evil," *San Francisco Chronicle*, July 25, 1881, p. 3.
111. "Philadelphia's Opium Parlor," *New-York Times*, August 29, 1882, p. 2.
112. "Opium Joints," *Massachusetts Ploughman* 42, no. 33 (May 19, 1883), 2.
113. "Opium Joints: How Life Is Dreamed Away in One of Them," *Brooklyn Daily Eagle*, July 8, 1882, p. 1.
114. [Crane], "Opium's Varied Dreams," 27.
115. Gilfoyle, *A Pickpocket's Tale*, 153.
116. "The 'Big Flat' Raided," *New-York Times*, December 8, 1884, p. 2.
117. Leslie E. Keeley, *The Morphine Eater: Or, From Bondage to Freedom* (Dwight, Ill.: C. L. Palmer and Co., 1881), 176.
118. "Topics in the Sagebrush," p. 1.
119. Quoted in Florence C. Lister and Robert H. Lister, "Chinese Sojourners in Territorial Prescott," *Journal of the Southwest* 31, no. 1 (Spring 1989), 39.
120. H. H. Kane, "Opium Smoking: A New Form of the Opium Habit Amongst Americans," *Gaillard's Medical Journal* 33, no. 2 (February 1882), 112.
121. Quoted in Ahmad, *Opium Debate and Chinese Exclusion Laws*, 62.
122. Karen A. Keely, "Sexual Slavery in San Francisco's Chinatown: 'Yellow Peril' and 'White Slavery' in Frank Norris's Early Fiction," *Studies in American Naturalism* 2, no. 2 (Winter 2007), 132.

123. California State Senate, Special Committee on Chinese Immigration, *Chinese Immigration: The Social, Moral, and Political Effect of Chinese Immigration* (Sacramento, Calif.: State Printing Office, 1876), 152.

124. Gabriel, "Gods and Monsters," 409.

125. Wong, "The Chinese in New York," 308.

126. Roland G. Fryer Jr., "Guess Who's Been Coming to Dinner? Trends in Interracial Marriage over the 20th Century," *Journal of Economic Perspectives* 21, no. 2 (Spring 2007), 74.

127. Ahmad, "Opium Smoking, Anti-Chinese Attitudes, and the American Medical Community," 61.

128. [Wright], "Opium Problem," 45; Timothy A. Hickman, *The Secret Leprosy of Modern Days: Narcotic Addiction and Cultural Crisis in the United States, 1870–1920* (Amherst: University of Massachusetts Press, 2007), 104.

129. Courtwright, *Dark Paradise*, 63.

130. Mrs. M. M. Mathews, *Ten Years in Nevada: Or, Life on the Pacific Coast* (Buffalo: Baker, Jones and Co., 1880), 259.

131. Kane, *Opium-Smoking in America and China*, 3.

132. Quoted in *Knoxville Daily Chronicle*, June 22, 1881, p. 2.

133. "Chinese Vices," *Virginia City* [Nev.] *Territorial Enterprise*, April 7, 1877.

134. Quoted in Gregory Yee Mark, "Opium in America and the Chinese," in *Chinese America: History and Perspectives* (Brisbane, Calif.: Fong Brothers, 1997), 61.

135. Williams, *Demon of the Orient*, 42.

136. "Chinese in New-York: How They Live, and Where," *New-York Times*, December 26, 1873, p. 3.

137. "Oriental Vice," *Herald* [Los Angeles, Calif.], June 19, 1897, p. 1.

138. Williams, *Demon of the Orient*, 35.

139. "Mott Street Picketed," *Sun* [New York], May 11, 1883, p. 1.

140. Costello, *Our Police Protectors*, 524.

141. "Victim of a Chinese Opium Den," *Record-Union* [Sacramento, Calif.], June 10, 1886, p. 4; Washington M. Ryer, *The Conflict of Races* (San Francisco: P. J. Thomas, 1886), 56, 3, 80.

142. Jeff Goldberg and Dean Latimer, *Flowers in the Blood: The Story of Opium* (Skyhorse, 2014), 212.

143. Williams, *Demon of the Orient*, 30–31, 44.

144. [Allen S. Williams], "A New Charge," *New-York Times*, May 13, 1883.

145. Scott D. Seligman, *The First Chinese American: The Remarkable Life of Wong Chin Foo* (Hong Kong: University of Hong Kong Press, 2013), 111–12; John Kuo Wei Tchen, "Quimbo Appo's Fear of Fenians: Chinese-Irish-Anglo Relations in New York City," in Ronald H. Bayor and Timothy J. Meagher, eds., *The New York Irish* (Baltimore: Johns Hopkins University Press, 1996), 139–40.

146. Kathleen Auerhahn, "The Split Labor Market and the Origins of Antidrug Legislation in the United States," *Law & Social Inquiry* 24, no. 2 (1999), 414, 415, 417–19, 423–36.

147. "The Opium Dens," *San Francisco Chronicle* (November 16, 1875), p. 3.

148. *The Revised Statutes of Idaho Territory. Enacted at the Fourteenth Session of the Legislative Assembly* (Boise City, Idaho, 1887), 736–37.

149. Ronald Hamowy, "Introduction: Illicit Drugs and Government Control," in Ronald Hamowy, ed., *Dealing with Drugs: Consequences of Government Control* (Lexington, Mass.: D. C. Heath and Company, 1987), 12–13.

150. Marion S. Goldman, *Gold Diggers and Silver Miners: Prostitution and Social Life on the Comstock Lode* (Ann Arbor: University of Michigan Press, c. 1981), 133.

151. *Ex parte Yung Jon*, 28 F. 308 (D. Ore. 1886).

152. Davenport-Hines, *Pursuit of Oblivion*, 127.

153. Ahmad, *Opium Debate and Chinese Exclusion Laws*, 57, 59, 67.

154. "A Growing Evil," p. 3.

155. [Crane], "Opium's Varied Dreams."

156. Wong, "The Chinese in New York," 311.

157. Adelaide Mellier Nevin, *The Social Mirror: A Character Sketch of the Women of Pittsburg and Vicinity* ... (Pittsburgh, Pa.: T. W. Nevin, 1888), 93; Margaret Henderson Floyd, *Architecture*

*After Richardson: Regionalism Before Modernism* (Chicago: University of Chicago Press, 1994), xvii, 149, 347, 350.

158. William L. White, "Addiction as a Disease: Birth of a Concept," *Counselor* 1 (2000), 49.

## Chapter 8

1. [David W. Cheever], "Narcotics," *North American Review* 95, no. 197 (October 1862), 399, 375.
2. [Cheever], "Narcotics," 415.
3. Horace B. Day, *The Opium Habit, with Suggestions as to the Remedy* (Harper & Brothers, 1868), 32–36; Stephen R. Kandall, *Substance and Shadow: Women and Addiction in the United States* (Cambridge, Mass.: Harvard University Press, 1999), 54.
4. "General Facts About the Use of Opium in This Country," *Quarterly Journal of Inebriety* 2, no. 4 (September 1878), 216.
5. [D. W. Nolan], "The Opium Habit," *Catholic World* 33 (September 1881), 835.
6. David T. Courtwright, *Dark Paradise: A History of Opiate Addiction in America* (Cambridge, Mass.: Harvard University Press, 2001), 26–28.
7. H. Wayne Morgan, *Drugs in America: A Social History, 1800–1980* (Syracuse, N. Y.: Syracuse University Press, 1981), 2–3; Timothy A. Hickman, "'Mania Americana': Narcotic Addiction and Modernity in the United States, 1870–1920," *Journal of American History* 90, no. 4 (March 2004), 1276–77, 1270.
8. Jeffrey Clayton Foster, "The Rocky Road to a 'Drug Free Tennessee': A History of the Early Regulation of Cocaine and the Opiates, 1897–1913," *Journal of Social History* 29, no. 3 (Spring 1996), 548.
9. Richard Davenport-Hines, *The Pursuit of Oblivion: A Global History of Narcotics* (New York: W. W. Norton, 2002), 100.
10. Byron Stinson, "The Army Disease," *American History Illustrated* 6, no. 8 (1971), 13; Courtwright, *Dark Paradise*, 46.
11. Courtwright, *Dark Paradise*, 47–51.
12. Henry Gibbons, M.D., *Letheomania: The Result of the Hypodermic Injection of Morphia* (San Francisco: F. Clarke, 1869), 1. Louise M. Darling Biomedical Library, UCLA.
13. Gibbons, *Letheomania*, 1, 2, 4–5.
14. David F. Musto, *The American Disease: Origins of Narcotic Control* (New York: Oxford University Press, 1999), 3.
15. "The Opium Eaters of New York," *New York Herald* (July 14, 1869), 10.
16. Charles C. Cranmer, M.D., and Ed. Reporter, "Correspondence: The Use and Abuse of Opium," *Medical and Surgical Reporter* 33 (November 6, 1875), 378.
17. S. F. McFarland, "Opium Inebriety and the Hypodermic Syringe," *Transactions of the Medical Society of the State of New York for the Year 1877* (Albany, N.Y.: 1877), 289–90.
18. Morgan, *Drugs in America*, 104.
19. Musto, *American Disease*, 4, 9, 5.
20. Courtwright, *Dark Paradise*, 51.
21. "Morphine Drinking," *American Agriculturist* 37, no. 7 (July 1878), 263.
22. Timothy A. Hickman, *The Secret Leprosy of Modern Days: Narcotic Addiction and Cultural Crisis in the United States, 1870–1920* (Amherst: University of Massachusetts Press, 2007), 47.
23. [Fitz Hugh Ludlow], "What Shall They Do to Be Saved?" *Harper's New Monthly Magazine* 35, no. 207 (August 1867), 377–87; James Coulter Layard, "Morphine," *Atlantic Monthly* 33 (June 1874), 697–712.
24. American Association for the Study and Cure of Inebriety, *The Disease of Inebriety from Alcohol, Opium and Other Narcotic Drugs . . .* (New York: E. B. Treat, 1893), v–vi.
25. "Opium," *Old and New* 3, no. 3 (March 1871), 351.
26. "Washington News and Gossip," *Evening Star* [Washington, D. C.], September 10, 1880, p. 1.
27. "Opium-Eating Did It," *Boston Daily Globe*, May 4, 1887, 1.
28. "An Unhappy Household," *New-York Times*, June 18, 1887; Charles J. Rosebault, "The Opium Habit," *Fort Worth Daily Gazette*, July 11, 1887, p. 6.

29. "Remarks on the Opium Habit," *Medical and Surgical Reporter* 37, no. 22 (December 1, 1877), 436.

30. Susan Zieger, "Impostors of Freedom: Southern White Manhood, Hypodermic Morphine, and E. P. Roe's *Without a Home*," *American Literature* 80, no. 3 (September 2008), 527.

31. Edward P. Roe, *Without a Home* (New York: Dodd, Mead, & Company, 1881), 411, 490.

32. Susanne George Bloomfield, "'The Boy's Mother': Nineteenth-Century Drug Dependence in the Life of Kate M. Cleary," *Great Plains Quarterly* 20, no. 1 (Winter 2000), 4.

33. "The Boy's Mother," *Chicago Daily Tribune*, February 8, 1900, p. 7.

34. Old Cap Collier, *Old Tramp, the Hermit Detective; or, Tracking the Opium Smugglers of San Francisco* (New York, 1896); "Hop Lee, the Chinese Slave Dealer; or, Old and Young King Brady and the Opium Fiends," *Secret Service* 13 (April 21, 1899); Chas. E. Blaney, *The King of the Opium Ring* (New York: J. S. Ogilvie Publishing, 1905), 40, 96.

35. Kandall, *Substance and Shadow*, 65.

36. "Our Book Table: The Opium Habit," *Old Guard* 6, no. 11 (November 1868), 876–77.

37. H. H. Kane, "The Opium Habit Among American Women," *Harper's Bazar* 16, no. 43 (October 27, 1883), 673–74.

38. S. T. Morton, "An Experience with Opium," *Popular Science Monthly* (July 1885), 334.

39. Lorine Swainston Goodwin, *The Pure Food, Drink, and Drug Crusaders, 1879–1914* (Jefferson, N. C.: McFarland, 2006), 47.

40. Kandall, *Substance and Shadow*, 2; Caroline Jean Acker, "Take as Directed: The Dilemmas of Regulating Addictive Analgesics and Other Psychoactive Drugs," in Marcia L. Meldrum, ed., *Opioids and Pain Relief: A Historical Perspective* (Seattle: IASP Press, 2003), 38; David F. Musto, "Opium, Cocaine and Marijuana in American History," *Scientific American* 265, no. 1 (July 1991), 40.

41. Goodwin, *Pure Food, Drink, and Drug Crusaders*, 47–48; David Armstrong and Elizabeth Metzger Armstrong, *The Great American Medicine Show* (New York: Prentice Hall, 1991), 163.

42. Hickman, *Secret Leprosy of Modern Days*, 141–42.

43. "Opium-Eating," *Lippincott's Magazine* 1, no. 4 (April 1868), 407.

44. *Opium Eating: An Autobiographical Sketch by an Habituate* (Philadelphia: Claxton, Remsen & Haffelfinger, 1876), 20, 66.

45. "Opium. A 'Fiend' Talks to a Reporter About It," *Stockton Daily Independent*, August 28, 1883.

46. "The Opium Habit," *Medical and Surgical Reporter* 20 (May 8, 1869), 364.

47. Day, *Opium Habit*, 221–22.

48. Henry G. Cole, *Confessions of an American Opium Eater: From Bondage to Freedom* (Boston: James H. Earle, 1895), 168–69.

49. "Periscope: Gangrene Following Morphine Injections," *Medical and Surgical Reporter* 62, no. 12 (March 22, 1890), 346.

50. H. H. Kane, M.D., *Drugs That Enslave: The Opium, Morphine, Chloral and Hashisch Habits* (Philadelphia: Presley Blackiston, 1881), 71, 73.

51. Alonzo Calkins, M.D., *Opium and the Opium-Appetite* (Philadelphia: J. B. Lippincott & Co., 1871), 57–58.

52. Judson B. Andrews, M.D., "Case of Excessive Hypodermic Use of Morphia. Three Hundred Needles Removed from the Body of an Insane Woman," *American Journal of Insanity* 29 (1872), 13–20.

53. Col. D. F. MacMartin, *Thirty Years in Hell: or, The Confessions of a Drug Fiend* (Topeka, Kan.: Capper, 1921), 116.

54. Annie C. Meyers, *Eight Years in Cocaine Hell* (Chicago: St. Luke Society, 1902), 64.

55. "The Opium Fiend," *Montana Standard*, October 9, 1877, p. 1.

56. "A Victim of Morphia," *Chicago Daily Tribune*, August 20, 1877, p. 3.

57. Leslie E. Keeley, *Opium: Its Use, Abuse and Cure; or, From Bondage to Freedom* (Dwight, Ill.: Leslie E. Keeley Co., 1892), 13.

58. Dr. Fred. Heman Hubbard, M.D., *The Opium Habit and Alcoholism* (New York: A. S. Barnes & Co., 1881), 4.

59. "Literary Notices," *Godey's Lady's Book and Magazine* 77 (November 1868), 451.

60. "Books and Authors," *Christian Union* 25, no. 5 (February 2, 1882), 113.

61. Timothy J. Gilfoyle, *A Pickpocket's Tale: The Underworld of Nineteenth-Century New York* (New York: W. W. Norton, 2006), 155.

62. Quoted in Donald P. Dulchinos, *Pioneer of Inner Space: The Life of Fitz Hugh Ludlow, Hasheesh Eater* (Brooklyn, N. Y.: Autonomedia, 1998), 262.

63. Day, *Opium Habit*, 6, 15.

64. David T. Courtwright, "The Hidden Epidemic: Opiate Addiction and Cocaine Use in the South, 1860–1920," *Journal of Southern History* 49, no. 1 (February 1983), 72.

65. Calkins, *Opium and the Opium-Appetite*, 152.

66. William Rosser Cobbe, *Doctor Judas: A Portrayal of the Opium Habit* (Chicago: S. C. Griggs and Company, 1895), 61.

67. "Book Table: The Opium Habit," *Independent* 21, no. 1067 (May 13, 1869), 6.

68. Quoted in Henry O. Whiteside, "The Drug Habit in Nineteenth-Century Colorado," *Colorado Magazine* 55, no. 1 (1978), 57.

69. "Opium," *Inter Ocean* [Chicago, Ill.] (August 17, 1874), 4.

70. Asa P. Meylert, *Notes on the Opium Habit* (New York: G. P. Putnam's Sons, 1884), 20.

71. Fred L. Israel, ed., *1897 Sears Roebuck Catalogue* (New York: Chelsea House, 1968), insert section, p. 32.

72. Roe, *Without a Home*, 278.

73. Gibbons, *Letheomania*, 10–11.

74. Charles Edward French diaries, Massachusetts Historical Society, journal 14, Sunday, May 25, 1883, p. 111.

75. Quoted in Whiteside, "The Drug Habit in Nineteenth-Century Colorado," 58.

76. Cobbe, *Doctor Judas*, 171.

77. Hubbard, *Opium Habit and Alcoholism*, 21, 34; T. J. Happel, "The Opium Curse and Its Prevention," *Quarterly Journal of Inebriety* 17, no. 3 (July 1895), 239; Courtwright, *Dark Paradise*, 56.

78. Gary G. Shattuck, "Opium Eating in Vermont: 'A Crying Evil of the Day,'" *Vermont History* 83 (Summer/Fall 2015), 181.

79. Quoted in H. H. Kane, *The Hypodermic Injection of Morphia: Its History, Advantages and Dangers* (New York: Chas. L. Bermingham & Co., 1880), 277.

80. W. D. Wilhite, M.D., "The Opium Habit: A Narrative of Personal Experience," *Southern Medical Record* 13, no. 7 (July 20, 1883), 247, 248.

81. Leslie E. Keeley, *The Morphine Eater: Or, From Bondage to Freedom* (Dwight, Ill.: C. L. Palmer & Co., 1881), 112.

82. Edward R. Squibb, Edward H. Squibb, and Charles F. Squibb, *An Ephemeris of Materia Medica, Pharmacy, Therapeutics and Collateral Information* (Brooklyn, N. Y., 1885), II: 763–64.

83. Charles Warrington Earle, "The Opium Habit," *Chicago Medical Review* 2, no. 9 (November 5, 1880), 494–95.

84. T. D. Crothers, M.D., *Morphinism and Narcomanias from Other Drugs: Their Etiology, Treatment, and Medicolegal Relations* (Philadelphia: W. B. Saunders & Company, 1902), 32.

85. Cobbe, *Doctor Judas*, 312–13.

86. Ernest S. Bishop, M.D., "Narcotic Addiction—A Systemic Disease Condition," *Journal of the American Medical Association* 60, no. 6 (February 8, 1913), 431.

87. Jonathan Lewy, "The Army Disease: Drug Addiction and the Civil War," *War in History* 21, no. 1 (January 2014), 109.

88. Edward Levinstein, M.D., *Morbid Craving for Morphia*, trans. Charles Harrer (London: Smith, Elder, & Co., 1878), 3.

89. Terry M. Parssinen and Karen Kerner, "Development of the Disease Model of Drug Addiction in Britain, 1870–1926," *Medical History* 24, no. 3 (July 1980), 278–79.

90. S. W. Gould, "The Opium Habit," *Medical and Surgical Reporter* 38, no. 25 (June 22, 1878), 496–97.

91. George E. Pettey, M.D., "A Rational Basis for the Treatment of Narcotic Drug Addiction," *New York Medical Journal* 92, no. 19 (November 5, 1910), 916.

92. Marcus Aurin, "Chasing the Dragon: The Cultural Metamorphosis of Opium in the United States, 1825–1935," *Medical Anthropology Quarterly* 14, no. 3 (September 2000), 435–36.

93. Lars-Winfried Seiler, "The Development of an Anti-Opium Ideology in Late Nineteenth Century America" (PhD diss., University of South Carolina, 2004), 269–70; Hickman, *Secret Leprosy of Modern Days*, 46.

94. H. Wayne Morgan, *Yesterday's Addicts: American Society and Drug Abuse, 1865–1920* (Norman: University of Oklahoma Press, 1974), 17.

95. E.g., H. H. Kane, "Rapid and Easy Cure of Morphine Habit of Twelve Years' Standing," *Physicians and Surgeons' Investigator* 2, no. 10 (October 15, 1881), 300.

96. Dr. C. H. Hughes, "The Opium Psycho-Neurosis—Chronic Meconism or Papaverism," *Alienist and Neurologist* 5 (1884), 134–37.

97. David Paulson, M.D., "Management of the Victims of Drug Habits," *Medical Standard* 24, no. 3 (March 1901), 131.

98. Calkins, *Opium and the Opium-Appetite*, 248.

99. "Remarks on the Opium Habit," 437.

100. Kane, *Drugs That Enslave*, 116.

101. E. W. Mitchell, M.D., "Treatment of Morphio-Mania," *Cincinnati Lancet-Clinic* (December 12, 1891), 760.

102. Kandall, *Substance and Shadow*, 64; "Poorer Drug Users in Pitiful Plight," *New York Times*, April 15, 1915, p. 7.

103. Calkins, *Opium and the Opium-Appetite*, 238–39, 210.

104. Crothers, *Morphinism and Narcomanias*, 55.

105. Mark Sullivan, *Our Times: The United States, 1900–1925* (New York: C. Scribner's Sons, 1927), II: 508–9.

106. Joseph L. Zentner, "Opiate Use in America During the Eighteenth and Nineteenth Centuries: The Origins of a Modern Scourge," *Studies in History & Society* 5, no. 2 (1974), 51n15, 42.

107. Bryan Denham, "Magazine Journalism in the Golden Age of Muckraking: Patent-Medicine Exposures Before and After the Pure Food and Drug Act of 1906," *Journalism & Communication Monographs* 22, no. 2 (2020), 104.

108. Goodwin, *Pure Food, Drink, and Drug Crusaders*, 41.

109. Kandall, *Substance and Shadow*, 62.

110. Morgan, *Drugs in America*, 66.

111. Thomas Dormandy, *Opium: Reality's Dark Dream* (New Haven, Conn.: Yale University Press, 2012), 190.

112. *Theriaki and Their Last Dose: Letters of Fitz Hugh Ludlow and Others, to Dr. Samuel B. Collins* (Chicago: Evening Journal Print, 1870), 36, 39, 69.

113. "'Opium Antidotes' Exposed," *Boston Medical and Surgical Journal* 95, no. 17 (October 26, 1876), 500–501.

114. "Opium," *Public Opinion* 21, no. 9 (August 27, 1896), 260; B. M. Woolley, *The Opium Habit and Its Cure* (1879).

115. Samuel Hopkins Adams, *The Great American Fraud: Articles on the Nostrum Evil and Quacks Reprinted from Collier's Weekly*, 4th ed. (P. F. Collier & Son: Chicago, Ill., 1905, 1906, 1907), 120.

116. Goodwin, *Pure Food, Drink, and Drug Crusaders*, 55; Adams, *The Great American Fraud*, 5.

117. Allan Chapman, *Physicians, Plagues and Progress: The History of Western Medicine from Antiquity to Antibiotics* (Oxford: Lion Books, 2016), 311; Stephen Snelders, Charles Kaplan, and Toine Pieters, "On Cannabis, Chloral Hydrate, and Career Cycles of Psychotropic Drugs in Medicine," *Bulletin of the History of Medicine* 80, no. 1 (Spring 2006), 98.

118. "The New Anæsthetic Chloral," *Scientific American* 22, no. 24 (June 11, 1870), 377.

119. Kane, *Drugs That Enslave*, 200, 150, 163.

120. "Morphia Disease," *New York Times*, April 30, 1876, p. 2.

121. "The Chloral Habit," *Demorest's Monthly Magazine* 21, no. 6 (April 1885), 385.

122. Cobbe, *Doctor Judas*, 135.

123. I. A. Watson, M.D., "Caution in the Use of Chloral Hydrate," *Medical and Surgical Reporter* 26, no. 4 (January 27, 1872), 77–79.

124. *Los Angeles Herald*, May 20, 1875, p. 4.

125. Itinerant, "Nervous Disease—Insomnia," *Ladies' Repository* 36 (January 1876), 9.

126. "Sayings and Doings," *Harper's Bazar* 4 (April 22, 1871), 251.

127. "Taking Physic," *Hall's Journal of Health* 8, no. 10 (October 1861), 241–42; "Editors' Table: A Warning," *Godey's Lady's Book and Magazine* 83, no. 495 (September 1871), 280.

128. Kane, *Drugs That Enslave*, 153.

129. Reprinted as "Home Medication," *Friend* 63, no. 23 (January 4, 1890), 178.

130. *Sixth Annual Report of the Secretary of the State Board of Health of the State of Michigan, for the Fiscal Year Ending Sept. 30, 1878* (Lansing: W. S. George & Co., 1878), 72.

131. Louis Weiss, Ph.G., "A Drug Store in the Far West," *American Journal of Pharmacy* (November 1877), 563.

132. Cole, *Confessions of an American Opium Eater*, 49.

133. American Association for the Study and Cure of Inebriety, *Disease of Inebriety*, 218–19.

134. Keeley, *Opium: Its Use, Abuse and Cure*, 164.

135. George Miller Beard, *American Nervousness: Its Causes and Consequences* (New York: Putnam, 1881), 22–23, 92.

136. Hickman, *Secret Leprosy of Modern Days*, 10.

137. Quoted in "The Opium Madness," *Arthur's Illustrated Home Magazine* 47, no. 2 (February 1879), 80.

138. American Association for the Study and Cure of Inebriety, *Disease of Inebriety*, 19–20.

139. Beard, *American Nervousness*, 114.

140. David E. Nye, "Shaping Communication Networks: Telegraph, Telephone, Computer," *Social Research* 64, no. 3 (Fall 1997), 1068.

141. Beard, *American Nervousness*, 99–100, 136–37, 97.

142. Anna Hayward Johnson, A. M., "Neurasthenia," *Philadelphia Medical Times* 11, no. 24 (August 27, 1881), 737.

143. Courtwright, *Dark Paradise*, 125.

144. "Cartoons and Comments: The Drug-Eaters," *Puck*, October 10, 1900, p. 7; "The Age of Drugs," *Puck*, October 10, 1900, pp. 8–9.

145. George M. Beard, M.D., *Stimulants and Narcotics; Medically, Philosophically, and Morally Considered* (New York: G. P. Putnam & Sons, 1871), 25, 39.

146. Edward P. Thwing, M.D., Ph.D., "American Life as Related to Inebriety," *Quarterly Journal of Inebriety* 10, no. 1 (January 1888), 46.

147. W. F. Waugh, M.D., "Opium Inebriety," *Quarterly Journal of Inebriety* 16, no. 4 (October 1894), 310.

148. "The Opium Habit's Power," *New-York Times*, December 30, 1877, p. 8.

149. [Nolan], "The Opium Habit," 832.

150. "The Opium Habit," *Memphis Avalanche*, August 23, 1885.

151. Hickman, *Secret Leprosy of Modern Days*, 127.

152. Alan Trachtenberg, *The Incorporation of America: Culture and Society in the Gilded Age* (New York: Hill and Wang, 2007), 90.

153. Allan Forman, "Some Adopted Americans," *American Magazine* 9, no. 1 (November 1888), 52.

154. Trachtenberg, *Incorporation of America*, 89–91; Harold R. Kerbo and Richard A. Shaffer, "Unemployment and Protest in the United States, 1890–1940: A Methodological Critique and Research Note," *Social Forces* 64, no. 4 (June 1986), 1048.

155. Brian Kelly, "No Easy Way Through: Race Leadership and Black Workers at the Nadir," *Labor* 7, no. 3 (Fall 2010), 79.

156. Lisa G. Materson and Joe William Trotter Jr., "African American Urban Electoral Politics in the Age of Jim Crow," *Journal of Urban History* 44, no. 2 (March 2018), 124; U.S. Department of Commerce, Bureau of the Census, *We the Americans: Blacks* (Washington, D. C.: U.S. Government Printing Office, 1993), 2.

157. Richard White, *The Republic for Which It Stands: The United States During Reconstruction and the Gilded Age, 1865–1896* (New York: Oxford University Press, 2017), 149–50, 156–57, 856.

158. Day, *Opium Habit*, 7.

159. "The Victims of Morphine," *Daily Republican* [Monongahela City, Pa.], September 13, 1883, p. 3.

160. James C. Wilson, "The Opium Habit and Kindred Affections," in William Pepper, ed., *A System of Practical Medicine* (Philadelphia: Lea Brothers & Co., 1886), 649.

161. American Association for the Study and Cure of Inebriety, *Disease of Inebriety*, 73.

162. "What Is, and What Might Be," *American Socialist* 4, no. 11 (March 13, 1879), 81.

163. Charles Warrington Earle, M.D., "The Opium Habit," *Chicago Medical Review* 2, no. 7 (October 5, 1880), 443, 444.

164. Calkins, *Opium and the Opium-Appetite*, 164.

165. Courtwright, *Dark Paradise*, 49.

166. Virgil G. Eaton, "How the Opium-Habit Is Acquired," *Popular Science Monthly* 33 (September 1888), 665.

167. Charles B. Towns, *Habits That Handicap: The Menace of Opium, Alcohol, and Tobacco, and the Remedy* (New York: Century Co., 1916), 27–28.

## Chapter 9

1. [David W. Cheever], "Narcotics," *North American Review* 95, no. 197 (October 1862), 401–2.

2. Annie C. Meyers, *Eight Years in Cocaine Hell* (Chicago: St. Luke Society, 1902), 10–13, 25–26.

3. Meyers, *Eight Years in Cocaine Hell*, 27.

4. "Mrs. Meyers Fined for Theft," *Daily Inter Ocean* [Chicago, Ill.], August 24, 1899.

5. Meyers, *Eight Years in Cocaine Hell*, 68, 7–8.

6. "Yankee Medico to Attend Opium Meet," *Bristol* [Tenn.] *Herald Courier*, October 29, 1908, p. 1.

7. Dr. Mantegazza, "On the Dietetic and Medicinal Properties of Erythroxylon Coca," *American Journal of Pharmacy* 32 (September 1860), 417.

8. Joseph F. Spillane, *Cocaine: From Medical Marvel to Modern Menace in the United States, 1884–1920* (Baltimore: Johns Hopkins University Press, 2002), 91; Mantegazza, "On the Dietetic and Medicinal Properties of Erythroxylon Coca," 417–18.

9. Howard Markel, *An Anatomy of Addiction: Sigmund Freud, William Halsted, and the Miracle Drug, Cocaine* (New York: Vintage, 2012), 53.

10. Joseph Michael Gabriel, "Gods and Monsters: Drugs, Addiction, and the Origins of Narcotic Control in the Nineteenth-Century Urban North" (PhD diss., Rutgers University, 2006), 444; Catherine Carstairs, "'The Most Dangerous Drug': Images of African-Americans and Cocaine Use in the Progressive Era," *Left History* 7 (May 2000), 48.

11. Richard Davenport-Hines, *The Pursuit of Oblivion: A Global History of Narcotics* (New York: W. W. Norton, 2002), 164; Spillane, *Cocaine*, 8, 14–16, 22.

12. Spillane, *Cocaine*, 21; Davenport-Hines, *Pursuit of Oblivion*, 152.

13. American Association for the Study and Cure of Inebriety, *The Disease of Inebriety from Alcohol, Opium and Other Narcotic Drugs* ... (New York: E. B. Treat, 1893), 357.

14. Walter Woodman, M.D., "Cocaine for Sleeplessness," *Boston Medical and Surgical Journal* 112, no. 12 (March 19, 1885), 287.

15. D. R. Brower, "The Effects of Cocaine on the Central Nervous System," *Medical Age* 4, no. 2 (January 25, 1886), 29.

16. Albert Doerschuk, Ph.G., "The Cocaine Habit," *Bulletin of Pharmacy* 9, no. 4 (April 1895), 154.

17. "Negro Cocaine Fiends," *New York Sun*, November 2, 1902, p. 35; Michael M. Cohen, "Jim Crow's Drug War: Race, Coca Cola, and the Southern Origins of Drug Prohibition," *Southern Cultures* 12, no. 3 (2006), 70.

18. Spillane, *Cocaine*, 92–93; C. P. Ambler, M.D., "Cocaine—Its Uses and Abuses," *Cleveland Medical Gazette* 10, no. 2 (December 1894), 60; Henry O. Whiteside, "The Drug Habit in Nineteenth-century Colorado," *Colorado Magazine* 55, no. 1 (Winter 1978), 64; Thomas G. Simonton, "The Increase of the Use of Cocaine Among the Laity of Pittsburg," *Philadelphia Medical Journal* 11, no. 13 (March 28, 1903), 556.

19. David Smith, "Hail Mariani: The Transformation of Vin Mariani from Medicine to Food in American Culture, 1886–1910," *Social History of Alcohol and Drugs* 23, no. 1 (Fall 2008), 42, 45–48.

20. Steven B. Karch, M.D., *A Brief History of Cocaine* (Boca Raton, Fla.: CRC Press, 1998), 106; Mark Pendergrast, *For God, Country, and Coca-Cola: The Unauthorized History of the Great American Soft Drink and the Company That Makes It* (New York: Charles Scribner's Sons, 1993), 422, 56n.

21. Lorine Swainston Goodwin, *The Pure Food, Drink, and Drug Crusaders, 1879–1914* (Jefferson, N. C.: McFarland, 2006), 45–46, 219.

22. Joseph L. Zentner, "Opiate Use in America During the Eighteenth and Nineteenth Centuries: The Origins of a Modern Scourge," *Studies in History & Society* 5, no. 2 (1974), 43, 52n23.

23. Samuel Hopkins Adams, *The Great American Fraud: Articles on the Nostrum Evil and Quacks Reprinted from Collier's Weekly*, 4th ed. (P. F. Collier and Son: Chicago, Ill., 1905, 1906, 1907), 3, 111–12.

24. Goodwin, *Pure Food, Drink, and Drug Crusaders*, 256; Adams, *Great American Fraud*, 177.

25. Adams, *Great American Fraud*, 111.

26. David F. Musto, *The American Disease: Origins of Narcotic Control* (New York: Oxford University Press, 1999), 94, 22, 309n52.

27. Adams, *Great American Fraud*, 157–59.

28. Jorge Durand, Douglas S. Massey, and Fernando Charvet, "The Changing Geography of Mexican Immigration to the United States: 1910–1996," *Social Science Quarterly* 81, no. 1 (March 2000), 4–5; Isaac Campos, "Mexicans and the Origins of Marijuana Prohibition in the United States: A Reassessment," *Social History of Alcohol & Drugs* 32, no. 1 (December 2018), 7.

29. "Voice of the Press: A Spurious Article," *Record-Union* [Sacramento, Calif.], December 31, 1897, p. 2.

30. "Two Republics," *Citrograph* [Redlands, Calif.], January 13, 1900, p. 9.

31. "Mexico Makes War on Brain-Destroying Weed," *Independent* [Santa Barbara, Calif.], June 3, 1907, p. 3; "Effects of Mexican Loco Weeds," *Californian* [Salinas, Calif.], March 2, 1905, p. 2.

32. "Policeman Lassoes a Drug Crazed Mexican," *El Paso Herald*, January 28, 1914, p. 4; "Poisonous Weeds of Mexico Cause Death," *El Paso Herald*, May 9, 1914, p. 32.

33. Campos, "Mexicans and the Origins of Marijuana Prohibition," 23–24, 26–28; "Legality of Sale of Cannabis Question," *Oregon Journal*, March 14, 1915, p. 6.

34. Campos, "Mexicans and the Origins of Marijuana Prohibition," 19, 20, 22.

35. Isaac Campos, *Home Grown: Marijuana and the Origins of Mexico's War on Drugs* (Chapel Hill: University of North Carolina Press, 2012), 22, 124, 155, 205.

36. "Crazed by a Weed, Man Murders," *El Paso Herald*, January 2, 1913, p. 2; Bob Chessey, "El Paso's 1915 Marihuana Ordinance: Myth and Reality," *Password* 58, no. 1 (2014), 34–35.

37. Richard J. Bonnie and Charles H. Whitebread II, "The Forbidden Fruit and the Tree of Knowledge: An Inquiry into the Legal History of American Marijuana Prohibition," *Virginia Law Review* 56, no. 6 (October 1970), 1056 and 1056n34.

38. "Opium Delegate Named," *San Francisco Examiner*, March 21, 1911, p. 6; Bruce La Brack, "Occupational Specialization among Rural California Sikhs: The Interplay of Culture and Economics," *Amerasia Journal* 9, no. 2 (1982), 29; Juan L. Gonzales Jr., "Asian Indian Immigration Patterns: The Origins of the Sikh Community in California," *International Migration Review* 20, no. 1 (Spring 1986), 42–44; Dale H. Gieringer, "The Forgotten Origins of Cannabis Prohibition in California," *Contemporary Drug Problems* 26 (Summer 1999), 251–53; Musto, *American Disease*, 218.

39. "Hindu Blames Cigaret for Prison Sentence," *Los Angeles Express*, February 21, 1913, p. 17.

40. Martin Booth, *Cannabis: A History* (New York: St. Martin's Press, 2003), 161.

41. Daniel C. Swan, *Peyote Religious Art: Symbols of Faith and Belief* (Jackson: University Press of Mississippi, 1999), 10.

42. James Mooney, "The Mescal Plant and Ceremony," *Therapeutic Gazette* 12, no. 1 (January 15, 1896), 7–9.

43. Alexander S. Dawson, *The Peyote Effect: From the Inquisition to the War on Drugs* (Berkeley: University of California Press, 2018), 2.

44. William Willard, "The First Amendment, Anglo-Conformity and American Indian Religious Freedom," *Wicazo Sa Review* 7, no. 1 (Spring 1991), 29–30; Mooney, "The Mescal Plant and Ceremony," 9; Joseph D. Calabrese, "The Therapeutic Use of Peyote in the Native American Church," in Michael J. Winkelman and Thomas B. Roberts, eds., *Psychedelic Medicine: New Evidence for Hallucinogenic Substances as Treatments* (Westport, Conn.: Praeger, 2007), II: 30.

45. D. W. Prentiss and Francis P. Morgan, "Mescal Buttons," *Transactions of the Association of American Physicians* 11 (Philadelphia, 1896), 306–7.

46. Hillary S. Webb, "The Use of Peyote as Treatment for Alcoholism within the NAC Community. Reflections on a Study: An Interview with John Halpern, M.D.," *Anthropology of Consciousness* 22, no. 2 (September 2011), 235, 240; John Horgan, "Tripping on Peyote in Navajo Nation," *Scientific American* (July 5, 2017), https://blogs.scientificamerican.com/cross-check/tripping-on-peyote-in-navajo-nation/.

47. Mooney, "The Mescal Plant and Ceremony," 7–11; quote p. 7.

48. D. W. Prentiss and Francis P. Morgan, "Anhalonium Lewinii (Mescal Buttons)," *Therapeutic Gazette* 11, no. 9 (September 16, 1895), 580, 583.

49. Havelock Ellis, "Mescal: A Study of a Divine Plant," *Popular Science Monthly* (May 1902), 64, 60, 65.

50. *Prohibition of Use of Peyote*, House of Representatives, 65th Congress, 2d Session, Report No. 560 (May 13, 1918), 21–22.

51. *Annual Report of the Commissioner of Indian Affairs to the Secretary of the Interior for the Year 1886* (Washington, D. C.: Government Printing Office, 1886), 130.

52. *Fifty-Seventh Annual Report of the Commissioner of Indian Affairs to the Secretary of the Interior* (Washington, D. C.: Government Printing Office, 1888), 99.

53. Quoted in Omer C. Stewart, "Origin of the Peyote Religion in the United States," *Plains Anthropologist* 19, no. 65 (August 1974), 214.

54. Benjamin R. Kracht, *Religious Revitalization Among the Kiowas: The Ghost Dance, Peyote, and Christianity* (Lincoln: University of Nebraska Press, 2018), 160; Omer C. Stewart, *Peyote Religion: A History* (Norman: University of Oklahoma Press, 1987), 134.

55. Gertrude Seymour, "Peyote Worship—An Indian Cult and a Powerful Drug," *Red Man* 8, no. 10 (June 1916), 345, 346.

56. Kracht, *Religious Revitalization Among the Kiowas*, 70, 158–59.

57. Mrs. Delavan L. Pierson, "Indian Peyote Worship," *Southern Workman* 44, no. 4 (April 1915), 242.

58. Martin Terry and Keeper Trout, "Regulation of Peyote (*Lophophora Williamsii*: Cactaceae) in the U.S.A.: A Historical Victory of Religion and Politics over Science and Medicine," *Journal of the Botanical Research Institute of Texas* 11, no. 1 (2017), 150–51.

59. Kracht, *Religious Revitalization Among the Kiowas*, 162.

60. Dawson, *Peyote Effect*, 5, 4.

61. Pierson, "Indian Peyote Worship," 241.

62. Seymour, "Peyote Worship—An Indian Cult and a Powerful Drug," 346, 347, 349.

63. Kracht, *Religious Revitalization Among the Kiowas*, 165, 71, 74.

64. Pierson, "Indian Peyote Worship," 245.

65. Dawson, *Peyote Effect*, 44, 163.

66. "Senate Passes Narcotic Bill," [Price, Utah] *News-Advocate*, January 25, 1917, p. 8.

67. Kracht, *Religious Revitalization Among the Kiowas*, 75–76, 148.

68. Dawson, *Peyote Effect*, 6.

69. E. G. Eberle and Frederick T. Gordon, "Report of Committee on the Acquirement of Drug Habits," *American Journal of Pharmacy* 75 (October 1903), 480.

70. Thomas S. Blair, M.D., "The Relation of Drug Addiction to Industry," *Journal of Industrial Hygiene* 1, no. 6 (October 1919), 289.

71. Stephen R. Kandall, *Substance and Shadow: Women and Addiction in the United States* (Cambridge, Mass.: Harvard University Press, 1999), 69; John Helmer, *Drugs and Minority Oppression* (New York: Seabury Press, 1975), 50; H. Wayne Morgan, *Drugs in America: A Social History, 1800–1980* (Syracuse, N. Y.: Syracuse University Press, 1981), 92.

72. "His Own Story," *Daily Inter Ocean* [Chicago, Ill.], December 31, 1887, p. 24.

73. Jonathan Lewy, *Drugs in Germany and the United States, 1919–1945: The Birth of Two Addictions* (Baden-Baden, Germany: Nomos Verlagsgesellschaft, 2017), 196–97.

74. *Banner-Democrat* [Lake Providence, La.], December 22, 1900, p. 3.

75. "Cocaine User Shoots 7," *New York Times*, December 6, 1907.

76. "Negro Was Crazed by Cocaine," [Meriden, Conn.] *Record-Journal*, April 20, 1909, p. 1; "Wild Negro Runs Amuck," *Baltimore Sun*, April 20, 1909, p. 11.

77. "The Cocain Habit," *Journal of the American Medical Association* 34, no. 25 (June 23, 1900), 1637.

78. "Rendered Insane by Cocaine," *Daily City News* [New Castle, Pa.], June 27, 1888, p. 1.

79. Brower, "Effects of Cocaine on the Central Nervous System," 29–30.

80. Douglas J. Flowe, "'Tell the Whole White World': Crime, Violence, and Black Men in Early Migration New York City, 1890–1917" (PhD diss., University of Rochester, 2014), 104.

81. Pendergrast, *For God, Country, and Coca-Cola*, 42; Cohen, "Jim Crow's Drug War," 73.

82. *Importation and Use of Opium: Hearings Before the Committee on Ways and Means of the House of Representatives*, 61st Congress, 3d Session, on H. R. 25240, H. R. 25241, H. R. 25242, and H. R. 28971 (December 14, 1910 and January 11, 1911) (statement of Dr. Christopher Koch, Vice President, State Pharmaceutical Examining Board of Pennsylvania; Chairman, Legislative Committee, Philadelphia Association of Retail Druggists) (Washington, D. C.: Government Printing Office, 1911), 72.

83. Musto, *American Disease*, 42–44; Hamilton Wright, *Report on the International Opium Commission and on the Opium Problem as Seen Within the United States and Its Possessions*. S. Doc. No. 377, 61st Congress, 2d session, 1909–1910 (Washington, D. C.: Government Printing Office, 1910), 50.

84. Musto, *American Disease*, 31–32.

85. "Tocsin of Battle Is Sounded," *Daily Missoulian* [Mont.], November 7, 1909, p. 13; "Publisher's Desk," *Rural New-Yorker* 68, no. 3099 (June 19, 1909), 618.

86. *Evening Times* [Grand Forks, N. D.], March 25, 1909, p. 4.

87. Charles W. Collins and John Day, "The Eighth Deadly Sin," *Everyday Life*, July 1909, 29.

88. Harris Dickson, "The Negro in Politics," *Hampton's Magazine* 23, no. 2 (August 1909), 236; Harris Dickson, "Exit the Black Man," *Hampton's Magazine* 23, no. 4 (October 1909), 497–505.

89. Collins and Day, "The Eighth Deadly Sin," 29; Harris Dickson, "The Unknowable Negro," *Hampton's Magazine* 22, no. 6 (June 1909), 734, 737. Emphasis in original.

90. Quoted in "Cocaine Curse of the South," *Leavenworth* [Kan.] *Post*, July 23, 1909, p. 1. Articles about the Currier Commission's report include, but are not limited to "Cocaine Habit American Curse," *Evening Times* [Grand Forks, N. D.], July 19, 1909, p. 1; "Cocaine Habit Race Menace," *Iola* [Kan.] *Daily Register*, July 20, 1909, p. 7; "Cocaine a Menace to Southern Negroes," *Jackson* [Miss.] *Daily News*, July 20, 1909, p. 8; and "Specter Among Negroes of South Now Cocaine," *Bridgeport* [Conn.] *Times and Evening Farmer*, July 20, 1909, p. 9.

91. "The Cocaine Habit," *Burlington* [Vt.] *Daily News*, July 6, 1909, p. 4.

92. Quoted in Flowe, "'Tell the Whole White World,'" 118–19; Spillane, *Cocaine*, 93.

93. E.g., "Abolish the Dives; Jail the Vagrants," *Tampa Tribune*, September 25, 1906, p. 4; "Southern View of Race Riot," *Long Branch* [N. J.] *Record*, October 19, 1906, p. 4; "Stripes for Cocaine Sellers," *Atlanta Constitution*, November 15, 1907, p. 6; "Carnival of Negro Crime," *Great Falls* [Mont.] *Tribune*, February 4, 1909, p. 1; "Negro Given Five Years in Jail," *Staunton* [Va.] *Daily Leader*, August 11, 1908, p. 1.

94. In searching for articles that reported cases of African American men accused of raping women as a result of cocaine use, I searched the Newspapers.com database for US newspapers between 1899 and 1910 where the words "negro," "cocaine," and "rape" appeared on the same page. The database includes thousands of newspapers, many of them local papers that reported local crimes. Three hundred ninety pages contained all three words, but not a single article alleged that an African American man had committed a rape after using cocaine. Database accessed July 16–30, 2019.

95. Cohen, "Jim Crow's Drug War," 76.

96. Denise A. Herd, "Prohibition, Racism and Class Politics in the Post-Reconstruction South," *Journal of Drug Issues* (Winter 1983), 82–83, 77–79; "Who Killed Margaret Lear?" *Nashville Tennessean* (June 17, 1908), p. 6; "To the Manhood of Tennessee," *Nashville Tennessean* (June 17, 1908), pp. 6–7; "The Negro Vote an Annoying Factor," *Nashville Tennessean* (July 28, 1911), 6.

97. Anne L. Foster, "Prohibition as Superiority: Policing Opium in South-East Asia, 1898–1925," *International History Review* 22, no. 2 (2000), 257; Gabriel, "Gods and Monsters," 507.

98. Foster, "Prohibition as Superiority," 255–56.

99. Foster, "Prohibition as Superiority," 257.

100. Anne L. Foster, "The Philippines, the United States, and the Origins of Global Narcotics Prohibition," *Social History of Alcohol and Drugs* 33, no. 1 (Spring 2019), 30; Anne L. Foster, "Medicine to Drug: Opium's Transimperial Journey," in *Crossing Empires: Taking U.S. History into Transimperial Terrain*, ed. Kristin L. Hoganson and Jay Sexton (Durham, N. C.: Duke University Press, 2020), 123–24.

101. Daniel J. P. Wertz, "Idealism, Imperialism, and Internationalism: Opium Politics in the Colonial Philippines, 1898–1925," *Modern Asian Studies* 47, no. 2 (March 2013), 473–74.

102. "Summary of Events," *Friend* 78, no. 12 (October 1, 1904), 96.

103. Quoted in Foster, "The Philippines, the United States, and the Origins of Global Narcotics Prohibition," 19; Gabriel, "Gods and Monsters," 507–8; Luke Messac, "No Opiates for the Masses: Untreated Pain, International Narcotics Control, and the Bureaucratic Production of Ignorance," *Journal of Policy History* 28, no. 2 (2016), 196.

104. Wertz, "Idealism, Imperialism, and Internationalism," 478.

105. "Opium in the Philippines," *Watchman* 86, no. 34 (August 25, 1904), 5.

106. Richard Harvey Brown, "The Opium Trade and Opium Policies in India, China, Britain, and the United States: Historical Comparisons and Theoretical Interpretations," *Asian Journal of Social Science* 30 (2002), 642; "Summary of Events," *Friend* 78, no. 12 (October 1, 1904), 96.

107. Wertz, "Idealism, Imperialism, and Internationalism," 484.

108. Brown, "Opium Trade and Opium Policies," 642.

109. Rosa Pendleton Chiles, "The Passing of the Opium Traffic," *Forum* 46 (July 1911), 27–31.

110. David T. Courtwright, *Forces of Habit: Drugs and the Making of the Modern World* (Cambridge, Mass.: Harvard University Press, 2001), 183; Lars-Winfried Seiler, "The Development of an Anti-Opium Ideology in Late Nineteenth Century America" (PhD diss., University of South Carolina, 2004), 238.

111. Musto, *American Disease*, 31; Brown, "Opium Trade and Opium Policies," 643.

112. Diana L. Ahmad, *The Opium Debate and Chinese Exclusion Laws in the Nineteenth-Century American West* (Reno: University of Nevada Press, 2007), 82; Hamilton Wright, *Report on the International Opium Commission*, 52.

113. David T. Courtwright, *Dark Paradise: A History of Opiate Addiction in America* (Cambridge, Mass.: Harvard University Press, 2001), 81.

114. "Congress Acts in the Nick of Time," *Outlook* 91 (February 13, 1909), 316.

115. Quoted in Gabriel, "Gods and Monsters," 512.

116. Ahmad, *Opium Debate and Chinese Exclusion Laws*, 70.

117. Helena Barop, "Building the 'Opium Evil' Consensus—The International Opium Commission of Shanghai," *Journal of Modern European History* 13, no. 1 (2015), 115.

118. William O. Walker, *Opium and Foreign Policy: The Anglo-American Search for Order in Asia, 1912–1954* (Chapel Hill: University of North Carolina Press, 1991), 16; "The International Anti-Opium Conference," *Outlook* 91, no. 12 (March 20, 1909), 611.

119. "The World-Wide Kingdom," *Baptist Missionary Magazine* 89, no. 5 (May 1909), 159.

120. Seiler, "Development of an Anti-Opium Ideology," 257; Ahmad, *Opium Debate and Chinese Exclusion Laws*, 83.

121. *Report of the International Opium Commission, Shanghai, China, February 1 to February 26, 1909* (Shanghai: North-China Daily News and Herald, Ltd., 1909), I: 47.

122. Musto, *American Disease*, 35–37; Martin Booth, *Opium* (New York: St. Martin's Griffin, 1996), 181.

123. Seiler, "Development of an Anti-Opium Ideology," 257.

124. Ernest L. Abel, *Marihuana: The First Twelve Thousand Years* (New York: Plenum Press, 1980), 194.

125. Foster, "Prohibition as Superiority," 255.

126. James Barr Ames, *A Selection of Cases on the Law of Torts* (Cambridge, Mass.: Harvard Law Review Publishing Association, 1893), I: 594–97.

127. B.F.D., "Annotation: Right of Action Against One Selling Habit-forming Drug to Child or Spouse," in *American Law Reports Annotated*, vol. 3, ed. Burdett A. Rich and M. Blair Wailes (Rochester, N. Y.: Lawyers Co-operative Publishing Company, 1919), 1152–53.

128. "Is Narcotism Drunkenness?" *Quarterly Journal of Inebriety* 12 (1890), 175; "Youngs v. Youngs," *Northeastern Reporter* 22 (August 9, 1889–January 24, 1890), 806.

129. *Acts of the General Assembly of the Commonwealth of Kentucky* (Frankfort: Kentucky Yeoman Office, 1872), 56.

130. "Order No. 1254—Prohibiting Opium Smoking Dens," *San Francisco Examiner*, November 24, 1875, p. 2.

131. "The Opium Dens," *San Francisco Chronicle*, November 16, 1875, p. 3.

132. Gieringer, "The Forgotten Origins of Cannabis Prohibition in California," 237; Ronald Hamowy, "Introduction: Illicit Drugs and Government Control," in Ronald Hamowy, ed., *Dealing with Drugs: Consequences of Government Control* (Lexington, Mass.: D.C. Heath and Company, 1987), 13; Audrey Redford and Benjamin Powell, "Dynamics of Intervention in the War on Drugs: The Buildup to the Harrison Act of 1914," *Independent Review* 20, no. 4 (Spring 2016), 519.

133. Hamowy, "Introduction: Illicit Drugs and Government Control," 9–10.

134. Musto, *American Disease*, 9.

135. "Vermont Should Have Stringent Drug Law," *Middlebury Register*, January 22, 1915, p. 2.

136. Courtwright, *Dark Paradise*, 52–53; L. F. Kebler, "Existing Laws Regulating the Sale of Habit-Forming Drugs and the Necessity for Additional Legislation," *American Journal of Pharmacy* (April 1909), 194; "Evolution of Current Law," *Congressional Digest* (November 2003), 260.

137. Thomas Dormandy, *Opium: Reality's Dark Dream* (New Haven, Conn.: Yale University Press, 2012), 205.

138. Musto, *American Disease*, 4, 5; Morgan, *Drugs in America*, 41; Courtwright, *Dark Paradise*, 2, 26–28, 50–51, 53, 110.

139. Dick Griffin, "Opium Addiction in Chicago: 'The Noblest and the Best Brought Low,'" *Chicago History* 6, no. 2 (July 1977), 114; Foster, "Prohibition as Superiority," 256.

140. Henry G. Cole, *Confessions of an American Opium Eater: From Bondage to Freedom* (Boston: James H. Earle, 1895), 25, 6.

141. "Boy Cocaine Snuffers Hunted by the Police," *New York Times*, January 8, 1907.

142. Louise Foxcroft, *The Making of Addiction: The 'Use and Abuse' of Opium in Nineteenth-Century Britain* (Burlington, Vt.: Ashgate, 2007), 10; Courtwright, *Dark Paradise*, 85, 91; Redford and Powell, "Dynamics of Intervention in the War on Drugs," 518–19.

143. Zentner, "Opiate Use in America," 49; William J. Cruikshank, "The Substitution of Drugs in the Dispensing of the Physician's Prescription," *Medical News* 87, no. 23 (December 2, 1905), 1071.

144. Courtwright, *Dark Paradise*, 90.

145. "Heroin and Its Advantages," *Medical News* 76, no. 1 (January 6, 1900), 20.

146. H. Wayne Morgan, *Yesterday's Addicts: American Society and Drug Abuse, 1865–1920* (Norman: University of Oklahoma Press, 1974), 28–30; "Say Drug Habit Grips the Nation," *New York Times*, December 5, 1913, p. 8; "Caught Using Heroin," *New York Times*, June 3, 1913, p. 18.

147. Caroline Jean Acker, "Take as Directed: The Dilemmas of Regulating Addictive Analgesics and Other Psychoactive Drugs," in Marcia L. Meldrum, ed., *Opioids and Pain Relief: A Historical Perspective* (Seattle: IASP Press, 2003), 38–39.

148. *Exploring the Dangerous Trades: The Autobiography of Alice Hamilton, M.D.* (Boston: Little, Brown, 1943), 100.

149. Simonton, "The Increase of the Use of Cocaine Among the Laity of Pittsburg," 556.

150. Joseph Spillane, "The Making of an Underground Market: Drug Selling in Chicago, 1900–1940," *Journal of Social History* 32, no. 1 (1998), 29; Helmer, *Drugs and Minority Oppression*, 42; David T. Courtwright, "The Female Opiate Addict in Nineteenth-Century America," *Essay in Arts and Sciences* 10 (March 1982), 166–67.

151. Patricia G. Erickson, "The Law, Social Control, and Drug Policy: Models, Factors, and Processes," *International Journal of the Addictions* 28 (1993), 1164.

152. Musto, *American Disease*, 40.

153. Marcus Aurin, "Chasing the Dragon: The Cultural Metamorphosis of Opium in the United States, 1825–1935," *Medical Anthropology Quarterly* 14, no. 3 (September 2000), 432.

154. Musto, *American Disease*, 41–42, 45, 46, 48; *Importation and Use of Opium: Hearings Before the Committee on Ways and Means of the House of Representatives* (Washington: Government Printing Office, 1911), 66.

155. Courtwright, *Dark Paradise*, 102.

156. Booth, *Cannabis*, 162.

157. Courtwright, *Dark Paradise*, 102; Musto, *American Disease*, 59.

158. Davenport-Hines, *Pursuit of Oblivion*, 213.

159. Musto, *American Disease*, 65.

160. "A Law That Is Cruel Only to Be Kind," *Chicago Tribune*, March 11, 1915, p. 6.

161. Courtwright, *Dark Paradise*, xi–xii, 29.

162. Hamilton Wright, "The International Opium Commission," *American Journal of International Law* 3, no. 3 (July 1909), 672.

163. Edward Huntington Williams, "The Drug-Habit Menace in the South," *Medical Record* (February 7, 1914), 247.

164. Spillane, *Cocaine*, 119–21.

165. Joel Williamson, *The Crucible of Race: Black-White Relations in the American South Since Emancipation* (New York: Oxford University Press, 1984), 210.

166. Cohen, "Jim Crow's Drug War," 74.

167. "Cocaine Gets in Its Deadly Work," *Lancaster* [South Carolina] *News*, September 30, 1913; "Admits He Led Mob," *Marion* [Ohio] *Daily Star*, September 30, 1913, p. 3.

168. Gregory Yee Mark, "Political, Economic and Racial Influences on America's First Drug Laws" (PhD diss., University of California, Berkeley, 1978), 165; Courtwright, *Dark Paradise*, 165, 101; Welles A. Gray, "The Opium Problem," *Annals of the American Academy of Political and Social Science* 122 (November 1925), 150.

169. "Opium," *Outlook* 110, no. 1 (May 5, 1915), 8.

170. Musto, *American Disease*, 53.

171. Mark, "Political, Economic and Racial Influences," 166, 168; Booth, *Opium*, 182.

172. Diana S. Kim, *Empires of Vice: The Rise of Opium Prohibition Across Southeast Asia* (Princeton, N. J.: Princeton University Press, 2020), 64.

173. James Windle, "How the East Influenced Drug Prohibition," *International History Review* 35, no. 5 (2013), 1188.

174. Aurin, "Chasing the Dragon," 421–22.

175. Musto, *American Disease*, 65.

176. C. B. Pearson, M. D., "The Treatment of Morphinism," *Medical Times* (August 1914), 245.

177. Quoted in Morgan, *Drugs in America*, 116.

178. Charles B. Towns, *Habits That Handicap; The Menace of Opium, Alcohol, and Tobacco, and the Remedy* (New York: Century Co., 1916), 244.

179. Musto, *American Disease*, 79–82, 89–90; Booth, *Opium*, 94.

180. C. E. Terry, "Six Months of the Harrison Act," *American Journal of Public Health* 6, no. 10 (October 1916), 1088.

181. Doerschuk, "The Cocaine Habit," 155.

182. John Harrison Hughes, "The Autobiography of a Drug Fiend," *Medical Review of Reviews* 22, no. 2 (February 1916), 113.

183. Dr. C. E. Terry, "Drug Addictions, A Public Health Problem," *American Journal of Public Health* 4, no. 1 (January 1914), 28–30, 35.

184. Courtwright, *Dark Paradise*, 12–14.

185. Lucius P. Brown, "Enforcement of the Tennessee Anti-Narcotics Law," *American Journal of Public Health* 5 (April 1915), 323.

186. "A Law That Is Cruel Only to Be Kind," 6.

187. Musto, *American Disease*, 64.

188. Musto, *American Disease*, 66.

189. Violet McNeal, *Four White Horses and a Brass Band* (Garden City, N. Y.: Doubleday, 1947), 240, 248.

## Chapter 10

1. Donald McCaskey, M.D., "The Independent Attitude of the 'Dope User'—and What Are We Going to Do About It," *American Journal of Public Health* 5, no. 4 (April 1915), 335.

2. "Editorial Comment," *American Medicine* 21, no. 11 (November 1915), 799–800.

3. "Poorer Drug Users in Pitiful Plight," *New York Times*, April 15, 1915, p. 7.

4. David F. Musto, *The American Disease: Origins of Narcotic Control* (New York: Oxford University Press, 1999),153.

5. "The Harrison Narcotic Law," *Journal of the American Medical Association* 64, no. 25 (June 19, 1915), 2087; "Sanitary Legislation. Court Decisions," *Public Health Reports* 31, no. 19 (May 12, 1916), 1205; Musto, *American Disease*, 123.

6. "Can the Allies Endure the Strain of Total Abstinence from Alcohol?" *Current Opinion* 58, no. 6 (June 1915), 418.

7. "Editorial Comment," 800.

8. Cornelius F. Collins, "The Drug Evil and the Drug Law," *Monthly Bulletin of the Department of Health, City of New York* 9, no. 1 (January 1919), 23–24.

9. Kurt Hohenstein, "Just What the Doctor Ordered: The Harrison Anti-Narcotic Act, the Supreme Court, and the Federal Regulation of Medical Practice, 1915–1919," *Journal of Supreme Court History* 26, no. 3 (2001), 232, 237.

10. David F. Musto, "Opium, Cocaine and Marijuana in American History," *Scientific American* 265, no. 1 (July 1991), 44.

11. Musto, *American Disease*, 129; Hohenstein, "Just What the Doctor Ordered," 247.

12. Timothy A. Hickman, *The Secret Leprosy of Modern Days: Narcotic Addiction and Cultural Crisis in the United States, 1870–1920* (Amherst: University of Massachusetts Press, 2007), 128–29; *United States v. Jin Fuey Moy*, 241 U.S. 394 (1916).

13. Hohenstein, "Just What the Doctor Ordered," 250, 248.

14. "Expect Good from Drug Law Decision," *Evening Sun* [Baltimore, Md.], March 4, 1919, p. 20; *United States v. Doremus*, 249 U.S. 86 (1919); Hohenstein, "Just What the Doctor Ordered," 248, 251.

15. Stephen R. Kandall, *Substance and Shadow: Women and Addiction in the United States* (Cambridge, Mass.: Harvard University Press, 1999), 77; *United States v. Doremus*, 249 U.S. 86 (1919).

16. Catherine A. Charles, "Doctors and Addicts: A Case Study of Demedicalization" (PhD diss., Columbia University, 1979), 94n2; Musto, "Opium, Cocaine and Marijuana," 44; Musto, *American Disease*, 132; *Webb et al. v. United States*, 249 U.S. 96 (1919).

17. Kandall, *Substance and Shadow*, 77.

18. Charles, "Doctors and Addicts," 100.

19. Musto, *American Disease*, 61, 132.

20. S. Dana Hubbard, M. D., "The New York City Narcotic Clinic and Differing Points of View on Narcotic Addiction," *Monthly Bulletin of the Department of Health, City of New York* 10, no. 2 (February 1920), 45.

21. David F. Musto, ed., *Drugs in America: A Documentary History* (New York: New York University Press, 2002), 262; Sara Graham-Mulhall, "Experiences in Narcotic Drug Control in the State of New York," *New York Medical Journal* 113, no. 3 (January 15, 1921), 107; David T. Courtwright, *Dark Paradise: A History of Opiate Addiction in America* (Cambridge, Mass.: Harvard University Press, 2001), 100.

22. Courtwright, *Dark Paradise*, 100, 111.

23. Ethan A. Nadelmann, "Should We Legalize Drugs? History Answers: Yes," *American Heritage* 44, no. 1 (February–March 1993), 46.

24. Thomas S. Blair, M.D., "The Relation of Drug Addiction to Industry," *Journal of Industrial Hygiene* 1, no. 6 (October 1919), 289.

25. Patrick Renshaw, "The IWW and the Red Scare, 1917–24," *Journal of Contemporary History* 3, no. 4 (October 1968), 67.

26. "Proceedings of the New Orleans Session: Addendum: Report of the Committee on the Narcotic Drug Situation in the United States," *Journal of the American Medical Association* 74, no. 19 (May 8, 1920), 1326–27.

27. "Wants New Laws for Drug Traffic," *New York Times*, November 28, 1917, p. 20.

28. United States Internal Revenue, Treasury Department, *Traffic in Narcotic Drugs: Report of Special Committee of Investigation Appointed March 25, 1918, by the Secretary of the Treasury* (Washington, D. C.: Government Printing Office, 1919), 22.

29. Collins, "The Drug Evil and the Drug Law," 2.

30. Charles, "Doctors and Addicts," 101.

31. William H. James and Stephen L. Johnson, *Doin' Drugs: Patterns of African American Addiction* (Austin: University of Texas Press, 1996), 80.

32. Musto, *American Disease*, 139.

33. Susan L. Speaker, "'The Struggle of Mankind Against Its Deadliest Foe': Themes of Counter-Subversion in Anti-Narcotic Campaigns, 1920–1940," *Journal of Social History* 34, no. 3 (Spring 2001), 594; Jill Jonnes, *Hep-Cats, Narcs, and Pipe Dreams: A History of America's Romance with Illegal Drugs* (Baltimore: Johns Hopkins University Press, 1999), 53.

34. S. Dana Hubbard, "Municipal Narcotic Dispensaries," *Public Health Reports* 35, no. 13 (March 26, 1920), 771.

35. Jill Jonnes, "The Rise of the Modern Addict," *American Journal of Public Health* 85, no. 8 (August 1995), 1159.

36. Hubbard, "The New York City Narcotic Clinic and Differing Points of View," 34.

37. Musto, *American Disease*, 148; Charles, "Doctors and Addicts," 141.

38. Courtwright, *Dark Paradise*, 127–28.

39. United States Internal Revenue, Treasury Department, *Traffic in Narcotic Drugs*, 19.

40. Quoted in Graham-Mulhall, "Experiences in Narcotic Drug Control," 110.

41. Graham-Mulhall, "Experiences in Narcotic Drug Control," 108–9.

42. Dr. C. E. Terry, "Drug Addictions, a Public Health Problem," *American Journal of Public Health* 4, no. 1 (January 1914), 31, 35.

43. McCaskey, "The Independent Attitude of the 'Dope User,'" 336; Graham-Mulhall, "Experiences in Narcotic Drug Control," 107.

44. Elizabeth Fee, "Charles E. Terry (1878–1945): Early Campaigner Against Drug Addiction," *American Journal of Public Health* 101, no. 3 (March 2011), 451; Charles E. Terry, M. D., "Narcotic Drug Addiction and Rational Administration," *American Medicine* 26, no. 1 (January 1920), 33–34; Charles, "Doctors and Addicts," 64–65.

45. Charles, "Doctors and Addicts," 136–37, 129.

46. Thos. S. Blair, "Making the Narcotic Laws Help the Doctor and Not Hinder Him in His Work," *American Medicine* (July 1920), 376.

47. "State Rights, State Duties, and the Harrison Narcotic Law," *Journal of the American Medical Association* 67, no. 1 (July 1, 1916), 37–38.

48. Charles, "Doctors and Addicts," 100.

49. Hubbard, "The New York City Narcotic Clinic and Differing Points of View," 43.

50. "Proceedings of the New Orleans Session," 1326.

51. Musto, *American Disease*, 84, 83.

52. Solomon H. Snyder, "Opiate Receptors and Internal Opiates," *Scientific American* 236, no. 3 (March 1977), 53.

53. Charles, "Doctors and Addicts," 123.

54. Marcus Aurin, "Chasing the Dragon: The Cultural Metamorphosis of Opium in the United States, 1825–1935," *Medical Anthropology Quarterly* 14, no. 3 (September 2000), 436.

55. U.S. Congress. Senate. *Illicit Narcotics Traffic, New York, N. Y. Hearings Before the Subcommittee on Improvements in the Federal Criminal Code of the Committee on the Judiciary, United States*

*Senate, 84th Congress, 1st session, on the Causes, Treatment, and Rehabilitation of Drug Addicts, Pursuant to S. Res. 67. September 19, 20, and 21, 1955, Part 5* (Washington, D. C.: Government Printing Office, 1956), 1957.

56. "Drug Habits," *Youth's Companion* 93, no. 50 (December 11, 1919), 716.

57. United States Internal Revenue, Treasury Department, *Traffic in Narcotic Drugs*, 24.

58. Courtwright, *Dark Paradise*, 126.

59. Lucius P. Brown, "Enforcement of the Tennessee Anti-Narcotics Law," *American Journal of Public Health* 5, no. 4 (April 1915), 333.

60. United States Internal Revenue, Treasury Department, *Traffic in Narcotic Drugs*, 22.

61. *Journal of the Assembly of the State of New York*, 140th sess. 3 (Albany: J. B. Lyon, 1917), 3445–49, 3451, 3452.

62. Charles, "Doctors and Addicts," 102, 105; Musto, *American Disease*, 84.

63. Louis Vyhnanek, "'Muggles,' 'Inchy,' and 'Mud': Illegal Drugs in New Orleans During the 1920s," *Louisiana History* 22, no. 3 (July 1981), 272–73.

64. Erich Goode, *Drugs in American Society* (New York: McGraw-Hill, 1989), 234. Emphasis in original.

65. Theodore H. Price and Richard Spillane, "The Commissioner of Internal Revenue as a Policeman," *Outlook* (November 27, 1918), 505.

66. Richard Davenport-Hines, *The Pursuit of Oblivion: A Global History of Narcotics* (New York: W. W. Norton, 2002), 17.

67. United States Internal Revenue, Treasury Department, *Traffic in Narcotic Drugs*, 7, 20.

68. Price and Spillane, "The Commissioner of Internal Revenue as a Policeman," 504.

69. "Habit-Forming Drugs," *Outlook* 110, no. 1 (May 5, 1915), 8–9.

70. Frederick R. Bechdolt, "The Hydra's Heads," *Sunset* 46, no. 4 (April 1921), 25.

71. Hickman, *Secret Leprosy of Modern Days*, 130, 10. Emphases in original.

72. United States Internal Revenue, Treasury Department, *Traffic in Narcotic Drugs*, 23.

73. S. Dana Hubbard, M.D., "Some Fallacies Regarding Narcotic Drug Addiction," *Journal of the American Medical Association* 74, no. 21 (May 22, 1920), 1439.

74. "Proceedings of the New Orleans Session," 1325–26.

75. Lawrence Kolb, M.D., "Pleasure and Deterioration from Narcotic Addiction," *Mental Hygiene* 9 (October 1925), 712–13.

76. "Solving the Narcotic Problem," *Druggists Circular* 67, no. 4 (April 1923), 141; Joseph F. Spillane, *Cocaine: From Medical Marvel to Modern Menace in the United States, 1884–1920* (Baltimore, Md.: Johns Hopkins University Press, 2002), 103.

77. C. B. Pearson, M.D., "Is Morphine 'Happy Dust' to the Addict?" *Medical Council* 23, no. 12 (December 1918), 919, 921.

78. Terry, "Narcotic Drug Addiction and Rational Administration," 34.

79. Gilbert G. Weigle, "Cupid Guides Addicts' Way to New Life," *San Francisco Examiner*, October 19, 1920, p. 5; Jim Baumohl, "The 'Dope Fiend's Paradise' Revisited: Notes from Research in Progress on Drug Law Enforcement in San Francisco, 1875–1915," *Drinking and Drug Practices Surveyor* 24 (June 1992), 4.

80. Blair, "The Relation of Drug Addiction to Industry," 285–86.

81. *Oxford English Dictionary*, s.v. "psychopath" (n. 2), updated September 2007, https://www-oed-com.proxy-tu.researchport.umd.edu/view/Entry/153920?redirected From=psychopath#eid.

82. Kolb, "Pleasure and Deterioration," 699, 701; Robert B. Livingston, M.D., ed., *Narcotic Drug Addiction Problems* (Washington, D.C.: Government Printing Office, 1963), 45; Courtwright, *Dark Paradise*, 132.

83. Kolb, "Pleasure and Deterioration," 705.

84. Douglas Clark Kinder, "Shutting Out the Evil: Nativism and Narcotics Control in the United States," *Journal of Policy History* 3, no. 4 (October 1991), 118–22.

85. "Senate Votes Stiffer Dope Penalties," *Los Angeles Times*, June 8, 1953, p. 6; Matthew D. Lassiter, "Impossible Criminals: The Suburban Imperatives of America's War on Drugs," *Journal of American History* 102, no. 1 (June 2015), 127, 129, 133, 135–36.

86. Julilly Kohler-Hausmann, "'The Attila the Hun Law': New York's Rockefeller Drug Laws and the Making of a Punitive State," *Journal of Social History* 44, no. 1 (Fall 2010), 71, 75–76.

87. Jessica Neptune, "Harshest in the Nation: The Rockefeller Drug Laws and the Widening Embrace of Punitive Politics," *Social History of Alcohol & Drugs* 26, no. 1 (Summer 2012), 185.

88. Quoted in Susan N. Herman, "Measuring Culpability by Measuring Drugs? Three Reasons to Reevaluate the Rockefeller Drug Laws," *Albany Law Review* 63, no. 3 (2000), 781; Neptune, "Harshest in the Nation," 184.

89. Kohler-Hausmann, " 'The Attila the Hun Law,' " 83.

90. Herman, "Measuring Culpability by Measuring Drugs?" 782.

91. Neptune, "Harshest in the Nation," 182, 185.

92. Kohler-Hausmann, " 'The Attila the Hun Law,' " 88.

93. Neptune, "Harshest in the Nation," 175.

94. C. Gerald Fraser, "Harlem Response Mixed," *New York Times* (January 5, 1973), 38.

95. LaJuana Davis, "Rock, Powder, Sentencing—Making Disparate Impact Evidence Relevant in Crack Cocaine Sentencing," *Journal of Gender, Race, and Justice* 14, no. 2 (Spring 2011), 382, 384, 385, 388–89.

96. Troy Duster, "Pattern, Purpose, and Race in the Drug War: The Crisis of Credibility in Criminal Justice," in Craig Reinarman and Harry G. Levine, eds., *Crack in America: Demon Drugs and Social Justice* (Berkeley: University of California Press, 1997), 265, 261–62, 282.

97. Katharine A. Neill, "Tough on Drugs: Law and Order Dominance and the Neglect of Public Health in U.S. Drug Policy," *World Medical & Health Policy* 6, no. 4 (December 2014), 387–88.

98. Katharine Q. Seelye, "In Heroin Crisis, White Families Seek Gentler War on Drugs," *New York Times*, October 30, 2015.

99. Michael Shaw, "Photos Reveal Media's Softer Tone on Opioid Crisis," *Columbia Journalism Review* (July 26, 2017), https://www.cjr.org/criticism/opioid-crisis-photos.php?link.

100. "The Opium Dens," *San Francisco Chronicle*, November 16, 1875, p. 3.

101. Michael J. Hayde, *My Name's Friday: The Unauthorized but True Story of* Dragnet *and the Films of Jack Webb* (Nashville, Tenn.: Cumberland House, 2001), 18–19, 23–24.

102. *Dragnet*, season 2, episode 4, "The Big Seventeen," written by James E. Moser, directed by Jack Webb, aired November 6, 1952.

103. Matthew D. Lassiter, "Pushers, Victims, and the Lost Innocence of White Suburbia: California's War on Narcotics During the 1950s," *Journal of Urban History* 41, no. 5 (September 2015), 787, 788, 797, 798.

104. "Can't Take Care of Themselves," *Colored American* (New York, N. Y.), March 15, 1838, p. 30.

105. "Our Brethren in the Free States," *Colored American* (New York, N. Y.), April 22, 1837.

106. Jonathan Rothwell, "How the War on Drugs Damages Black Social Mobility," Brookings Institution, September 30, 2014, https://www.brookings.edu/blog/social-mobility-memos/2014/09/30/how-the-war-on-drugs-damages-black-social-mobility/; "Rates of Drug Use and Sales, by Race; Rates of Drug Related Criminal Justice Measures, by Race," Hamilton Project, Brookings Institution, last modified October 21, 2016, https://www.hamiltonproject.org/charts/rates_of_drug_use_and_sales_by_race_rates_of_drug_relat ed_criminal_justice.

107. Michael L. Rosino and Matthew W. Hughey, "The War on Drugs, Racial Meanings, and Structural Racism: A Holistic and Reproductive Approach," *American Journal of Economics & Sociology* 77, no. 3/4 (May–September 2018), 871, 881, 868, 878, 875; Lassiter, "Impossible Criminals," 127.

# BIBLIOGRAPHY

## Secondary Sources

Abel, Ernest L. *Marihuana: The First Twelve Thousand Years.* New York: Plenum Press, 1980.

Ahmad, Diana L. *The Opium Debate and Chinese Exclusion Laws in the Nineteenth-Century American West.* Reno: University of Nevada Press, 2007.

Alatas, Syed Hussein. *The Myth of the Lazy Native: A Study of the Image of the Malays, Filipinos and Javanese from the 16th to the 20th Century and Its Function in the Ideology of Colonial Capitalism.* London: Frank Cass, 1977.

Ambrose, Stephen E. *Nothing Like It in the World: The Men Who Built the Transcontinental Railroad, 1863–1869.* New York: Simon & Schuster, 2000.

Armstrong, David, and Elizabeth Metzger Armstrong. *The Great American Medicine Show: Being an Illustrated History of Hucksters, Healers, Health Evangelists and Heroes from Plymouth Rock to the Present.* New York: Prentice Hall, 1991.

Baumler, Alan, ed. *Modern China and Opium: A Reader.* Ann Arbor: University of Michigan Press, 2001.

Beidler, Anne E. *The Addiction of Mary Todd Lincoln.* Seattle: Coffeetown Press, 2009.

Belenko, Stephen R., ed. *Drugs and Drug Policy in America: A Documentary History.* Westport, Conn.: Greenwood Press, 2000.

Berridge, Virginia. *Demons: Our Changing Attitudes to Alcohol, Tobacco, and Drugs.* Oxford: Oxford University Press, 2013.

Berridge, Virginia, and Griffith Edwards. *Opium and the People: Opiate Use in Nineteenth-Century England.* New Haven, Conn.: Yale University Press, 1987.

Booth, Martin. *Cannabis: A History.* New York: St. Martin's Press, 2003.

Booth, Martin. *Opium: A History.* New York: St. Martin's Griffin, 1996.

Bordman, Gerald, and Thomas S. Hischak. *The Oxford Companion to American Theatre.* New York: Oxford University Press, 2004.

Breen, Benjamin. *The Age of Intoxication: Origins of the Global Drug Trade.* Philadelphia: University of Pennsylvania Press, 2019.

Campbell, James Dykes. *Samuel Taylor Coleridge: A Narrative of the Events of His Life.* London: Macmillan and Co., 1896.

Campos, Isaac. *Home Grown: Marijuana and the Origins of Mexico's War on Drugs.* Chapel Hill: University of North Carolina Press, 2012.

Chapman, Allan. *Physicians, Plagues and Progress: The History of Western Medicine from Antiquity to Antibiotics.* Oxford: Lion Books, 2016.

Clinton, Catherine. *The Plantation Mistress: Woman's World in the Old South.* New York: Pantheon Books, 1982.

Cobb, Paul M. *The Race for Paradise: An Islamic History of the Crusades*. New York: Oxford University Press, 2014.

Coetzee, J. M. *White Writing: On the Culture of Letters in South Africa*. New Haven, Conn.: Yale University Press, 1988.

Cole, Juan. *Napoleon's Egypt: Invading the Middle East*. New York: Palgrave Macmillan, 2008.

Collier, Christopher, and James Lincoln Collier. *Decision in Philadelphia: The Constitutional Convention of 1787*. New York: Ballantine Books, 1986.

Courtwright, David T. *The Age of Addiction: How Bad Habits Became Big Business*. Cambridge, Mass.: Belknap Press of Harvard University Press, 2019.

Courtwright, David T. *Dark Paradise: A History of Opiate Addiction in America*. Cambridge, Mass.: Harvard University Press, 2001.

Courtwright, David T. *Forces of Habit: Drugs and the Making of the Modern World*. Cambridge, Mass.: Harvard University Press, 2002.

Dabney, Richard Heath. *John Randolph: A Character Sketch*. Chicago: University Association, 1898.

Daftary, Farhad. *The Assassin Legends: Myths of the Isma'ilis*. London: I. B. Tauris, 1994.

Daftary, Farhad. *Historical Dictionary of the Ismailis*. Lanham, Md.: Scarecrow Press, 2012.

Daftary, Farhad. *The Ismā'īlīs: Their History and Doctrines*. Cambridge: Cambridge University Press, 2007.

Davenport-Hines, Richard. *The Pursuit of Oblivion: A Global History of Narcotics*. New York: W. W. Norton, 2002.

Davidson, Cathy N. *Revolution and the Word: The Rise of the Novel in America*. New York: Oxford University Press, 1986.

Davis, Marni. *Jews and Booze: Becoming American in the Age of Prohibition*. New York: New York University Press, 2012.

Dawson, Alexander S. *The Peyote Effect: From the Inquisition to the War on Drugs*. Berkeley: University of California Press, 2018.

Dennett, Tyler. *John Hay: From Poetry to Politics*. New York: Dodd, Mead, 1934.

Derks, Hans. *History of the Opium Problem: The Assault on the East, ca. 1600–1950*. Leiden: Brill, 2012.

Dikötter, Frank, Lars Laamann, and Zhou Xun. *Narcotic Culture: A History of Drugs in China*. Chicago: University of Chicago Press, 2004.

Dormandy, Thomas. *Opium: Reality's Dark Dream*. New Haven, Conn.: Yale University Press, 2012.

Downs, Jacques M. *The Golden Ghetto: The American Commercial Community at Canton and the Shaping of American China Policy, 1784–1844*. Bethlehem, Pa: Lehigh University Press, 1997.

Downs, Jim. *Sick from Freedom: African-American Illness and Suffering During the Civil War and Reconstruction*. New York: Oxford University Press, 2012.

Dulchinos, Donald P. *Pioneer of Inner Space: The Life of Fitz Hugh Ludlow, Hasheesh Eater*. Brooklyn, N. Y.: Autonomedia, 1998.

Duvall, Chris S. *The African Roots of Marijuana*. Durham, N. C.: Duke University Press, 2019.

East, Robert A. *John Quincy Adams: The Critical Years: 1785–1794*. New York: Bookman, 1962.

Ellis, Joseph J. *Founding Brothers: The Revolutionary Generation*. New York: Vintage Books, 2000.

Estes, J. Worth. *Hall Jackson and the Purple Foxglove: Medical Practice and Research in Revolutionary America, 1760–1820*. Hanover, N. H.: University Press of New England, 1979.

Fay, Peter Ward. *The Opium War, 1840–1842: Barbarians in the Celestial Empire in the Early Part of the Nineteenth Century and the War by Which They Forced Her Gates Ajar*. Chapel Hill: University of North Carolina Press, 1998.

Finnie, David H. *Pioneers East: The Early American Experience in the Middle East*. Cambridge, Mass.: Harvard University Press, 1967.

Flexner, James Thomas. *States Dyckman: American Loyalist*. Boston: Little, Brown, 1980.

Floyd, Margaret Henderson. *Architecture After Richardson: Regionalism Before Modernism*. Chicago: University of Chicago Press, 1994.

Foxcroft, Louise. *The Making of Addiction: The 'Use and Abuse' of Opium in Nineteenth-Century Britain*. Burlington, Vt.: Ashgate, 2007.

Genovese, Eugene D. *Roll, Jordan, Roll: The World the Slaves Made*. New York: Vintage, 1976.

Gilfoyle, Timothy J. *A Pickpocket's Tale: The Underworld of Nineteenth-Century New York*. New York: W. W. Norton, 2006.

Goldberg, Jeff, and Dean Latimer. *Flowers in the Blood: The Story of Opium*. New York: Skyhorse, 2014.

Goldman, Marion S. *Gold Diggers and Silver Miners: Prostitution and Social Life on the Comstock Lode*. Ann Arbor: University of Michigan Press, c. 1981.

Goldsmith, Margaret. *The Trail of Opium: The Eleventh Plague*. London: Robert Hale, 1939.

Goldstein, Jonathan. *Philadelphia and the China Trade, 1682–1846: Commercial, Cultural, and Attitudinal Effects*. University Park: Pennsylvania State University Press, 1978.

Goode, Erich. *Drugs in American Society*. New York: McGraw-Hill, 1989.

Goodwin, Lorine Swainston. *The Pure Food, Drink, and Drug Crusaders, 1879–1914*. Jefferson, N. C.: McFarland, 2006.

Greenberg, Michael. *British Trade and the Opening of China 1800–42*. Cambridge: Cambridge University Press, 1969.

Grob, Gerald N. *Mental Institutions in America: Social Policy to 1875*. London: Routledge, 2009.

Gruen, J. Philip. *Manifest Destinations: Cities and Tourists in the Nineteenth-Century American West*. Norman: University of Oklahoma Press, 2014.

Haddad, John R. *America's First Adventure in China: Trade, Treaties, Opium, and Salvation*. Philadelphia: Temple University Press, 2013.

Hahn, Barbara. *Making Tobacco Bright: Creating an American Commodity, 1617–1937*. Baltimore, Md.: Johns Hopkins University Press, 2011.

Haller, John S. Jr., and Robin M. Haller. *The Physician and Sexuality in Victorian America*. Urbana: University of Illinois Press, 1974.

Hawthorne, Julian. *Nathaniel Hawthorne and His Wife: A Biography*. 2 vols. Boston: James R. Osgood and Company, 1885.

Hayde, Michael J. *My Name's Friday: The Unauthorized but True Story of Dragnet and the Films of Jack Webb*. Nashville, Tenn.: Cumberland House, 2001.

Hayter, Alethea. *Opium and the Romantic Imagination*. Berkeley: University of California Press, 1968.

Helmer, John. *Drugs and Minority Oppression*. New York: Seabury Press, 1975.

Herndl, Diane Price. *Invalid Women: Figuring Feminine Illness in American Fiction and Culture, 1840–1940*. Chapel Hill: University of North Carolina Press, 1993.

Hickman, Timothy A. *The Secret Leprosy of Modern Days: Narcotic Addiction and Cultural Crisis in the United States, 1870–1920*. Amherst: University of Massachusetts Press, 2007.

Hoffman, Ronald, and Sally D. Mason. *Princes of Ireland, Planters of Maryland: A Carroll Saga, 1500–1782*. Chapel Hill: University of North Carolina Press, 2000.

Holmes, Richard. *Coleridge: Darker Reflections, 1804–1834*. New York: Pantheon Books, 1998.

Holmes, Richard. *Coleridge: Early Visions, 1772–1804*. New York: Pantheon Books, 1989.

Isenberg, Nancy. *Fallen Founder: The Life of Aaron Burr*. New York: Penguin, 2007.

James, Lawrence. *Raj: The Making and Unmaking of British India*. New York: St. Martin's Griffin, 1997.

James, William H., and Stephen L. Johnson. *Doin' Drugs: Patterns of African American Addiction*. Austin: University of Texas Press, 1996.

Johnson, David. *John Randolph of Roanoke*. Baton Rouge: Louisiana State University Press, 2012.

Jonnes, Jill. *Hep-Cats, Narcs, and Pipe Dreams: A History of America's Romance with Illegal Drugs*. Baltimore, Md.: Johns Hopkins University Press, 1999.

Kamieński, Lukasz. *Shooting Up: A Short History of Drugs and War*. New York: Oxford University Press, 2016.

Kandall, Stephen R. *Substance and Shadow: Women and Addiction in the United States*. Cambridge, Mass.: Harvard University Press, 1999.

Karch, Steven B. *A Brief History of Cocaine*. Boca Raton, Fla.: CRC Press, 1998.

Kim, Diana S. *Empires of Vice: The Rise of Opium Prohibition Across Southeast Asia*. Princeton, N. J.: Princeton University Press, 2020.

Kirschke, James J. *Gouverneur Morris: Author, Statesman, and Man of the World.* New York: St. Martin's Press, 2005.

Kleiman, Mark A. R., Jonathan P. Caulkins, and Angela Hawken. *Drugs and Drug Policy: What Everyone Needs to Know.* New York: Oxford University Press, 2011.

Kracht, Benjamin R. *Religious Revitalization Among the Kiowas: The Ghost Dance, Peyote, and Christianity.* Lincoln: University of Nebraska Press, 2018.

Kremers, Edward, George Urdang, and Glenn Sonnedecker. *Kremers and Urdang's History of Pharmacy.* 4th ed. Madison, Wisc.: American Institute of the History of Pharmacy, 1976.

Kulikoff, Allan. *Tobacco and Slaves: The Development of Southern Cultures in the Chesapeake, 1680– 1800.* Chapel Hill: University of North Carolina Press, 1986.

Layton, Thomas N. *The Voyage of the 'Frolic': New England Merchants and the Opium Trade.* Stanford, Calif.: Stanford University Press, 1997.

Lefebure, Molly. *Samuel Taylor Coleridge: A Bondage of Opium.* Briarcliff Manor, N. Y.: Stein & Day, 1974.

Lewin, Louis. *Phantastica.* Rochester, Vt.: Park Street Press, 1998.

Lewy, Jonathan. *Drugs in Germany and the United States, 1919–1945: The Birth of Two Addictions.* Baden-Baden, Germany: Nomos Verlagsgesellschaft, 2017.

Livingston, Robert B., ed. *Narcotic Drug Addiction Problems.* Washington, D. C.: Government Printing Office, 1963.

Logan, Peter Melville. *Nerves and Narratives: A Cultural History of Hysteria in Nineteenth-Century British Prose.* Berkeley: University of California Press, 1997.

Lowe, Lisa. *The Intimacies of Four Continents.* Durham, N. C.: Duke University Press, 2015.

Löwy, Michael, and Robert Sayre. *Romanticism Against the Tide of Modernity.* Translated by Catherine Porter. Durham, N. C.: Duke University Press, 2001.

Markel, Howard. *An Anatomy of Addiction: Sigmund Freud, William Halsted, and the Miracle Drug Cocaine.* New York: Vintage, 2012.

Martin, Scott C. *Devil of the Domestic Sphere: Temperance, Gender, and Middle-Class Ideology, 1800– 1860.* DeKalb: Northern Illinois University Press, 2008.

McCullough, David. *John Adams.* New York: Simon & Schuster, 2001.

McMahon, Keith. *The Fall of the God of Money: Opium Smoking in Nineteenth-Century China.* Lanham, Md.: Rowman & Littlefield, 2002.

McMillen, Sally G. *Motherhood in the Old South: Pregnancy, Childbirth, and Infant Rearing.* Baton Rouge: Louisiana State University Press, 1990.

Metrick-Chen, Lenore. *Collecting Objects/Excluding People: Chinese Subjects and American Visual Culture, 1830–1900.* Albany: State University of New York Press, 2012.

Miller, Stuart Creighton. *The Unwelcome Immigrant: The American Image of the Chinese, 1785– 1882.* Berkeley: University of California Press, 1969.

Morgan, H. Wayne. *Drugs in America: A Social History, 1800–1980.* Syracuse, N. Y.: Syracuse University Press, 1981.

Morgan, H. Wayne, ed. *Yesterday's Addicts: American Society and Drug Abuse, 1865–1920.* Norman: University of Oklahoma Press, 1974.

Mortimer, W. Golden. *Peru: History of Coca, "The Divine Plant" of the Incas.* New York: J. H. Vail, 1901.

Mott, Frank Luther. *A History of American Magazines, 1741–1850.* Cambridge, Mass.: Harvard University Press, 1966.

Murdock, Catherine Gilbert. *Domesticating Drink: Women, Men, and Alcohol in America, 1870– 1940.* Baltimore, Md.: Johns Hopkins University Press, 1998.

Musto, David F. *The American Disease: Origins of Narcotic Control.* New York: Oxford University Press, 1999.

Musto, David F., ed. *Drugs in America: A Documentary History.* New York: New York University Press, 2002.

Nagel, Paul C. *The Lees of Virginia: Seven Generations of an American Family.* New York: Oxford University Press, 1990.

Nance, Susan. *How the Arabian Nights Inspired the American Dream, 1790–1935*. Chapel Hill, N. C.: University of North Carolina Press, 2009.

Norling, Lisa. *Captain Ahab Had a Wife: New England Women and the Whalefishery, 1720–1870.* Chapel Hill: University of North Carolina Press, 2000.

O'Neal, Tatum. *A Paper Life.* New York: Harper Entertainment, 2004.

Osborn, Matthew Warner. *Rum Maniacs: Alcoholic Insanity in the Early American Republic.* Chicago: University of Chicago Press, 2014.

Ostrowsky, Michael K. *Self-Medication and Violent Behavior.* El Paso, Tex.: LFB Scholarly Publishing LLC, 2009.

Padwa, Howard. *Social Poison: The Culture and Politics of Opiate Control in Britain and France, 1821–1926.* Baltimore, Md.: Johns Hopkins University Press, 2012.

Palmer, Cynthia, and Michael Horowitz, eds. *Shaman Woman, Mainline Lady: Women's Writings on the Drug Experience.* New York: Quill, 1982.

Palmer, Cynthia, and Michael Horowitz, eds. *Sisters of the Extreme: Women Writing on the Drug Experience.* Rochester, Vt.: Park Street Press, 2000.

Pendergrast, Mark. *For God, Country, and Coca-Cola: The Unauthorized History of the Great American Soft Drink and the Company That Makes It.* New York: Charles Scribner's Sons, 1993.

Perrine, Daniel M. *The Chemistry of Mind-Altering Drugs: History, Pharmacology, and Cultural Context.* Washington, D. C.: American Chemical Society, 1996.

Phillips, Mackenzie. *High on Arrival: A Memoir.* New York: Gallery Books, 2009.

Pratt, Mary Louise. *Imperial Eyes: Travel Writing and Transculturation.* London: Routledge, 1992.

Ricci, James V. *The Development of Gynæcological Surgery and Instruments.* San Francisco: Norman Publishing, 1990.

Rimner, Steffen. *Opium's Long Shadow: From Asian Revolt to Global Drug Control.* Cambridge, Mass.: Harvard University Press, 2018.

Rorabaugh, W. J. *The Alcoholic Republic: An American Tradition.* New York: Oxford University Press, 1979.

Rosenberg, Charles E. *The Cholera Years: The United States in 1832, 1849, and 1866.* Chicago: University of Chicago Press, 1987.

Rosenthal, Franz. *The Herb: Hashish Versus Medieval Muslim Society.* Leiden: E. J. Brill, 1971.

Sabin, Edwin L. *Building the Pacific Railway.* Philadelphia: J. B. Lippincott, 1919.

Said, Edward W. *Orientalism.* New York: Vintage Books, 1978.

Schaefer, Eric. *"Bold! Daring! Shocking! True!": A History of Exploitation Films, 1919–1959.* Durham, N. C.: Duke University Press, 1999.

Schneider, Elisabeth. *Coleridge, Opium and Kubla Khan.* Chicago: University of Chicago Press, 1953.

Seaburg, Carl, and Stanley Paterson. *Merchant Prince of Boston: Colonel T. H. Perkins, 1764–1854.* Cambridge, Mass.: Harvard University Press, 1971.

Seilhamer, George O. *History of the American Theatre: New Foundations.* Philadelphia: Globe Printing House, 1891.

Seligman, Scott D. *The First Chinese American: The Remarkable Life of Wong Chin Foo.* Hong Kong: University of Hong Kong Press, 2013.

Siegel, Frederick F. *The Roots of Southern Distinctiveness: Tobacco and Society in Danville, Virginia, 1780–1865.* Chapel Hill: University of North Carolina Press, 1987.

Sismondo, Christine. *America Walks into a Bar: A Spirited History of Taverns and Saloons, Speakeasies and Grog Shops.* New York: Oxford University Press, 2011.

Smith, Rev. George G. *The Life and Letters of James Osgood Andrew.* Nashville, Tenn.: Southern Methodist Publishing House, 1882.

Smith-Rosenberg, Carroll. *Disorderly Conduct: Visions of Gender in Victorian America.* New York: Oxford University Press, 1985.

Smithers, William W. *The Life of John Lofland, "The Milford Bard."* Philadelphia: Wallace M. Leonard, 1894.

Spillane, Joseph F. *Cocaine: From Medical Marvel to Modern Menace in the United States, 1884–1920.* Baltimore, Md.: Johns Hopkins University Press, 2002.

Spurr, David. *The Rhetoric of Empire: Colonial Discourse in Journalism, Travel Writing, and Imperial Administration.* Durham, N. C.: Duke University Press, 1993.

Sterling, Dorothy, ed. *We Are Your Sisters: Black Women in the Nineteenth Century.* New York: W. W. Norton, 1984.

Stern, Madeleine B. *Louisa May Alcott: A Biography.* Lebanon, N. H.: Northeastern University Press, 1996.

Stewart, Omer C. *Peyote Religion: A History.* Norman: University of Oklahoma Press, 1987.

Sturm-Lind, Lisa. *Actors of Globalization: New York Merchants in Global Trade, 1784–1812.* Leiden: Brill, 2018.

Sullivan, Mark. *Our Times: The United States, 1900–1925.* Vol. 2, *America Finding Herself.* New York: C. Scribner's Sons, 1927.

Swan, Daniel C. *Peyote Religious Art: Symbols of Faith and Belief.* Jackson: University Press of Mississippi, 1999.

Swanson, Drew A. *A Golden Weed: Tobacco and Environment in the Piedmont South.* New Haven, Conn.: Yale University Press, 2014.

Takaki, Ronald. *Iron Cages: Race and Culture in 19th-Century America.* New York: Oxford University Press, 1990.

Taliaferro, John. *All the Great Prizes: The Life of John Hay, from Lincoln to Roosevelt.* New York: Simon and Schuster, 2013.

Tate, Cassandra. *Cigarette Wars: The Triumph of "The Little White Slaver."* New York: Oxford University Press, 1999.

Terkel, Studs. *And They All Sang: Adventures of an Eclectic Disc Jockey.* New York: New Press, 2006.

Terrell, John Upton. *Furs by Astor.* New York: William Morrow, 1963.

Thayer, William Roscoe. *The Life and Letters of John Hay.* Vol. I. Boston: Houghton Mifflin, 1915.

Tice, Patricia M. *Altered States: Alcohol and Other Drugs in America.* Rochester, N. Y.: Strong Museum, 1992.

Trachtenberg, Alan. *The Incorporation of America: Culture and Society in the Gilded Age.* New York: Hill and Wang, 2007.

Tracy, Sarah W., and Caroline Jean Acker, eds. *Altering American Consciousness: The History of Alcohol and Drug Use in the United States, 1800–2000.* Amherst: University of Massachusetts Press, 2004.

Trocki, Carl A. *Opium, Empire and the Global Political Economy: A Study of the Asian Opium Trade, 1750–1950.* London: Routledge, 1999.

Unrau, William E. *White Man's Wicked Water: The Alcohol Trade and Prohibition in Indian Country, 1802–1892.* Lawrence: University Press of Kansas, 1996.

Walker, William O. *Opium and Foreign Policy: The Anglo-American Search for Order in Asia, 1912–1954.* Chapel Hill: University of North Carolina Press, 1991.

Warren, Leonard. *Adele Marion Fielde: Feminist, Social Activist, Scientist.* London: Routledge, 2002.

Wasson, R. Gordon. *Soma: Divine Mushroom of Immortality.* New York: Harcourt Brace Jovanovich, 1968.

White, Richard. *The Republic for Which It Stands: The United States During Reconstruction and the Gilded Age, 1865–1896.* New York: Oxford University Press, 2017.

Wild, Antony. *The East India Company: Trade and Conquest from 1600.* New York: Lyons Press, 2000.

Williamson, Joel. *The Crucible of Race: Black-White Relations in the American South Since Emancipation.* New York: Oxford University Press, 1984.

Zabin, Serena R. *Dangerous Economies: Status and Commerce in Imperial New York.* Philadelphia: University of Pennsylvania Press, 2009.

Zieger, Susan. *Inventing the Addict: Drugs, Race, and Sexuality in Nineteenth-Century British and American Literature.* Amherst: University of Massachusetts Press, 2008.

Zinberg, Norman E. *Drug, Set, and Setting: The Basis for Controlled Intoxicant Use.* New Haven, Conn.: Yale University Press, c.1984.

## Journal Articles

Ackerman, Eron. "Ruling Pleasures and Growing Pains: Drugs and Colonial Expansion in Southern Africa, 1652–1850." Alcohol and Drugs History Society, last modified July 12, 2013, https://alcoholanddrugshistorysociety.org.

Ahmad, Diana L. "The Campaign Against Smoking Opium: Nevada Journalists as Agents of Social Reform, 1875–1882." *Nevada Historical Society Quarterly* 46, no. 4 (December 2003): 243–56.

Ahmad, Diana L. "Opium Smoking, Anti-Chinese Attitudes, and the American Medical Community, 1850–1890." *American Nineteenth Century History* 1, no. 2 (Summer 2000): 53–68.

Ahmad, Diana L. "To Preserve Moral Virtue: Opium Smoking in Nevada and the Pressure for Chinese Exclusion." *Nevada Historical Society Quarterly* 41, no. 3 (September 1998): 141–68.

Auerhahn, Kathleen. "The Split Labor Market and the Origins of Antidrug Legislation in the United States." *Law & Social Inquiry* 24, no. 2 (1999): 411–40.

Aurin, Marcus. "Chasing the Dragon: The Cultural Metamorphosis of Opium in the United States, 1825–1935." *Medical Anthropology Quarterly* 14, no. 3 (September 2000): 414–41.

Aynur, Hatice, and Jan Schmidt. "A Debate Between Opium, Berş, Hashish, Boza, Wine and Coffee; The Use and Perception of Pleasurable Substances Among Ottomans." *Journal of Turkish Studies* 31, no. 1 (2007): 51–117.

Barop, Helena. "Building the 'Opium Evil' Consensus—The International Opium Commission of Shanghai." *Journal of Modern European History* 13, no. 1 (2015): 115–37.

Baumohl, Jim. "The 'Dope Fiend's Paradise' Revisited: Notes from Research in Progress on Drug Law Enforcement in San Francisco, 1875–1915." *Drinking and Drug Practices Surveyor* 24 (June 1992): 3–12.

Beitiks, Mikelis. "'Devilishly Uncomfortable': In the Matter of Sic—The California Supreme Court Strikes a Balance Between Race, Drugs and Government in 1880s California." *California Legal History* 6 (2011): 229–50.

Berglund, Barbara. "Chinatown's Tourist Terrain: Representation and Racialization in Nineteenth-Century San Francisco." *American Studies* 46, no. 2 (Summer 2005): 5–36.

Bloomfield, Susanne George. "'The Boy's Mother': Nineteenth-Century Drug Dependence in the Life of Kate M. Cleary." *Great Plains Quarterly* 20, no. 1 (Winter 2000): 3–18.

Bonnie, Richard J., and Charles H. Whitebread II. "The Forbidden Fruit and the Tree of Knowledge: An Inquiry into the Legal History of American Marijuana Prohibition." *Virginia Law Review* 56, no. 6 (October 1970): 971–1203.

Boulette, Matthew. "On the Inertia of Appetite: Transient Relations from the Chinatown Opium Scene." *American Quarterly* 71, no. 3 (September 2019): 813–34.

Brown, Richard Harvey. "The Opium Trade and Opium Policies in India, China, Britain, and the United States: Historical Comparisons and Theoretical Interpretations." *Asian Journal of Social Science* 30, no. 3 (2002): 623–56.

Bruhn, Jan G., and Bo Holmstedt. "Early Peyote Research: An Interdisciplinary Study." *Economic Botany* 28, no. 4 (October–December 1974): 353–90.

Butrica, James L. "The Medical Use of Cannabis Among the Greeks and Romans." *Journal of Cannabis Therapeutics* 2, no. 2 (2002): 51–70.

Campbell, Brad. "The Making of 'American': Race and Nation in Neurasthenic Discourse." *History of Psychiatry* 18, no. 2 (June 2007): 157–78.

Campos, Isaac. "Mexicans and the Origins of Marijuana Prohibition in the United States: A Reassessment." *Social History of Alcohol & Drugs* 32, no. 1 (December 2018): 6–37.

Caquet, P. E. "Notions of Addiction in the Time of the First Opium War." *Historical Journal* 58, no. 4 (December 2015): 1009–29.

Caric, Ric N. "The Man with the Poker Enters the Room: Delerium Tremens and Popular Culture in Philadelphia, 1828–1850." *Pennsylvania History* 74, no. 4 (Autumn 2007): 452–91.

Carstairs, Catherine. "'The Most Dangerous Drug': Images of African-Americans and Cocaine Use in the Progressive Era." *Left History* 7, no. 1 (May 2000): 46–61.

Chaplin, Joyce E. "Creating a Cotton South in Georgia and South Carolina, 1760–1815." *Journal of Southern History* 57, no. 2 (May 1991): 171–200.

Charles, Robert. "Olyphant and Opium: A Canton Merchant Who 'Just Said "No."'" *International Bulletin of Missionary Research* 16, no. 2 (April 1, 1992): 66–69.

Chepesiuk, Ron. "The United States' War Against Drugs, Its Early Evolution, 1840–1914." *Proceedings of the South Carolina Historical Association* (1999): 89–95.

Chessey, Bob. "El Paso's 1915 Marihuana Ordinance: Myth and Reality." *Password* 58, no. 1 (2014): 27–40.

Çirakman, Asli. "From Tyranny to Despotism: The Enlightenment's Unenlightened Image of the Turks." *International Journal of Middle East Studies* 33, no. 1 (2001): 49–68.

Cohen, Michael M. "Jim Crow's Drug War: Race, Coca Cola, and the Southern Origins of Drug Prohibition." *Southern Cultures* 12, no. 3 (Fall 2006): 55–79.

Courtwright, David. "Opiate Addiction in the American West, 1850–1920." *Journal of the West* 21, no. 3 (July 1982): 23–31.

Courtwright, David T. "The Female Opiate Addict in Nineteenth-Century America." *Essay in Arts and Sciences* 10, no. 2 (March 1982): 161–70.

Courtwright, David T. "The Hidden Epidemic: Opiate Addiction and Cocaine Use in the South, 1860–1920." *Journal of Southern History* 49, no. 1 (February 1983): 57–72.

Courtwright, David T. "Opiate Addiction as a Consequence of the Civil War." *Civil War History* 24, no. 2 (June 1978): 101–11.

Damania, A. B. "The Origin, History, and Commerce of the Opium Poppy (*Papaver somniferum*) in Asia and the United States." *Asian Agri-History* 15, no. 2 (April–June 2011): 109–23.

Davis, LaJuana. "Rock, Powder, Sentencing—Making Disparate Impact Evidence Relevant in Crack Cocaine Sentencing." *Journal of Gender, Race, and Justice* 14, no. 2 (Spring 2011): 375–404.

DeLyser, D. Y., and W. J. Kasper. "Hopped Beer: The Case for Cultivation." *Economic Botany* 48, no. 2 (April–June 1994): 166–70.

Denham, Bryan. "Magazine Journalism in the Golden Age of Muckraking: Patent-Medicine Exposures Before and After the Pure Food and Drug Act of 1906." *Journalism & Communication Monographs* 22, no. 2 (2020): 100–59.

Dickey, Colin. "The Addicted Life of Thomas De Quincey." *Lapham's Quarterly* 6, no. 1 (Winter 2013).

Dikötter, Frank, Lars Laamann, and Zhou Xun. "Narcotic Culture: A Social History of Drug Consumption in China." *British Journal of Criminology* 42, no. 2 (Spring 2002): 317–36.

Dimmock, Matthew. "Faith, Form and Faction: Samuel Purchas's *Purchas His Pilgrimage* (1613)." *Renaissance Studies* 28, no. 2 (April 2014): 262–78.

Donoghue, Keith. "Casualties of War: Criminal Drug Law Enforcement and Its Special Costs for the Poor." *New York University Law Review* 77 (December 2002): 1776–1804.

Downs, Jacques M. "American Merchants and the China Opium Trade, 1800–1840." *Business History Review* 42, no. 4 (Winter 1968): 418–42.

Downs, Jacques M. "Fair Game: Exploitive Role-Myths and the American Opium Trade." *Pacific Historical Review* 41, no. 2 (May 1972): 133–49.

Durand, Jorge, Douglas S. Massey, and Fernando Charvet. "The Changing Geography of Mexican Immigration to the United States: 1910–1996." *Social Science Quarterly* 81, no. 1 (March 2000): 1–15.

du Toit, Brian M. "Man and Cannabis in Africa: A Study of Diffusion." *African Economic History* 1 (Spring 1976): 17–35.

Erickson, Patricia G. "The Law, Social Control, and Drug Policy: Models, Factors, and Processes." *International Journal of the Addictions* 28, no. 12 (1993): 1155–76.

"Evolution of Current Law." *Congressional Digest* (November 2003): 260–61.

Fagan, Abigail. "The Citizen as Self-Abnegating: Othering the Drunkard in the Early Republic." *Amerikastudien/American Studies* 65, no. 4 (2020): 405–26.

Fee, Elizabeth. "Charles E. Terry (1878–1945): Early Campaigner Against Drug Addiction." *American Journal of Public Health* 101, no. 3 (March 2011): 451.

Footman, David. "The Riddle of Hassan II." *History Today* 1, no. 9 (September 1951): 65–70.

Ford, Chandra L., and Nina T. Harawa. "A New Conceptualization of Ethnicity for Social Epidemiologic and Health Equity Research." *Social Science & Medicine* 71, no. 2 (July 2010): 251–58.

Foster, Anne L. "The Philippines, the United States, and the Origins of Global Narcotics Prohibition." *Social History of Alcohol and Drugs* 33, no. 1 (Spring 2019): 13–36.

Foster, Anne L. "Prohibition as Superiority: Policing Opium in South-East Asia, 1898–1925." *International History Review* 22, no. 2 (June 2000): 253–73.

Foster, Jeffrey Clayton. "The Rocky Road to a 'Drug Free Tennessee': A History of the Early Regulation of Cocaine and the Opiates, 1897–1913." *Journal of Social History* 29, no. 3 (Spring 1996): 547–64.

Fryer, Roland G. Jr. "Guess Who's Been Coming to Dinner? Trends in Interracial Marriage over the 20th Century." *Journal of Economic Perspectives* 21, no. 2 (Spring 2007): 71–90.

Fye, W. Bruce. "H. Newell Martin—A Remarkable Career Destroyed by Neurasthenia and Alcoholism." *Journal of the History of Medicine and Allied Sciences* 40, no. 2 (April 1985): 133–66.

Gabriel, Joseph M. "Restricting the Sale of 'Deadly Poisons': Pharmacists, Drug Regulation, and Narratives of Suffering in the Gilded Age." *Journal of the Gilded Age and Progressive Era* 9, no. 3 (July 2010): 313–36.

Gieringer, Dale H. "The Forgotten Origins of Cannabis Prohibition in California." *Contemporary Drug Problems* 26 (Summer 1999): 237–88.

Gonzales, Juan L. Jr. "Asian Indian Immigration Patterns: The Origins of the Sikh Community in California." *International Migration Review* 20, no. 1 (Spring 1986): 40–54.

Gordon, David. "From Rituals of Rapture to Dependence: The Political Economy of Khoikhoi Narcotic Consumption, c. 1487–1870." *South African Historical Journal* 35 (November 1996): 62–88.

Gray, Elizabeth Kelly. "'Whisper to Him the Word "India"': Trans-Atlantic Critics and American Slavery, 1830–1860." *Journal of the Early Republic* 27, no. 3 (Fall 2008): 379–406.

Gray, Welles A. "The Opium Problem." *Annals of the American Academy of Political and Social Science* 122 (November 1925): 148–59.

Griffin, Dick. "Opium Addiction in Chicago: 'The Noblest and the Best Brought Low.'" *Chicago History* 6, no. 2 (July 1977): 107–16.

Griggs, Earl Leslie, and Seymour Teulon Porter. "Samuel Taylor Coleridge and Opium." *Huntington Library Quarterly* 17, no. 4 (August 1954): 357–78.

Guba, David A. "Antoine Isaac Silvestre de Sacy and the Myth of the Hachichins: Orientalizing Hashish in Nineteenth-century France." *Social History of Alcohol and Drugs* 30 (2016): 50–74.

Guerra, Francisco. "Sex and Drugs in the 16th Century." *British Journal of Addiction to Alcohol & Other Drugs* 69, no. 3 (September 1974): 269–90.

Harris, Victoria. "Intoxicating Trends." *History Today* 62, no. 4 (April 2012): 3–4.

Hemphill, Katie M. "'Driven to the Commission of This Crime': Women and Infanticide in Baltimore, 1835–1860." *Journal of the Early Republic* 32, no. 3 (Fall 2012): 437–61.

Herbet, Mariola, and Ewa Jagiełło-Wójtowicz. "Datura Stramonium L.—Its Use over the Ages." *Acta Toxicologica* 14, issno. 1/2 (2006): 5–9.

Herd, Denise A. "Prohibition, Racism and Class Politics in the Post-Reconstruction South." *Journal of Drug Issues* (Winter 1983): 77–94.

Herman, Susan N. "Measuring Culpability by Measuring Drugs? Three Reasons to Reevaluate the Rockefeller Drug Laws." *Albany Law Review* 63, no. 3 (2000): 777–98.

Herndl, Diane Price. "The Invisible (Invalid) Woman: African-American Women, Illness, and Nineteenth-Century Narrative." *Women's Studies* 24, no. 6 (September 1995): 553–72.

Herndon, G. Melvin. "Hemp in Colonial Virginia." *Agricultural History* 37, no. 2 (April 1963): 86–93.

Hess, Albert G. "Deviance Theory and the History of Opiates." *International Journal of the Addictions* 6, no. 4 (December 1971): 585–98.

Hickman, Timothy A. "Drugs and Race in American Culture: Orientalism in the Turn-of-the-Century Discourse of Narcotic Addiction." *American Studies* 41, no. 1 (Spring 2000): 71–91.

Hickman, Timothy A. "'Mania Americana': Narcotic Addiction and Modernity in the United States, 1870–1920." *Journal of American History* 90, no. 4 (March 2004): 1269–94.

Hohenstein, Kurt. "Just What the Doctor Ordered: The Harrison Anti-Narcotic Act, the Supreme Court, and the Federal Regulation of Medical Practice, 1915–1919." *Journal of Supreme Court History* 26, no. 3 (2001): 231–56.

Horrocks, Thomas A. "'The Poor Man's Riches, The Rich Man's Bliss': Regimen, Reform, and the *Journal of Health,* 1829–1833." *Proceedings of the American Philosophical Society* 139, no. 2 (June 1995): 115–34.

Humphreys, Keith. "Thomas de Quincey, Confessions of an English Opium Eater." *Addiction* 99, no. 9 (September 2004): 1221–22.

Imai, Hissei, Yusuke Ogawa, Kiyohito Okumiya, and Kozo Matsubayashi. "Amok: A Mirror of Time and People. A Historical Review of Literature." *History of Psychiatry* 30, no. 1 (March 2019): 38–57.

Jones, James B. Jr. "Selected Aspects of Drug Abuse in Nineteenth- and Early Twentieth-Century Tennessee History, ca. 1830–1920." *West Tennessee Historical Society Papers* 48 (1994): 1–23.

Jones, Jonathan S. "Opium Slavery: Civil War Veterans and Opiate Addiction." *Journal of the Civil War Era* 10, no. 2 (June 2020): 185–212.

Jones, Jonathan S. "Then and Now: How Civil War-Era Doctors Responded to Their Own Opiate Epidemic." *Civil War Monitor,* November 3, 2017. https://www.civilwarmonitor.com/blog/then-and-now-how-civil-war-era-doctors-responded-to-their-own-opiate-epidemic.

Jonnes, Jill. "The Rise of the Modern Addict." *American Journal of Public Health* 85, no. 8 (August 1995): 1157–62.

Jun, Helen H. "Black Orientalism: Nineteenth-Century Narratives of Race and U.S. Citizenship." *American Quarterly* 58, no. 4 (December 2006): 1047–66.

Kalant, H. "Opium Revisited: A Brief Review of Its Nature, Composition, Non-Medical Use and Relative Risks." *Addiction* 92, no. 3 (1997): 267–77.

Katcher, Brian S. "Benjamin Rush's Educational Campaign Against Hard Drinking." *American Journal of Public Health* 83, no. 2 (February 1993): 273–81.

Keely, Karen A. "Sexual Slavery in San Francisco's Chinatown: 'Yellow Peril' and 'White Slavery' in Frank Norris's Early Fiction." *Studies in American Naturalism* 2, no. 2 (Winter 2007): 129–49.

Keire, Mara L. "Dope Fiends and Degenerates: The Gendering of Addiction in the Early Twentieth Century." *Journal of Social History* 31, no. 4 (Summer 1998): 809–22.

Kelley, Sean M. "American Rum, African Consumers, and the Transatlantic Slave Trade." *African Economic History* 46, no. 2 (2018): 1–29.

Kelly, Brian. "No Easy Way Through: Race Leadership and Black Workers at the Nadir." *Labor* 7, no. 3 (Fall 2010): 79–93.

Kerbo, Harold R., and Richard A. Shaffer. "Unemployment and Protest in the United States, 1890–1940: A Methodological Critique and Research Note." *Social Forces* 64, no. 4 (June 1986): 1046–56.

Kinder, Douglas Clark. "Shutting Out the Evil: Nativism and Narcotics Control in the United States." *Journal of Policy History* 3, no. 4 (October 1991): 117–42.

Kohler-Hausmann, Julilly. "'The Attila the Hun Law': New York's Rockefeller Drug Laws and the Making of a Punitive State." *Journal of Social History* 44, no. 1 (Fall 2010): 71–95.

Komel, Mirt. "Re-orientalizing the Assassins in Western Historical-Fiction literature: Orientalism and Self-Orientalism in Bartol's *Alamut*, Tarr's *Alamut*, Boschert's *Assassins of Alamut* and Oden's *Lion of Cairo*." *European Journal of Cultural Studies* 17, no. 5 (2014): 525–48.

Kwakye, Gunnar F., et al. "*Atropa belladonna* Neurotoxicity: Implications to Neurological Disorders." *Food and Chemical Toxicology* 116 (2018): 346–53.

La Brack, Bruce. "Occupational Specialization Among Rural California Sikhs: The Interplay of Culture and Economics." *Amerasia Journal* 9, no. 2 (1982): 29–56.

Laliberte, Daniel A. "Hot on the Opium Smugglers' Trail." *Naval History* 30, no. 5 (October 2016): 40–46.

Lassiter, Matthew D. "Impossible Criminals: The Suburban Imperatives of America's War on Drugs." *Journal of American History* 102, no. 1 (June 2015): 126–40.

Lassiter, Matthew D. "Pushers, Victims, and the Lost Innocence of White Suburbia: California's War on Narcotics During the 1950s." *Journal of Urban History* 41, no. 5 (September 2015): 787–807.

Lazich, Michael C. "American Missionaries and the Opium Trade in Nineteenth-Century China." *Journal of World History* 17, no. 2 (June 2006): 197–223.

Lee, Harry F., and David D. Zhang. "A Tale of Two Population Crises in Recent Chinese History." *Climatic Change* 116 (2013): 285–308. https://doi.org/10.1007/s10584-012-0490-9.

Leshner, Alan I. "Addiction Is a Brain Disease, and It Matters." *Science* 278 (October 3, 1997): 45–47.

Levine, Harry Gene. "The Discovery of Addiction: Changing Conceptions of Habitual Drunkenness in America." *Journal of Studies on Alcohol* 39, no. 1 (1978): 143–74.

Lewy, Jonathan. "The Army Disease: Drug Addiction and the Civil War." *War in History* 21, no. 1 (January 2014): 102–19.

Lin, Man-Houng. "Late Qing Perceptions of Native Opium." *Harvard Journal of Asiatic Studies* 64, no. 1 (June 2004): 117–44.

Ling, Huping. "'Hop Alley': Myth and Reality of the St. Louis Chinatown, 1860s–1930s." *Journal of Urban History* 28, no. 2 (January 2002): 184–219.

Lister, Florence C., and Robert H. Lister. "Chinese Sojourners in Territorial Prescott." *Journal of the Southwest* 31, no. 1 (Spring 1989): 1–111.

Lloyd, James M. "Fighting Redlining and Gentrification in Washington, D.C.: The Adams-Morgan Organization and Tenant Right to Purchase." *Journal of Urban History* 42, no. 6 (November 2016): 1091–1109.

Lloyd, Margaret H. "The Forgotten Victims of the War on Drugs: An Analysis of U.S. Drug Policy and Reform from a Child Well-Being Perspective." *Journal of Policy Practice* 14, no. 2 (April–June 2015): 114–38.

Lui, Mary Ting Yi. "Saving Young Girls from Chinatown: White Slavery and Woman Suffrage, 1910–1920." *Journal of the History of Sexuality* 18, no. 3 (September 2009): 393–417.

Lynn, Vanessa. "Dialogues of the War on Drugs: Towards Restorative Reentry Initiatives." *Contemporary Justice Review* 21, no. 2 (June 2018): 159–84.

Mark, Gregory Yee. "Opium in America and the Chinese." *Chinese America: History and Perspectives* (1997): 61–74.

Marks, David F. "IQ Variations Across Time, Race, and Nationality: An Artifact of Differences in Literacy Skills." *Psychological Reports* 106, no. 3 (June 2010): 643–64.

Martin, Scott C. "'He Is an Excellent Doctor if Called when Sober': Temperance, Physicians and the American Middle Class, 1800–1860." *Social History of Alcohol and Drugs* 24, no. 1 (Winter 2010): 20–36.

Materson, Lisa G., and Joe William Trotter Jr., "African American Urban Electoral Politics in the Age of Jim Crow." *Journal of Urban History* 44, no. 2 (March 2018): 123–33.

McCarthy, Raymond G. "Alcoholism: Attitudes and Attacks, 1775–1935." *Annals of the American Academy of Political and Social Science* 315 (January 1958): 12–21.

McConnell, Torrey. "The War on Women: The Collateral Consequences of Female Incarceration." *Lewis & Clark Law Review* 21, no. 2 (June 2017): 493–524.

McMahon, Keith. "Opium Smoking and Modern Subjectivity." *Postcolonial Studies* 8, no. 2 (May 2005): 165–80.

Messac, Luke. "No Opiates for the Masses: Untreated Pain, International Narcotics Control, and the Bureaucratic Production of Ignorance." *Journal of Policy History* 28, no. 2 (2016): 193–220.

Miller, Laura. "The Romantics and the Opium-Eater." Slate.com. Last modified November 7, 2016. http://www.slate.com/articles/arts/books/2016/11/biography_of_thomas_de_quincey_guilty_thing_by_frances_wilson_reviewed.html

Milligan, Barry. "Morphine-Addicted Doctors, the English Opium-Eater, and Embattled Medical Authority." *Victorian Literature & Culture* 33, no. 2 (September 2005): 541–53.

Morgan, Patricia A. "The Political Economy of Drugs and Alcohol: An Introduction." *Journal of Drug Issues* 13, no. 1 (Winter 1983): 1–7.

Morrison, Robert. "De Quincey's Addiction." *Romanticism* 17, no. 3 (2011): 270–77.

Morrison, Robert. "Opium-Eaters and Magazine Wars: De Quincey and Coleridge in 1821." *Victorian Periodicals Review* 30, no. 1 (Spring 1997): 27–40.

Musto, David F. "Opium, Cocaine and Marijuana in American History." *Scientific American* 265, no. 1 (July 1991): 40–47.

Nadelmann, Ethan A. "Should We Legalize Drugs? History Answers: Yes." *American Heritage* 44, no. 1 (February–March 1993): 45–47.

Nahas, Gabriel G. "Hashish in Islam 9th to 18th century." *Bulletin of the New York Academy of Medicine* 58, no. 9 (December 1982): 814–31.

Neill, Katharine A. "Tough on Drugs: Law and Order Dominance and the Neglect of Public Health in U.S. Drug Policy." *World Medical & Health Policy* 6, no. 4 (December 2014): 375–94.

Neptune, Jessica. "Harshest in the Nation: The Rockefeller Drug Laws and the Widening Embrace of Punitive Politics." *Social History of Alcohol and Drugs* 26, no. 2 (Summer 2012): 170–91.

Netherland, Julie, and Helena B. Hansen. "The War on Drugs That Wasn't: Wasted Whiteness, 'Dirty Doctors,' and Race in Media Coverage of Prescription Opioid Misuse." *Culture, Medicine and Psychiatry: An International Journal of Cross-Cultural Health Research* 40, no. 4 (December 2016): 664–86.

Newman, R. K. "Opium Smoking in Late Imperial China: A Reconsideration." *Modern Asian Studies* 29, no. 4 (October 1995): 765–94.

Nichols, Emma Hitt. "Understanding Addiction: Dopamine and Brain Function." *MD Conference Express* 14, no. 8 (June 2014): 6–8.

Nye, David E. "Shaping Communication Networks: Telegraph, Telephone, Computer." *Social Research* 64, no. 3 (Fall 1997): 1067–91.

Osborn, Matthew Warner. "A Detestable Shrine: Alcohol Abuse in Antebellum Philadelphia." *Journal of the Early Republic* 29, no. 1 (Spring 2009): 101–32.

Osborn, Matthew Warner. "Diseased Imaginations: Constructing Delirium Tremens in Philadelphia, 1813–1832." *Social History of Medicine* 19, no. 2 (2006): 191–208.

Ou, Hsin-Yun. "Chinese Ethnicity and the American Heroic Artisan in Henry Grimm's *The Chinese Must Go* (1879)." *Comparative Drama* 44, no. 1 (2010): 63–84.

Pandey, Subhash C., Adip Roy, Huaibo Zhang, and Tiejun Xu. "Partial Deletion of the cAMP Response Element-Binding Protein Gene Promotes Alcohol-Drinking Behaviors." *Journal of Neuroscience* 24, no. 21 (May 26, 2004): 5022–30.

Parssinen, Terry M., and Karen Kerner. "Development of the Disease Model of Drug Addiction in Britain, 1870–1926." *Medical History* 24, no. 3 (July 1980): 275–96.

Paulson, George. "Illnesses of the Brain in John Quincy Adams." *Journal of the History of the Neurosciences* 13, no. 4 (December 2004): 336–44.

Philbrick, Nathaniel. "The Nantucket Sequence in Crèvecoeur's *Letters from an American Farmer*." *New England Quarterly* 64, no. 3 (September 1991): 414–32.

Philips, John Edward. "African Smoking and Pipes." *Journal of African History* 24, no. 4 (1983): 303–19.

Pickard, John B. "John Greenleaf Whittier and Mary Emerson Smith." *American Literature* 38, no. 4 (January 1967): 478–97.

Piomelli, Daniele, and Ethan B. Russo. "The *Cannabis sativa* Versus *Cannabis indica* Debate: An Interview with Ethan Russo, MD." *Cannabis and Cannabinoid Research* 1, no. 1 (January 1, 2016): 44–46. DOI: 10.1089/can.2015.29003.ebr.

Poor, Daryoush Mohammad. "Secular/Religious Myths of Violence: The Case of Nizārī Ismailis of the Alamūt Period." *Studia Islamica* 114, no. 1 (2019): 47–68.

Poroy, Ibrahim Ihsan. "Expansion of Opium Production in Turkey and the State Monopoly of 1828–1839." *International Journal of Middle East Studies* 13, no. 2 (May 1981): 191–211.

Pugsley, Andrea. "'As I Kill This Chicken So May I Be Punished if I Tell an Untruth': Chinese Opposition to Legal Discrimination in Arizona Territory." *Journal of Arizona History* 44, no. 2 (2003): 171–90.

Quinones, Mark A. "Drug Abuse During the Civil War (1861–1865)." *International Journal of the Addictions* 10, no. 6 (1975): 1007–20.

Redford, Audrey, and Benjamin Powell. "Dynamics of Intervention in the War on Drugs: The Buildup to the Harrison Act of 1914." *Independent Review* 20, no. 4 (Spring 2016): 509–30.

Renshaw, Patrick. "The IWW and the Red Scare, 1917–24." *Journal of Contemporary History* 3, no. 4 (October 1968): 63–72.

Rönnbäck, Klas. "The Idle and the Industrious—European Ideas About the African Work Ethic in Precolonial West Africa." *History in Africa* 41 (2014): 117–45.

Rosino, Michael L., and Matthew W. Hughey. "The War on Drugs, Racial Meanings, and Structural Racism: A Holistic and Reproductive Approach." *American Journal of Economics & Sociology* 77, no. 3/4 (May–September 2018): 849–92.

Ross, William G. "The Legal Career of John Quincy Adams." *Akron Law Review* 23, no. 3 (Spring 1990): 415–53.

Rotunda, Michele. "Savages to the Left of Me, Neurasthenics to the Right, Stuck in the Middle with You: Inebriety and Human Nature in American Society, 1855–1900." *Canadian Bulletin of Medical History* 24, no. 1 (Spring 2007): 49–65.

Rush, James R. "Opium in Java: A Sinister Friend." *Journal of Asian Studies* 44, no. 3 (May 1985): 549–60.

Sahu, A. C. "Genesis and Growth of Indo-Chinese Opium Monopoly Under East India Company." *Journal of Indian History* 57, no. 1 (April 1979): 163–69.

Shankman, Arnold. "Black on Yellow: Afro-Americans View Chinese-Americans, 1850–1935." *Phylon* 39, no. 1 (Spring 1978): 1–17.

Sharma, Jayeeta. "'Lazy' Natives, Coolie Labour, and the Assam Tea Industry." *Modern Asian Studies* 43, no. 6 (2009): 1287–1324.

Shattuck, Gary G. "Opium Eating in Vermont: 'A Crying Evil of the Day.'" *Vermont History* 83, no. 2 (Summer/Fall 2015): 157–92.

Shaw, Douglas V. "Infanticide In New Jersey: A Nineteenth-Century Case Study." *New Jersey History* 115, no. 1/2 (Spring/Summer 1997): 3–31.

Shaw, Michael. "Photos Reveal Media's Softer Tone on Opioid Crisis." *Columbia Journalism Review* (July 26, 2017). https://www.cjr.org/criticism/opioid-crisis-photos.php?link.

Shulman, Max. "Anatomy of an Addict: Junie McCree and the Vaudeville Dope Fiend." *Theatre Survey* 60, no. 2 (May 2019): 261–84.

Siegel, Stephen A. "Francis Wharton's Orthodoxy: God, Historical Jurisprudence, and Classical Legal Thought." *American Journal of Legal History* 46, no. 4 (October 2004): 422–46.

Smith, Benjamin T., and Wil G. Pansters. "US Moral Panics, Mexican Politics, and the Borderlands Origins of the War on Drugs, 1950–62." *Journal of Contemporary History* 55, no. 2 (April 2020): 364–87.

Smith, David. "Hail Mariani: The Transformation of Vin Mariani from Medicine to Food in American Culture, 1886–1910." *Social History of Alcohol and Drugs* 23, no. 1 (Fall 2008): 42–56.

Snelders, Stephen, Charles Kaplan, and Toine Pieters. "On Cannabis, Chloral Hydrate, and Career Cycles of Psychotropic Drugs in Medicine." *Bulletin of the History of Medicine* 80, no. 1 (Spring 2006): 95–114.

Snyder, Solomon H. "Opiate Receptors and Internal Opiates." *Scientific American* 236, no. 3 (March 1977): 44–57.

Sonnedecker, Glenn. "Emergence of the Concept of Opiate Addiction." *Journal mondial de pharmacie* 3 (1962): 275–90.

Speaker, Susan L. "'The Struggle of Mankind Against Its Deadliest Foe': Themes of Counter-Subversion in Anti-Narcotic Campaigns, 1920–1940." *Journal of Social History* 34, no. 3 (Spring 2001): 591–610.

Spillane, Joseph. "The Making of an Underground Market: Drug Selling in Chicago, 1900–1940." *Journal of Social History* 32, no. 1 (1998): 27–47.

Stelle, Charles C. "American Trade in Opium to China, Prior to 1820." *Pacific Historical Review* (December 1940): 425–44.

Stewart, Omer C. "Origin of the Peyote Religion in the United States." *Plains Anthropologist* 19, no. 65 (August 1974): 211–23.

Stinson, Byron. "The Army Disease." *American History Illustrated* 6, no. 5 (August 1971): 10–17.

Su, Alastair. "'The Cause of Human Freedom': John Quincy Adams and the Problem of Opium in the Age of Emancipation." *Journal of the Early Republic* 40, no. 3 (Fall 2020): 465–96.

Swann, John P. "FDA and the Practice of Pharmacy: Prescription Drug Regulation Before the Durham-Humphrey Amendment of 1951." *Pharmacy in History* 36, no. 2 (1994): 55–70.

Temin, Peter. "The Origin of Compulsory Drug Prescriptions." *Journal of Law & Economics* 22, no. 1 (April 1979): 91–105.

Terry, Martin, and Keeper Trout. "Regulation of Peyote (*Lophophora Williamsii*: Cactaceae) in the U.S.A.: A Historical Victory of Religion and Politics over Science and Medicine." *Journal of the Botanical Research Institute of Texas* 11, no. 1 (2017): 147–56.

Titcomb, Margaret. "Kava in Hawaii." *Journal of the Polynesian Society* 57, no. 2 (June 1948): 105–71.

Uhlman, James Todd. "Gas-Light Journeys: Bayard Taylor and the Cultural Work of the American Travel Lecturer in the Nineteenth Century." *American Nineteenth Century History* 13, no. 3 (September 2012): 371–401.

Van, Rachel Tamar. "Cents and Sensibilities: Fairness and Free Trade in the Early Nineteenth Century." *Diplomatic History* 42, no. 1 (January 2018): 72–89.

Viljoen, Russel. "Aboriginal Khoikhoi Servants and Their Masters in Colonial Swellendam, South Africa, 1745–1795." *Agricultural History* 75, no. 1 (Winter 2001): 28–51.

Vyhnanek, Louis. "'Muggles,' 'Inchy,' and 'Mud': Illegal Drugs in New Orleans During the 1920s." *Louisiana History* 22, no. 3 (July 1981): 253–79.

Ward, Geoffrey C., and Frederic Delano Grant Jr. "'A Fair, Honorable, and Legitimate Trade.'" *American Heritage* 37, no. 5 (August–September 1986), 49–64.

Warf, Barney. "High Points: An Historical Geography of Cannabis." *Geographical Review* 104, no. 4 (October 2014): 414–38.

Webb, Hillary S. "The Use of Peyote as Treatment for Alcoholism Within the NAC Community: Reflections on a Study. An Interview with John Halpern, M.D." *Anthropology of Consciousness* 22, no. 2 (September 2011): 234–44.

Wertz, Daniel J. P. "Idealism, Imperialism, and Internationalism: Opium Politics in the Colonial Philippines, 1898–1925." *Modern Asian Studies* 47, no. 2 (March 2013): 467–99.

White, Kenneth Michael, and Mirya R. Holman. "Marijuana Prohibition in California: Racial Prejudice and Selective-Arrests." *Race, Gender & Class* 19, no. 3–4 (2012): 75–92.

White, William L. "Addiction as a Disease: Birth of a Concept." *Counselor* 1, no. 1 (2000): 46–51, 73.

Whiteside, Henry O. "The Drug Habit in Nineteenth-century Colorado." *Colorado Magazine* 55, no. 1 (1978): 46–68.

Willard, William. "The First Amendment, Anglo-Conformity and American Indian Religious Freedom." *Wicazo Sa Review* 7, no. 1 (Spring 1991): 25–41.

Wilson, Sven E. "Prejudice and Policy: Racial Discrimination in the Union Army Disability Pension System, 1865–1906." *American Journal of Public Health* 100, no. S1 (April 2010): S56–S65.

Windle, James. "How the East Influenced Drug Prohibition." *International History Review* 35, no. 5 (2013): 1185–99.

Winkler, Allan M. "Drinking on the American Frontier." *Quarterly Journal of Studies on Alcohol* 29, no. 2 (1968): 413–45.

Wood, Ann Douglas. "'The Fashionable Diseases': Women's Complaints and Their Treatment in Nineteenth-Century America." *Journal of Interdisciplinary History* 4, no. 1 (Summer 1973): 25–52.

Woods, Louis Lee II. "The Federal Home Loan Bank Board, Redlining, and the National Proliferation of Racial Lending Discrimination, 1921–1950." *Journal of Urban History* 38, no. 6 (November 2012): 1036–59.

Youngquist, Paul. "Rehabilitating Coleridge: Poetry, Philosophy, Excess." *ELH* 66 (Winter 1999): 885–909.

Zentner, Joseph L. "Opiate Use in America During the Eighteenth and Nineteenth Centuries: The Origins of a Modern Scourge." *Studies in History & Society* 5, no. 2 (1974): 40–54.

Zieger, Susan. "Impostors of Freedom: Southern White Manhood, Hypodermic Morphine, and E. P. Roe's *Without a Home*." *American Literature* 80, no. 3 (September 2008): 527–54.

## Essays

Acker, Caroline Jean. "From All Purpose Anodyne to Marker of Deviance: Physicians' Attitudes Towards Opiates in the US from 1890 to 1940." In *Drugs and Narcotics in History*, edited by Roy Porter and Mikuláš Teich, 114–32. Cambridge: Cambridge University Press, 1995.

Acker, Caroline Jean. "Take as Directed: The Dilemmas of Regulating Addictive Analgesics and Other Psychoactive Drugs." In *Opioids and Pain Relief: A Historical Perspective*, edited by Marcia L. Meldrum, 35–55. Seattle: IASP Press, 2003.

Calabrese, Joseph D. "The Therapeutic Use of Peyote in the Native American Church." In *Psychedelic Medicine: New Evidence for Hallucinogenic Substances as Treatments*, edited by Michael J. Winkelman and Thomas B. Roberts, II: 29–42. Westport, Conn.: Praeger, 2007.

Chan, Loren B. "The Chinese in Nevada: An Historical Survey, 1856–1970." In *Chinese on the American Frontier*, edited by Arif Dirlik, 85–122. Lanham, Md.: Rowman and Littlefield, 2001.

Chan, Sucheng. "The Exclusion of Chinese Women, 1870–1943." In *Entry Denied: Exclusion and the Chinese Community in America, 1882–1943*, edited by Sucheng Chan, 94–146. Philadelphia: Temple University Press, 1994.

Chavigny, Katherine A. "Reforming Drunkards in Nineteenth-Century America: Religion, Medicine, Therapy." In *Altering American Consciousness: The History of Alcohol and Drug Use in the United States, 1800–2000*, edited by Sarah W. Tracy and Caroline Jean Acker, 108–23. Amherst: University of Massachusetts Press, 2004.

Coetzee, J. M. "Idleness in South Africa." In *The Violence of Representation: Literature and the History of Violence*, edited by Nancy Armstrong and Leonard Tennenhouse, 119–39. London: Routledge, 1989.

B.F.D. "Annotation: Right of Action Against One Selling Habit-forming Drug to Child or Spouse." In *American Law Reports Annotated*, vol. 3, edited by Burdett A. Rich and M. Blair Wailes, 1152–53. Rochester, N. Y.: Lawyers Co-operative Publishing, 1919.

Duster, Troy. "Pattern, Purpose, and Race in the Drug War: The Crisis of Credibility in Criminal Justice." In *Crack in America: Demon Drugs and Social Justice*, edited by Craig Reinarman and Harry G. Levine, 260–87. Berkeley: University of California Press, 1997.

Fagan, John L. "The Chinese Cannery Workers of Warrendale, Oregon, 1876–1930." In *Hidden Heritage: Historical Archaeology of the Overseas Chinese*, edited by Priscilla Wegars, 215–28. Amityville, N. Y.: Baywood, c. 1993.

Fairbank, John K. "America and China: The Mid-Nineteenth Century." In *American-East Asian Relations: A Survey*, edited by Ernest R. May and James C. Thomson Jr., 19–33. Cambridge, Mass.: Harvard University Press, 1972.

Foster, Anne L. "Medicine to Drug: Opium's Transimperial Journey." In *Crossing Empires: Taking U.S. History into Transimperial Terrain*, edited by Kristin L. Hoganson and Jay Sexton, 112–31. Durham, N. C.: Duke University Press, 2020.

Goldstein, Jonathan. "A Clash of Civilizations in the Pearl River Delta: Stephen Girard's Trade with China, 1787–1824." In *Americans and Macao: Trade, Smuggling, and Diplomacy on the South China Coast*, edited by Paul A. Van Dyke, 17–32. Hong Kong: Hong Kong University Press, 2012.

Gray, Elizabeth Kelly. "The Trade-Off: Chinese Opium Traders and Antebellum Reform in the United States, 1815–1860." In *Drugs and Empires: Essays in Modern Imperialism and Intoxication, c. 1500–c. 1930*, edited by James H. Mills and Patricia Barton, 220–42. Basingstoke, UK: Palgrave Macmillan, 2007.

Haenni, Sabine. "Filming 'Chinatown': Fake Visions, Bodily Transformations." In *Screening Asian Americans*, edited by Peter X. Feng, 21–52. New Brunswick, N. J.: Rutgers University Press, 2002.

Hamowy, Ronald. "Introduction: Illicit Drugs and Government Control." In *Dealing with Drugs: Consequences of Government Control*, edited by Ronald Hamowy, 1–34. Lexington, Mass.: D.C. Heath, 1987.

Loeser, John D. "Opiophobia and Opiophilia." In *Opioids and Pain Relief: A Historical Perspective*, edited by Marcia L. Meldrum, 1–4. Seattle: IASP Press, 2003.

Mancall, Peter C. "'I Was Addicted to Drinking Rum': Four Centuries of Alcohol Consumption in Indian Country." In *Altering American Consciousness: The History of Alcohol and Drug Use in the United States, 1800–2000*, edited by Sarah W. Tracy and Caroline Jean Acker, 91–107. Amherst: University of Massachusetts Press, 2004.

Nadelmann, Ethan A. "Drug Prohibition in the U.S.: Costs, Consequences, and Alternatives." In *Crack in America: Demon Drugs and Social Justice*, edited by Craig Reinarman and Harry G. Levine, 288–316. Berkeley: University of California Press, 1997.

Renard, Ronald D. "The Making of a Problem: Narcotics in Mainland Southeast Asia." In *Development or Domestication? Indigenous Peoples of Southeast Asia*, edited by Don McCaskill and Ken Kampe, 307–28. Chiang Mai, Thailand: Silkworm Books, 1997.

Tchen, John Kuo Wei. "Quimbo Appo's Fear of Fenians: Chinese-Irish-Anglo Relations in New York City." In *The New York Irish*, edited by Ronald H. Bayor and Timothy J. Meagher, 125–52. Baltimore, Md.: Johns Hopkins University Press, 1996.

Wylie, Jerry, and Richard E. Fike. "Chinese Opium Smoking Techniques and Paraphernalia." In *Hidden Heritage: Historical Archaeology of the Overseas Chinese*, edited by Priscilla Wegars, 255–306. Amityville, N. Y.: Baywood, c. 1993.

## Blog Posts and Data Visualization

Hamilton Project, Brookings Institution. "Rates of Drug Use and Sales, by Race; Rates of Drug Related Criminal Justice Measures, by Race." Last modified October 21, 2016. https://www.hamiltonproject.org/charts/rates_of_drug_use_and_sales_by_race_rates_of_drug_related_criminal_justice.

Horgan, John. "Tripping on Peyote in Navajo Nation." *Scientific American* (blog). July 5, 2017. https://blogs.scientificamerican.com/cross-check/tripping-on-peyote-in-navajo-nation/.

Rothwell, Jonathan. "How the War on Drugs Damages Black Social Mobility." Brookings Institution (blog). September 30, 2014. https://www.brookings.edu/blog/social-mobility-memos/2014/09/30/how-the-war-on-drugs-damages-black-social-mobility/.

## Primary Books

*Acts of the General Assembly of the Commonwealth of Kentucky*. Frankfort: Kentucky Yeoman Office, 1872.

Adams, Abigail. *The Quotable Abigail Adams.* Edited by John P. Kaminski. Cambridge, Mass.: Belknap Press of Harvard University Press, 2009.

Adams, John. *Letters of John Adams, Addressed to His Wife.* Vol. 2. Edited by Charles Francis Adams. Boston: Charles C. Little and James Brown, 1841.

Adams, John. *Statesman and Friend: Correspondence of John Adams with Benjamin Waterhouse, 1784–1822.* Edited by Worthington Chauncey Ford. Boston: Little, Brown, 1927.

Adams, John Quincy. *Life in a New England Town: 1787, 1788: Diary of John Quincy Adams.* Boston: Little, Brown, 1903.

Adams, Samuel Hopkins. *The Great American Fraud: Articles on the Nostrum Evil and Quacks Reprinted from Collier's Weekly.* 4th ed. Chicago, Ill.: P. F. Collier, 1907.

Addams, Jane. *Twenty Years at Hull-House with Autobiographical Notes.* New York: Macmillan, 1911.

[Africanus, Leo.] *A Geographical Historie of Africa.* Translated by John Pory. London, 1600.

Africanus, Leo. *The History and Description of Africa, and of the Notable Things Therein Contained.* Vol. 3. Translated by John Pory. Edited by Dr. Robert Brown. London: The Hakluyt Society, 1896.

Aikin, J. *Geographical Delineations, or A Compendious View of the Natural and Political State of All Parts of the Globe.* Philadelphia: F. Nichols, 1807.

Alcott, Louisa May. *Louisa May Alcott: Her Life, Letters, and Journals.* Edited by Ednah D. Cheney. Boston: Roberts Brothers, 1889.

Allen, Nathan. *An Essay on the Opium Trade.* Boston: John P. Jewett and Co., 1850.

American Association for the Study and Cure of Inebriety. *The Disease of Inebriety from Alcohol, Opium and Other Narcotic Drugs . . .* New York: E. B. Treat, 1893.

*The American Farmer's New and Universal Hand-book.* Philadelphia: Cowperthwait, Desilver, and Butler, 1854.

Ames, James Barr. *A Selection of Cases on the Law of Torts,* Vol. 1. Cambridge, Mass.: Harvard Law Review Publishing Association, 1893.

Awsiter, John. *An Essay on the Effects of Opium. Considered as a Poison.* London: G. Kearsly, 1763.

*Baltimore: Past and Present.* Baltimore: Richardson & Bennett, 1871.

Barnes, L. *Opium.* Cleveland: Beckwith and Co., 1868.

Barrow, John. *Travels in China . . .* London: A. Strahan, 1804.

Bartholow, Roberts. *Manual of Hypodermic Medication.* Philadelphia: J. B. Lippincott and Co., 1873.

Beard, George M. *Stimulants and Narcotics; Medically, Philosophically, and Morally Considered.* New York: G. P. Putnam and Sons, 1871.

Beard, George Miller. *American Nervousness: Its Causes and Consequences.* New York: Putnam, 1881.

Beasley, Henry. *The Book of Prescriptions, Containing 3000 Prescriptions.* Philadelphia: Lindsay and Blakiston, 1865.

Beck, Louis J. *New York's Chinatown.* New York: Bohemia Publishing Company, 1898.

Benezet, Anthony. *A Short Account of that Part of Africa, Inhabited by the Negroes.* Philadelphia: W. Dunlap, 1762.

*Biographies of Successful Philadelphia Merchants.* Philadelphia: James K. Simon, 1864.

Blaney, Chas. E. *The King of the Opium Ring.* New York: J. S. Ogilvie, 1905.

Blaney, Henry. *Journal of Voyages to China and Return.* Boston: Privately printed, 1913.

Boardman, H. A. *The Bible in the Counting-House: A Course of Lectures to Merchants.* Philadelphia: Lippincott, Grambo and Co., 1853.

Bonsal, Stephen Jr. *Morocco as It Is.* New York: Harper & Brothers, 1893.

Bowne, Eliza Southgate. *A Girl's Life Eighty Years Ago: Selections from the Letters of Eliza Southgate Bowne.* New York: Charles Scribner's Sons, 1887.

Brookes, R. *Brookes's General Gazetteer Improved; or, A New and Compendious Geographical Dictionary . . .* Philadelphia: Jacob Johnson, and Co., 1806.

Brown, Henry Collins, ed. *Valentine's Manual of the City of New York for 1916–7.* New York: Valentine Company, 1916.

Bryarly, Wakeman. *An Inaugural Essay, on the Lupulus Communis, or Gærtner; or the Common Hop.* Philadelphia: John H. Oswald, 1805.

Burns, John. *Popular Directions for the Treatment of the Diseases of Women and Children.* New-York: Thomas A. Ronalds, 1811.

Byrnes, Thomas. *Professional Criminals of America.* New York: Cassell and Company, 1886.

Cadogan, William. *A Dissertation on the Gout* . . . London: J. Dodsley, 1771.

Caldwell, Charles. *Medical & Physical Memoirs* . . . Philadelphia: Thomas and William Bradford, 1801.

[Calhoun, John C.]. *Speeches of John C. Calhoun.* New-York: Harper and Brothers, 1843.

Calkins, Alonzo. *Opium and the Opium-Appetite.* Philadelphia, J. B. Lippincott and Co., 1871.

Carpenter, George W. *Observations and Experiments on the Pharmaceutical Preparations and Constituent Principles of Opium.* Philadelphia: s.n. 1827.

Cheyne, George. *The English Malady.* London: G. Strahan, 1733.

Chipman, Samuel. *Report of an Examination of Poor-Houses, Jails, &c. in the State of New-York.* Albany: Hoffman and White, 1834.

Cobbe, William Rosser. *Doctor Judas: A Portrayal of the Opium Habit.* Chicago: S. C. Griggs and Company, 1895.

Cole, Henry G. *Confessions of an American Opium Eater: From Bondage to Freedom.* Boston: James H. Earle, 1895.

Collier, Old Cap. *Old Tramp, the Hermit Detective; or, Tracking the Opium Smugglers of San Francisco.* New York, 1896.

Colton, Rev. Walter, U.S.N. *Visit to Constantinople and Athens.* New-York: Leavitt, Lord and Co., 1836.

Combe, George. *A System of Phrenology.* Edinburgh: MacLachlan and Stewart, 1836.

*The Continental Almanac, For the Year of our Lord, 1780.* Philadelphia: Francis Bailey, [1779].

Cooke, M. C. *The Seven Sisters of Sleep: Popular History of the Seven Prevailing Narcotics of the World.* London: James Blackwood, 1860.

Cooper, Thomas, Esq. M. D. *Tracts on Medical Jurisprudence.* Philadelphia: James Webster, 1819.

Costello, Augustine E. *Our Police Protectors: History of the New York Police.* New York, 1885.

Crèvecoeur, J. Hector St. John de. *Letters from an American Farmer* and *Sketches of Eighteenth-Century America.* New York: Penguin Books, 1981. First published 1782 by T. Davies.

Crothers, T. D. *Morphinism and Narcomanias from Other Drugs: Their Etiology, Treatment, and Medicolegal Relations.* Philadelphia: W. B. Saunders, 1902.

Crumpe, Samuel, M. D. *An Inquiry into the Nature and Properties of Opium.* London: G. G. and J. Robinson, 1793.

Cummins, Ella Sterling. *The Story of the Files: A Review of Californian Writers and Literature.* San Francisco: Co-operative Printing Co., 1893.

Dame Shirley [Mrs. Louise Amelia Knapp Smith Clappe]. *The Shirley Letters from California Mines in 1851–52.* San Francisco: Thomas C. Russell, 1922.

[Darwin, Erasmus], *The Botanic Garden. A Poem, in Two Parts. Part 2, The Loves of the Plants.* New-York: T. and J. Swords, 1807.

Day, Horace. *The Opium Habit, With Suggestions as to the Remedy.* New York: Harper and Brothers, 1868.

De Quincey, Thomas. *Confessions of an English Opium-Eater* and *Suspiria de Profundis.* Boston: Ticknor, Reed, and Fields, 1850.

Drinker, Elizabeth. *The Diary of Elizabeth Drinker: The Life Cycle of an Eighteenth-Century Woman.* Edited and abridged by Elaine Forman Crane. Boston: Northeastern University Press, 1994.

*The Druggist's Manual, Being a Price Current of Drugs, Medicines, Paints, Dye-Stuffs, Glass, Patent Medicines, &c. . . .* Philadelphia: Solomon W. Conrad, 1826.

Dumas, Alexandre. *The Count of Monte-Cristo.* 5 vols. London: George Routledge and Sons, 1888.

Dunglison, Robley, M. D. *Medical Lexicon: A New Dictionary of Medical Science . . .* Philadelphia: Lea and Blanchard, 1842.

Ellet, Mrs. *The Queens of American Society.* New York: Charles Scribner and Company, 1867.

Field, Henry M. *From Egypt to Japan.* New York: Scribner, Armstrong and Co., 1877.

Forbes, Robert B. *Personal Reminiscences.* Boston: Little, Brown, and Company, 1882.

Forbes, Robert Bennet. *Letters from China: The Canton-Boston Correspondence of Robert Bennet Forbes, 1838–1840.* Edited by Phyllis Forbes Kerr. Mystic, Conn.: Mystic Seaport Museum, Inc., c. 1996.

Franklin, Benjamin. *The Writings of Benjamin Franklin,* vol. 10, *1789–1790.* Edited by Albert Henry Smyth. New York: MacMillan, 1907.

Gibbons, Henry, M. D. *Letheomania: The Result of the Hypodermic Injection of Morphia.* San Francisco: F. Clarke, 1869.

Gibson, Rev. O. [Otis] A. M. *The Chinese in America.* Cincinnati: Hitchcock and Walden, 1877.

Gove, Mrs. Mary S. *Lectures to Ladies on Anatomy and Physiology.* Boston: Saxton and Peirce, 1842.

Greeley, Horace. *An Overland Journey, from New York to San Francisco, in the Summer of 1859.* New York: C. M. Saxton, Barker and Co., 1860.

Greeley, Horace. *Recollections of a Busy Life.* New York: J. B. Ford and Co., 1868.

Grover, George Wheelock, M. D. *Shadows Lifted or Sunshine Restored in the Horizon of Human Lives.* Chicago: Stromberg, Allen & and Co., 1894.

Hamilton, Alexander. *A Treatise on the Management of Female Complaints, and of Children in Early Infancy.* New-York: Samuel Campbell, 1792.

Hamilton, Alice. *Exploring the Dangerous Trades: The Autobiography of Alice Hamilton, M.D.* Boston: Little, Brown, 1943.

Handy, Hast. *An Inaugural Dissertation on Opium . . .* Philadelphia: T. Lang, 1791.

Harriott, Lieut. John. *Struggles Through Life, Exemplified in the Various Travels and Adventures in Europe, Asia, Africa, and America . . .* Vol. 1. London: C. and W. Galabin, 1809.

Hawkesworth, John, ed. *A New Voyage Round the World, in the Years 1768, 1769, 1770, and 1771.* Vol. 1. New-York: James Rivington, 1774.

Hayward, John. *New-England and New-York Law-Register, for the Year 1835.* Boston: John Hayward, 1834.

Heermann, Lewis. *Directions for the Medicine Chest.* New-Orleans: John Mowry, and Co., 1811.

Hitchcock, Edward. *An Essay on Alcoholic & Narcotic Substances, as Articles of Common Use. Addressed Particularly to Students.* Amherst: J. S. and C. Adams, 1830.

Hitchcock, Edward. *An Essay on Temperance.* Amherst: J. S. and C. Adams, 1830.

Hodgkinson, John. *A Narrative of His Connection with the Old American Company . . .* New-York: J. Oram, 1797.

Hoffman, Ronald, Sally D. Mason, and Eleanor S. Darcy, eds. *Dear Papa, Dear Charley: The Peregrinations of a Revolutionary Aristocrat . . .* Chapel Hill: University of North Carolina Press, 2001.

Hollick, Frederick. *The Matron's Manual of Midwifery.* New-York: T. W. Strong, 1849.

Hough, Franklin B. *A History of Lewis County, in the State of New York . . .* Albany: Munsell and Rowland, 1860.

Howe, Julia Ward. *Words for the Hour.* Boston: Ticknor and Fields, 1857.

Hubbard, Dr. Fred. Heman. *The Opium Habit and Alcoholism.* New York: A. S. Barnes and Co., 1881.

Hunter, William. *Travels in the Year 1792 through France, Turkey, and Hungary, to Vienna.* London: Printed by J. Davis, for B. and J. White, 1796.

Israel, Fred L. ed. *1897 Sears Roebuck Catalogue.* New York: Chelsea House, 1968.

Jefferson, Thomas. *The Writings of Thomas Jefferson.* Edited by H. A. Washington. 9 vols. Washington, D. C.: Taylor and Maury, 1854.

Jennings, Samuel K. *The Married Lady's Companion, or, Poor Man's Friend . . .* Richmond: T. Nicolson, 1804.

Johnston, James F. *The Chemistry of Common Life.* New York: D. Appleton and Company, 1856.

Jones, Dr. John. *The Mysteries of Opium Reveal'd.* London: Printed for Richard Smith, 1701.

Kane, H. H. *Drugs That Enslave: The Opium, Morphine, Chloral and Hashisch Habits.* Philadelphia: Presley Blackiston, 1881.

Kane, H. H. *The Hypodermic Injection of Morphia: Its History, Advantages and Dangers.* New York: Chas. L. Bermingham and Co., 1880.

Kane, H. H. *Opium-Smoking in America and China*. New York: G. P. Putnam's Sons, 1882.

Keeley, Leslie E. *The Morphine Eater: Or, From Bondage to Freedom*. Dwight, Ill.: C. L. Palmer and Co., 1881.

Keeley, Leslie E. *Opium: Its Use, Abuse and Cure; or, From Bondage to Freedom*. Dwight, Ill.: Leslie E. Keeley Co., 1892.

Kesler, Abraham. *Trial and Execution of Abraham Kesler . . .* Albany, 1818.

Kolb, Peter. *The Present State of the Cape of Good-Hope*. London: W. Innys, 1731.

Langford, Nathaniel Pitt. *Vigilante Days and Ways: The Pioneers of the Rockies*. 2 vols. New York: D. D. Merrill Company, 1893.

Lee, Robert E., ed. *The Revolutionary War Memoirs of General Henry Lee*. New York: Da Capo Press, 1998.

Leigh, John. *An Experimental Inquiry into the Properties of Opium, and its Effects on Living Subjects*. Edinburgh: Printed for Charles Elliot, 1786.

Leslie, Mrs. Frank. *California: A Pleasure Trip from Gotham to the Golden Gate*. New York: G. W. Carleton and Co., 1877.

Levinstein, Edward. *Morbid Craving for Morphia*. Translated by Charles Harrer. London: Smith, Elder, and Co., 1878.

Lofland, John. *The Poetical and Prose Writings of Dr. John Lofland, the Milford Bard, Consisting of Sketches in Poetry and Prose*. Collected and arranged by J. N. M'Jilton. Baltimore: John Murphy and Co., 1853.

A Lover of Mankind [Anthony Benezet]. *The Mighty Destroyer Displayed, In some Account of the Dreadful Havock made by the mistaken Use as well as Abuse of Distilled Spirituous Liquors*. Philadelphia: Joseph Crukshank, 1774.

[Ludlow, Fitz Hugh]. *The Hasheesh Eater: Being Passages from the Life of a Pythagorean*. New York: Harper and Brothers, 1857.

MacMartin, Col. D. F. *Thirty Years in Hell: or, The Confessions of a Drug Fiend*. Topeka, Kan.: Capper Printing, 1921.

Madden, R. R. *Travels in Turkey, Egypt, Nubia, and Palestine, in 1824, 1825, 1826, and 1827*. Vol. 1. London: Henry Colburn, 1829.

Madison, Dolly. *Life and Letters of Dolly Madison*. Edited by Allen C. Clark. Washington, D.C.: W. F. Roberts, 1914.

Madison, James. *The Writings of James Madison*. Vol. 9, *1819–1836*. Edited by Gaillard Hunt. New York: G. P. Putnam's Sons, 1910.

Malcom, Howard. *Travels in South-Eastern Asia . . .* 2 vols. Boston: Gould, Kendall, and Lincoln, 1839.

Masson, David. *De Quincey*. New York: Harper and Brothers, 1882.

Mathews, Mrs. M. M. *Ten Years in Nevada: Or, Life on the Pacific Coast*. Buffalo: Baker, Jones and Co., 1880.

McNeal, Violet. *Four White Horses and a Brass Band*. Garden City, N. Y.: Doubleday, 1947.

Mead, Richard. *A Mechanical Account of Poisons in Several Essays*. London: J. R. for Ralph South, 1702.

Mease, James. *An Inaugural Dissertation on the Disease Produced by the Bite of a Mad Dog or other Rabid Animal*. Philadelphia: Thomas Dobson, 1792.

Meyers, Annie C. *Eight Years in Cocaine Hell*. Chicago: St. Luke Society, 1902.

Meylert, Asa P. *Notes on the Opium Habit*. New York: G. P. Putnam's Sons, 1884.

Morell, John Reynell. *Algeria: The Topography and History, Political, Social, and Natural, of French Africa*. London: Nathaniel Cooke, 1854.

Morris, Gouverneur. *The Diary and Letters of Gouverneur Morris*. Edited by Anne Cary Morris. 2 vols. New York: Da Capo Press, 1970.

Morse, Jedidiah. *The American Universal Geography . . .* 2 vols. Boston: J. T. Buckingham, 1805.

Nevin, Adelaide Mellier. *The Social Mirror: A Character Sketch of the Women of Pittsburg and Vicinity . . .* Pittsburg, Pa.: T. W. Nevin, 1888.

Olin, Stephen. *Greece, and the Golden Horn*. New York: J. C. Derby, 1854.

Olin, Stephen. *The Life and Letters of Stephen Olin, D.D., LL.D.* 2 vols. New York: Harper and Brothers, 1853–1854.

Olmsted, Frederick Law. *The Cotton Kingdom: A Traveller's Observations on Cotton and Slavery in the American Slave States.* New York: Mason Brothers, 1862.

*Opium Eating: An Autobiographical Sketch by an Habituate.* Philadelphia: Claxton, Remsen and Haffelfinger, 1876.

Ossoli, Margaret Fuller. *At Home and Abroad; Or, Things and Thoughts in America and Europe,* Edited by Arthur B. Fuller. Boston: Brown, Taggard and Chase, 1860.

Percival, Thomas. *A Father's Instructions . . .* Philadelphia: Printed for Thomas Dobson, 1788.

*The Porter Family. Proceedings at the Reunion of the Descendants of John Porter, of Danvers, Held at Danvers, Mass., July 17th, 1895.* Danvers, [Mass.]: Eben Putnam, 1897.

Prime, E. D. G. *Around the World: Sketches of Travel Through Many Lands and Over Many Seas.* New York: Harper and Brothers, 1874.

*Public Laws of the State of Maine, from 1853 to 1857 Inclusive.* Augusta: Fuller and Fuller, 1856.

Purchas, Samuel. *Purchas His Pilgrimage, or Relations of the World and the Religions Observed in All Ages . . .* 4 vols. London: William Stansby, 1614.

Ramsay, David. *The History of South-Carolina, from Its First Settlement in 1670, to the Year 1808.* Vol. 2. Charleston: David Longworth, 1809.

Reid, John. *Essays on Hypochondriacal and Other Nervous Affections.* Philadelphia: M. Carey and Son, 1817.

*The Revised Statutes of Idaho Territory. Enacted at the Fourteenth Session of the Legislative Assembly.* Boise City, Idaho, 1887.

Richardson, James D., ed. *A Compilation of the Messages and Papers of the Presidents, 1789–1897.* Vol. 8. Washington, D. C.: Government Printing Office, 1898.

Riis, Jacob August. *How the Other Half Lives: Studies Among the Tenements of New York.* New York: Charles Scribner's Sons, 1890.

Roe, Edward P. *Without a Home.* New York: Dodd, Mead, and Company, 1881.

Ruble, Thomas W. *American Medical Guide for the Use of Families.* Richmond, Ky.: E. Harris, 1810.

Rush, Benjamin. *An Inquiry into the Effects of Ardent Spirits upon the Human Body and Mind.* Philadelphia: Thomas Dobson, 1805.

Rush, Benjamin. *Medical Inquiries and Observations.* 4 vols. Philadelphia: J. Conrad and Co., 1805.

Rush, Benjamin. *Medical Inquiries and Observations, Upon the Diseases of the Mind.* Philadelphia: Kimber and Richardson, 1812.

Russell, Alex. *The Natural History of Aleppo, and Parts Adjacent.* London: A. Millar, 1756.

Ryer, Washington M. *The Conflict of Races.* San Francisco: P. J. Thomas, 1886.

Saunders, Richard. *Poor Richard Improved: Being an Almanack and Ephemeris of the Motions of the Sun and Moon . . .* Philadelphia: D. Hall and W. Sellers, 1767.

Scott, Franklin. *Experiments and Observations on the Means of Counteracting the Deleterious Effects of Opium . . .* Philadelphia: H. Maxwell, 1803.

Seaman, Valentine. *An Inaugural Dissertation on Opium.* Philadelphia: Johnston and Justice, 1792.

Shaw, Samuel. *The Journals of Major Samuel Shaw.* Boston: Wm. Crosby and H. P. Nichols, 1847.

Shuck, Mrs. Henrietta. *Scenes in China: or, Sketches of the Country, Religion, and Customs, of the Chinese.* Philadelphia: American Baptist Publication Society, 1852.

Simmons, William H. *An Essay on Some of the Effects of Contusions of the Head.* Philadelphia: Archibald Bartram, 1806.

*Sixth Annual Report of the Secretary of the State Board of Health of the State of Michigan, for the Fiscal Year Ending Sept. 30, 1878.* Lansing: W. S. George and Co., 1878.

Smithers, William W. *The Life of John Lofland, "The Milford Bard."* Philadelphia: Wallace M. Leonard, 1894.

Smollett, Tobias. *The Miscellaneous Works of Tobias Smollett, M. D.* Vol. 3. Edinburgh: Mundell, Doig and Stevenson, 1806.

Squibb, E. H. "Brief Comments on the Materia Medica, Pharmacy, and Therapeutics of the Year Ending October 1, 1891, Alphabetically Arranged." In *Transactions of the New York*

*State Medical Association, for the Year 1891*, edited by E. D. Ferguson, M.D., 508–37. Vol. 8. New York City: The Association, 1892.

Squibb, Edward R., Edward H. Squibb, and Charles F. Squibb. *An Ephemeris of Materia Medica, Pharmacy, Therapeutics and Collateral Information*. Vol. 2, 1884 and 1885. Brooklyn, N. Y., 1885.

Strong, George Templeton. *The Diary of George Templeton Strong*. Vol. 1, *Young Man in New York, 1835–1849*. Edited by Allan Nevins and Milton Halsey Thomas. New York: The MacMillan, 1952.

Tavernier, Jean-Baptiste. *The Six Voyages of John Baptista Tavernier, Baron of Aubonne* . . . Vol. 1. London: Robert Littlebury and Moses Pitt, 1677.

Taylor, Bayard. *The Lands of the Saracen; or, Pictures of Palestine, Asia Minor, Sicily, and Spain*. New York: G. P. Putnam & Co., 1855.

Tennent, John. *Every Man His Own Doctor: OR, The Poor Planter's Physician*. Williamsburg: William Parks, 1734.

Theobald, John. *Every Man His Own Physician*. London: W. Griffin, and Boston: Cox and Berry, 1767.

*Theriaki and Their Last Dose: Letters of Fitz Hugh Ludlow and Others, to Dr. Samuel B. Collins*. Chicago: Evening Journal Print, 1870.

Thoreau, Henry David. *The Writings of Henry David Thoreau: Journal*. Vol. 2, *1850–September 15, 1851*. Edited by Bradford Torrey. Boston: Houghton Mifflin, 1906.

Towns, Charles B. *Habits That Handicap; The Menace of Opium, Alcohol, and Tobacco, and the Remedy*. New York: Century, 1916.

Train, Geo. Francis. *An American Merchant in Europe, Asia, and Australia* . . . New York: G. P. Putnam & Co., 1857.

*Transactions of the Medical Society of the State of Pennsylvania, at its Twentieth Annual Session, Held at Erie, June, 1869*. 2 vols. Philadelphia: Collins, 1869.

Trotter, Thomas. *An Essay, Medical, Philosophical, and Chemical, on Drunkenness, and Its Effects on the Human Body*. London: T. N. Longman, 1804.

Trotter, Thomas. *A View of the Nervous Temperament* . . . London: Longman, Hurst, Rees, and Orme, 1807.

Twain, Mark. *Roughing It*. New York: Penguin Books, 1985.

Walling, George W. *Recollections of a New York Chief of Police*. New York: Caxton Book Concern, 1887.

Walsh, The Rev. R. *A Residence at Constantinople* . . . 2 vols. London: Frederick Westley and A. H. Davis, 1836.

Wesley, John. *Primitive Physick* . . . Philadelphia: Andrew Steuart, 1764.

White, Moses Clark. *Dissertation on the Abuses of Opium*. M.D. thesis, Yale University, 1854. Harvey Cushing/John Hay Whitney Medical Library, Yale University.

Williams, Allen S. *The Demon of the Orient, and His Satellite Fiends of the Joints*. New York: The Author, 1883.

Williams, S. Wells. *The Middle Kingdom* . . . 2 vols. London: Kegan Paul, 2005.

Williams, Samuel. *The City of the Golden Gate: A Description of San Francisco in 1875*. San Francisco: Book Club of California, 1921.

Willis, N. P. *Pencillings by the Way*. Vol. 2. London: John Macrone, 1835.

Wilson, Daniel. *An Inaugural Dissertation on the Morbid Effects of Opium Upon the Human Body*. Philadelphia: Solomon W. Conrad, 1803.

Wilson, James C. "The Opium Habit and Kindred Affections." In *A System of Practical Medicine*, edited by William Pepper, 647–77. Philadelphia: Lea Brothers and Co., 1886.

Woolley, B. M. *The Opium Habit and Its Cure. And What Others Say of His Cures*. [Atlanta?]: Atlanta Constitution Print, [1879?].

Woolson, Abba Goold. *Woman in American Society*. Boston: Roberts Brothers, 1873.

*Yearbook of the United States Department of Agriculture. 1908*. Washington, D. C.: Government Printing Office, 1909.

Young, George. *A Treatise on Opium, Founded Upon Practical Observations*. London: Printed for A. Millar, 1753.


## Primary Journal and Magazine Articles

L. M. A. "Perilous Play." *Frank Leslie's Chimney Corner*, February 13, 1869, 180–91.

Adams, W. I. Lincoln. "Flash Light Photography." *Outing*, December 1890, 177–83.

Adams, W. I. Lincoln. "Flash Light Photography." *Outing*, January 1891, 259–64.

"The Age of Drugs." *Puck*, October 10, 1900, 8–9.

Alcott, William A. "On the Study of Physiology as a Branch of General Education." *American Annals of Education and Instruction* 3, no. 9 (September 1833): 385–403.

Allen, Nathan. "Abuse of Opiates." *Friends' Intelligencer*, February 18, 1871, 813–15.

Ambler, C. P. "Cocaine—Its Uses and Abuses." *Cleveland Medical Gazette* 10, no. 2 (December 1894): 54–62.

Andrews, Judson B. "Case of Excessive Hypodermic Use of Morphia. Three Hundred Needles Removed from the Body of an Insane Woman." *American Journal of Insanity* 29 (1872): 13–20.

"Another Dose of Physic." *Friends' Review*, August 20, 1859, 796.

Anthony, Milton. "Observations on the Cultivation of the Poppy and the Formation of Opium." *Philadelphia Medical Museum*, n.s. 1, no. 3 (1810): 142–46.

"Artificial Stimulation." *Popular Science*, February 1899, 47–48.

J. B., "Oil of Turpentine in Burns." *New-England Journal of Medicine and Surgery* 1, no. 2 (April 1812): 195–96.

Bacon, John E. "Kava Kava in Gonorrhea." *American Therapist* 1, no. 12 (June 15, 1893): 304–6.

Barnes, L. "Opium–Morphine." *Ohio Medical and Surgical Reporter* 2, no. 3 (May 1868): 65–77.

Beard, George M. "Certain Symptoms of Nervous Exhaustion." *Virginia Medical Monthly* 5, no. 3 (June 1878): 161–85.

Bechdolt, Frederick R. "The Hydra's Heads." *Sunset*, April 1921, 24–26, 86.

"Biographical Memoir of Dr. Samuel Bard." *American Medical Recorder* 4, no. 4 (October 1821): 609–33.

Bishop, Ernest S. "Narcotic Addiction—A Systemic Disease Condition." *Journal of the American Medical Association* 60, no. 6 (February 8, 1913): 431–34.

Blair, Thos. S. "Making the Narcotic Laws Help the Doctor and Not Hinder Him in His Work." *American Medicine* (July 1920): 373–80.

Blair, Thomas S. "The Relation of Drug Addiction to Industry." *Journal of Industrial Hygiene* 1, no. 6 (October 1919): 284–96.

Blair, William. "An Opium-Eater in America." *Knickerbocker*, July 1842, 47–57.

"Books and Authors." *Christian Union*, February 2, 1882, 112–13.

"Boston, June 28, 1788." *New-Haven Gazette, and the Connecticut Magazine*, July 31, 1788, 2–5.

Briggs, G. W. "Hog Plague." *American Farmer*, May 1877, 168–69.

Brooks, Will. "A Fragment of China." *Californian*, July 1882, 6–15.

Brower, D. R. "The Effects of Cocaine on the Central Nervous System." *Medical Age* 4, no. 2 (January 25, 1886): 27–32.

Brown, Charles H. "Correspondence. The Opium Habit." *Medical News* 78, no. 11 (March 16, 1901): 433–34.

Brown, Lucius P. "Enforcement of the Tennessee Anti-Narcotics Law." *American Journal of Public Health* 5, no. 4 (April 1915): 323–33.

Brown, Wm. A. "An Interesting Case of Malingering." *Ohio Medical and Surgical Journal* 12 (March 1860): 285–90.

"Cafe and Divan at Algiers." *Flag of Our Union*, April 11, 1857, 116.

"Can the Allies Endure the Strain of Total Abstinence from Alcohol?" *Current Opinion*, June 1915, 418.

Carpenter, George W. "Observations and Experiments on Opium." *American Journal of Science* 13, no. 1 (January 1828): 17–32.

"Carpenter on Opium." *Philadelphia Journal of the Medical and Physical Sciences* 5, no. 10 (1827): 239–53.

Carson, J. "Note upon India Opium." *American Journal of Pharmacy* (July 1849): 193–206.

"Cartoons and Comments: The Drug-Eaters." *Puck*, October 10, 1900, 7.

Carver, J. "Veterinary Pharmacopœia." *Farrier's Magazine*, June 1, 1818, 99–118.

"Cases of Insanity." *American Journal of Insanity* 3 (January 1847): 193–99.

Chadbourne, Tho. "Cases of Uterine Polypi." *Boston Medical and Surgical Journal* 21, no. 18 (December 11, 1839): 289–92.

[Cheever, David W.]. "Narcotics." *North American Review* 95, no. 197 (October 1862): 374–415.

Cheever, David W. "A Reminiscence of My Professional Life." *Boston Medical and Surgical Journal* 165, no. 13 (September 28, 1911), 483–87.

[Cheever, David W.]. "Tobacco." *Atlantic Monthly*, August 1860, 187–202.

"The Chemistry of Common Life." *Ladies' Repository*, May 1855, 289–93.

Chiles, Rosa Pendleton. "The Passing of the Opium Traffic." *Forum*, July 1911, 22–39.

"China." *Advocate of Peace*, December 1839, 79–83.

"The Chinamen." *Massachusetts Ploughman*, August 14, 1886, 3.

A Chinese Missionary. "The Opium Trade in the East." *National Magazine*, January 1855, 40–47.

A Chinese Missionary. "The Opium Trade in the East." *National Magazine*, May 1855, 432–39.

"The Chinese Opium Pipe as a Therapeutic Agent." *Quarterly Epitome of American Practical Medicine and Surgery* 9 (March 1882): 5–6.

"The Chloral Habit." *Demorest's Monthly Magazine*, April 1885, 385.

"The Chloroform Habit as Described by One of Its Victims." *Detroit Lancet* 8, no. 6 (December 1884): 251–54.

"The City of the Golden Gate." *Scribner's Monthly*, July 1875, 266–85.

Clark, Helen F. "The Chinese of New York; Contrasted with Their Foreign Neighbors." *Century Magazine*, November 1896, 104–13.

"The Cocain Habit." *Journal of the American Medical Association* 34, no. 25 (June 23, 1900): 1637.

Cocke, James. "Rules for the Recovery of the Apparently Dead." *Baltimore Medical and Physical Recorder* 1, no. 1 (1809): 6–11.

"Coleridge." *Princeton Review* 20, no. 2 (April 1848): 143–86.

Collins, Charles W., and John Day. "The Eighth Deadly Sin." *Everyday Life*, July 1909, 3–4, 29.

Collins, Cornelius F. "The Drug Evil and the Drug Law." *Monthly Bulletin of the Department of Health, City of New York* 9, no. 1 (January 1919): 1–24.

"Commerce and the Opium Trade at Hong Kong." *Hunt's Merchants' Magazine*, January 1847, 122.

"Confessions of a Medicine-Chest." *Merry's Museum*, January 1846, 19–22.

"Confessions of an English Opium-Eater." *Christian Examiner*, November 1841, 274.

"Confessions of an English Opium-Eater." *Saturday Magazine*, January 5, 1822; January 12, 1822, 34–38; January 19, 1822, 63–68; January 26, 1822, 90–94; February 2, 1822, 110–14; February 9, 1822, 134–37; February 16, 1822, 157–60; February 23, 1822, 171–74; March 23, 1822, 257–61; April 6, 1822, 309–13; April 13, 1822, 332–35; April 20, 1822, 356–60; May 4, 1822, 394–99; May 11, 1822, 427–30; May 18, 1822, 456–60; May 25, 1822, 477–83.

"Confessions of an English Opium-eater." *United States Literary Gazette* (May 15, 1824): 38–40.

"Congress Acts in the Nick of Time." *Outlook*, February 13, 1909, 316–17.

Crane, Rev. J. Townley. "Drugs as an Indulgence." *Methodist Quarterly Review*, October 1858, 551–66.

Cranmer, Charles C., and Ed. Reporter. "Correspondence: The Use and Abuse of Opium." *Medical and Surgical Reporter* 33 (November 6, 1875): 378.

Cress, James Conquest. "Case of Poisoning by Opium, Successfully Treated by Cold Affusions." *Philadelphia Journal of the Medical and Physical Sciences* 8, no. 16 (1824): 398–400.

"The Cruelty of Avarice—The Opium Smokers of China." *National Magazine*, April 1855, 314–20.

Cruikshank, William J. "The Substitution of Drugs in the Dispensing of the Physician's Prescription." *Medical News* 87, no. 23 (December 2, 1905): 1071–81.

Culin, Stewart. "Opium Smoking by the Chinese in Philadelphia." *American Journal of Pharmacy* (October 1891): 497–502.

"Curious Facts: Opium." *New-York Mirror, and Ladies' Literary Gazette*, May 6, 1826, 322–23.

"Curious Historical and Descriptive Particulars Respecting the Inhabitants of the Kingdom of Canary on the Coast of Malabar." *Massachusetts Magazine: or, Monthly Museum*, June 1796, 313–20.

Dickson, Harris. "Exit the Black Man." *Hampton's Magazine*, October 1909, 497–505.

Dickson, Harris. "The Negro in Politics." *Hampton's Magazine*, August 1909, 225–36.

Dickson, Harris. "The Unknowable Negro." *Hampton's Magazine*, June 1909, 729–42.

Diver, Wm. B. "Facts Concerning the Opium Trade." *Christian Observer*, March 11, 1842, 38.

Doerschuk, Albert N., Ph.G. "The Cocaine Habit." *Bulletin of Pharmacy* 9, no. 4 (April 1895): 154–55.

"Domestic Opium." *New England Journal of Medicine and Surgery* 1, no. 3 (July 1812): 315.

"The Dreams of a Hasheesh Smoker." *Cincinnati Medical Journal* 4, no. 1 (January 1889): 30–31.

"Drug Habits." *Youth's Companion*, December 11, 1919, 716.

"Drunkenness." *Hall's Journal of Health* 9, no. 3 (March 1862): 61–67.

B. E. "Chinese Materia Medica." *Journal of the Philadelphia College of Pharmacy* 1, no. 2 (July 1829): 150–53.

Earle, Charles Warrington. "The Opium Habit." *Chicago Medical Review* 2, no. 7 (October 5, 1880): 442–46.

Earle, Charles Warrington. "The Opium Habit." *Chicago Medical Review* 2, no. 9 (November 5, 1880): 493–98.

"Eating Opium." *New York Evangelist*, April 11, 1840, 60.

Eaton, Virgil G. "How the Opium-Habit Is Acquired." *Popular Science Monthly*, September 1888, 663–67.

Eberle, E. G., and Frederick T. Gordon. "Report of Committee on the Acquirement of Drug Habits." *American Journal of Pharmacy* 75 (October 1903): 474–88.

"Editorial Comment." *American Medicine* 10, no. 11 (November 1915): 799–801.

"Editorial Miscellany." *De Bow's Review*, October 1860, 488–94.

"Editors' Book Table." *Godey's Magazine and Lady's Book*, December 1849, 464–66.

"Editor's Table." *Southern Literary Messenger*, January 1860, 72–78.

"Editors' Table: A Warning." *Godey's Lady's Book and Magazine*, September 1871, 280.

"Effects of Opium." *Scientific American* 4, no. 47 (August 11, 1849): 371.

"Effects of Opium Eating." *Boston Medical and Surgical Journal* 6, no. 8 (April 4, 1832): 128–31.

Ellis, C. "Patent Medicines." *American Journal of Pharmacy* 5, no. 1 (April 1839): 67–74.

Ellis, Havelock. "Mescal: A Study of a Divine Plant." *Popular Science Monthly*, May 1902, 52–71.

Ely, [Albert Welles]. "China in One Thousand Eight Hundred and Fifty-Three." *DeBow's Review*, April 1853, 339–73.

"England and China." *United States Magazine and Democratic Review*, June 1840, 516–29.

Fielde, A. M. "An Experience in Hasheesh-Smoking." *Therapeutic Gazette*, July 16, 1888, 449–51.

Fitch, George H. "A Night in Chinatown." *Cosmopolitan*, February 1887, 349–58.

"Fluid and Solid Extracts, Resinoids and Sugar-Coated Pills." *Pharmacist and Chemist* 13, no. 1 (January 1880): 490.

Forman, Allan. "Celestial Gotham." *Arena*, April 1893, 620–28.

Forman, Allan. "Some Adopted Americans." *American Magazine*, November 1888, 46–53.

H. J. G. "New Remedy for the Bots." *Southern Planter*, January 1849, 4–5.

"General Facts About the Use of Opium in This Country." *Quarterly Journal of Inebriety*, September 1878, 214–17.

[Gilmor, Robert]. "The Diary of Robert Gilmor." *Maryland Historical Magazine*, September 1922, 231–68.

Gould, S. W. "The Opium Habit." *Medical and Surgical Reporter* 38, no. 25 (June 22, 1878): 496–97.

Graham-Mulhall, Sara. "Experiences in Narcotic Drug Control in the State of New York." *New York Medical Journal* 113, no. 3 (January 15, 1921): 106–11.

Greenwood, Grace. "The Chinese in San Francisco." *Youth's Companion,* July 24, 1873, 236.

"Habit-Forming Drugs." *Outlook,* May 5, 1915, 8–9.

"Habitual Use of Opium." *American Journal of the Medical Sciences* 20 (October 1850): 498–503.

Happel, T. J. "The Opium Curse and Its Prevention." *Quarterly Journal of Inebriety* 17, no. 3 (July 1895): 237–47.

"Hasheesh." *Frank Leslie's Popular Monthly,* January 1882, 110–11.

"Hasheesh and Its Smokers and Eaters." *Scientific American,* October 23, 1858, 49.

Haskins, Dr. E. B. "Clinical Observations in Private Practice." *Western Journal of Medicine and Surgery* 7 (January 1851): 1–10.

"Heermann's Case of Anomalous Disease." *New-York Medical Magazine* 1 (January 1814): 130–34.

"Heroin and Its Advantages." *Medical News* 76, no. 1 (January 6, 1900): 20.

Holder, C. F. "The Opium Industry in America." *Scientific American* 78, no. 10 (March 5, 1898): 147.

"Hop Lee, the Chinese Slave Dealer; or, Old and Young King Brady and the Opium Fiends." *Secret Service* 13 (April 21, 1899): 1–31.

"Horrors of Opium Eating." *Water-Cure Journal,* January 1, 1846, 39.

"How Opium Is Smoked." *Christian Recorder,* October 14, 1875, 7.

"How Opium Is Smoked." *Saturday Evening Post,* October 2, 1875, 7.

Hubbard, S. Dana. "Municipal Narcotic Dispensaries." *Public Health Reports* 35, no. 13 (March 26, 1920): 771–73.

Hubbard, S. Dana. "The New York City Narcotic Clinic and Differing Points of View on Narcotic Addiction." *Monthly Bulletin of the Department of Health, City of New York* 10, no. 2 (February 1920): 33–49.

Hubbard, S. Dana. "Some Fallacies Regarding Narcotic Drug Addiction." *Journal of the American Medical Association* 74, no. 21 (May 22, 1920): 1439–41.

Hughes, C. H. "The Opium Psycho-Neurosis—Chronic Meconism or Papaverism." *Alienist and Neurologist* 5 (1884): 123–45.

Hughes, John Harrison. "The Autobiography of a Drug Fiend." *Medical Review of Reviews* 22, no. 2 (February 1916): 105–20.

Hungerford, Mary C. "An Overdose of Hasheesh." *Popular Science Monthly,* February 1884, 509–15.

"Hypodermic Administration of Certain Medicines." *American Journal of the Medical Sciences* 50, no. 99 (July 1865): 206–8.

"Improper Use of Laudanum." *Scientific American,* June 23, 1855, 325.

"India: Part First—Ancient India." *Christian Review,* July 1859, 458–80.

"Indictment for Murder: Commonwealth vs. John Pinchback." *Hazard's Register of Pennsylvania* 8, no. 25 (December 17, 1831): 395–96.

"The International Anti-Opium Conference." *Outlook,* March 20, 1909, 611–12.

"Is Narcotism Drunkenness?" *Quarterly Journal of Inebriety* 12 (1890): 175.

Itinerant. "Nervous Disease—Insomnia." *Ladies' Repository,* January 1876, 6–11.

Johnson, Anna Hayward. "Neurasthenia." *Philadelphia Medical Times* 11, no. 24 (August 27, 1881): 737–44.

Jones, Dr. Alexander. "Observations Relative to the Culture of the Poppy." *Southern Agriculturist,* April 1831, 188–89.

Jones, Dr. Alexander. "On the Culture of the Persian Poppy." *Southern Agriculturist,* November 1830, 567–72.

K. "Literary Notices: The Complete Works of Samuel Taylor Coleridge." *Universalist Quarterly and General Review,* July 1853, 321–22.

Kane, H. H. "American Opium-Smokers." *Harper's Weekly,* September 24, 1881, 646–47.

Kane, H. H. "American Opium-Smokers." *Harper's Weekly,* October 8, 1881, 682–83.

Kane, H. H. "The Chinese Opium-Pipe as a Therapeutic Agent." *Medical Record* 20, no. 19 (November 5, 1881): 511–15.

Kane, H. H. "The Opium Habit Among American Women." *Harper's Bazaar,* October 27, 1883, 673–74.

Kane, H. H. "Opium Smoking: A New Form of the Opium Habit Amongst Americans." *Gaillard's Medical Journal* 33, no. 2 (February 1882): 101–16.

Kane, H. H. "Rapid and Easy Cure of Morphine Habit of Twelve Years' Standing." *Physicians and Surgeons' Investigator* 2, no. 10 (October 15, 1881): 300–304.

Kebler, L. F. "Existing Laws Regulating the Sale of Habit-Forming Drugs and the Necessity for Additional Legislation." *American Journal of Pharmacy* 81 (April 1909): 186–95.

Kolb, Lawrence. "Pleasure and Deterioration from Narcotic Addiction." *Mental Hygiene* 9 (October 1925): 699–724.

H. L. "Evils of Opium in South-Eastern Asia." *Episcopal Recorder*, September 13, 1834, 97.

[Lathrop, George Parsons]. "The Sorcery of Madjoon." *Scribner's Monthly*, July 1880, 416–22.

"The Laudanum Bottle, or 'I've Killed it!'" *Parley's Magazine*, January 1844, 357–58.

Layard, James Coulter. "Morphine." *Atlantic Monthly*, June 1874, 697–712.

"Life and Writings of Coleridge." *American Review*, November 1849, 532–39.

"Life of the late Dr. John Jones." *American Medical and Philosophical Register* 3 (January 1813): 325–37.

"Literary Notices." *Godey's Lady's Book and Magazine*, November 1868, 451–53.

"Literary Notices." *Russell's Magazine*, January 1858, 377–84.

"Literary Notices: The Hasheesh-Eater." *Knickerbocker*, February 1858, 197–98.

Lobernheim, Dr. "Forms of Disease in Which Opiates Are Indicated." *The Half-Yearly Abstract of the Medical Sciences* 1 (January–June 1845): 88–92.

[Ludlow, Fitz Hugh]. "Hasheesh and Hasheesh Eaters." *Harper's New Monthly Magazine*, April 1858, 653–58.

Mantegazza, Dr. "On the Dietetic and Medicinal Properties of Erythroxylon Coca." *American Journal of Pharmacy* 32 (September 1860): 417–21.

Masters, Frederick J. "The Opium Traffic in California." *Chautauquan*, October 1896, 54–61.

Mattison, J. B. "The Ethics of Opium Habitués." *Medical and Surgical Reporter* 59 (September 8, 1888): 296–98.

Mattison, J. B. "Opium Addiction Among Medical Men." *Medical Record* 23, no. 23 (June 9, 1883): 621.

Mattison, Rich. V. "Opium Smoking Among the Celestials." *American Journal of Pharmacy* (April 1879): 209–10.

McCaskey, Donald. "The Independent Attitude of the 'Dope User'—and What Are We Going to Do About It." *American Journal of Public Health* 5, no. 4 (April 1915): 334–36.

McFarland, S. F. "Opium Inebriety and the Hypodermic Syringe." In *Transactions of the Medical Society of the State of New York for the Year 1877*, 289–93. Albany, N. Y.: 1877.

"Medical and Surgical Society of Baltimore: Opium Poisoning." *Medical and Surgical Reporter* 37, no. 4 (July 28, 1877): 68–69.

"Medical Jurisprudence." *American Medical Recorder* 1, no. 3 (July 1818): 386–98.

A Member of the Party. "The Opium Den Pictures—How They Were Taken." *Californian Illustrated Magazine*, May 1892, 627–30.

"Mental Science: Psychic Effects of Hasheesh," *Science*, October 12, 1888, 175.

Meriwether, Lee. "The Labor Question on the Pacific Coast." *Harper's Weekly*, October 13, 1888, 778–79.

"Miscellaneous Intelligence: Effects of Opium Eating," *Western Journal of the Medical and Physical Sciences* 5, no. 4 (January–March 1832): 627–30.

"Miscellany: Opium Smuggling." *American Journal of Pharmacy* 14 (January 1848): 74–78.

"Mission to the Sandwich Islands." *Missionary Herald*, April 1821, 110–24.

"Mission to the Sandwich Islands." *Religious Intelligencer*, April 14, 1821, 737–42.

"Missionary: Foreign: Sandwich Islands." *Latter Day Luminary*, June 1825, 177–81.

Mitchell, Mrs. Ellen M. "Thomas De Quincey." *Arthur's Illustrated Home Magazine*, April 1877, 183–86.

"Monthly Commercial Chronicle." *Hunt's Merchants' Magazine*, January 1845, 74–80.

Mooney, James. "The Mescal Plant and Ceremony." *Therapeutic Gazette* 12, no. 1 (January 15, 1896): 7–11.

"Morphine Drinking." *American Agriculturist*, July 1878, 263.

Morton, S. T. "An Experience with Opium." *Popular Science Monthly*, July 1885, 334–39.

"Mr. Cottle and His Friends." *Harper's New Monthly Magazine*, December 1853, 68–76.

"Narcotics." *Friend*, December 6, 1862, 110–11.

"The Necessity of Caution in Prescribing Opiates." *Medical and Surgical Reporter* 33 (November 13, 1875): 396–98.

Nelson, Thomas Calhoun. "An Inaugural Dissertation on the Effects of Emetics in Mercurial Salivation." *Transylvania Journal of Medicine and the Associate Sciences* 3, no. 2 (May 1830): 232–48.

"The New Anæsthetic Chloral." *Scientific American*, June 11, 1870, 377.

"New Remedies." *Pharmacist* 11, no. 6 (June 1878), 200.

[Nolan, D. W.]. "The Opium Habit." *Catholic World*, September 1881, 827–35.

"North Carolina." *Baltimore Weekly Magazine*, December 31, 1800, 164.

"Notes and Notices." *Godey's Lady's Book and Magazine*, March 1871, 288–89.

"Notices of New Works, and Literary Intelligence." *Southern Literary Messenger*, November 1841, 807–16.

"Notices of New Works: Confessions of an Opium Eater." *Southern Literary Messenger*, December 1850, 764.

"Notices of Recent Publications." *Christian Examiner and Religious Miscellany*, March 1855, 297–316.

"Novel Case." *Monthly Traveller*, June 1836, 205–6.

Noyes, Dr. J. Oscar. "Intemperance in Europe and the East." *Ohio Medical and Surgical Journal* 9, no. 3 (January 1857): 241–46.

"Of the Oriental Learning and Philosophy." *Port Folio*, February 7, 1807, 93–95.

"On Making Opium." *Archives of Useful Knowledge*, October 1811, 169–77.

"On the Influence of Opium-eating on Health and Longevity." *American Journal of the Medical Sciences* 10 (May 1832): 252–54.

"Opiologia; or Confessions of an English Opium-Eater." *American Medical Recorder* 5 (July 1822): 542–60.

"Opium." *Boston Medical and Surgical Journal* 16, no. 1 (February 8, 1837): 5–11.

"Opium." *Boston Medical and Surgical Journal* 16, no. 7 (March 22, 1837): 101–4.

"Opium." *Old and New*, March 1871, 351.

"Opium." *Outlook*, May 5, 1915. 8.

"Opium." *Public Opinion*, August 27, 1896, 260.

"'Opium Antidotes' Exposed." *Boston Medical and Surgical Journal* 95, no. 17 (October 26, 1876): 500–501.

"The Opium Eater." *New-England Magazine*, March 1, 1833, 217–29.

"Opium Eaters." *Spirit of the English Magazines*, June 1, 1824, 205.

"Opium Eaters." *Boston Medical and Surgical Journal* 2, no. 32 (September 22, 1829): 503–4.

"Opium-Eaters and Snuff-Chewers." *Journal of Health* 1, no. 19 (June 9, 1830): 297–99.

"Opium-Eaters and the Opium Trade." *Flag of Our Union*, May 23, 1857, 164.

"Opium Eating." *Boston Medical and Surgical Journal* 9, no. 4 (September 4, 1833): 66–67.

"Opium-Eating." *Boston Medical and Surgical Journal* 18, no. 8 (March 28, 1838): 128–29.

"Opium-Eating." *Lippincott's Magazine*, April 1868, 404–09.

"Opium Eating in England." *Water-Cure Journal, and Herald of Reforms*, August 1849, 56.

"Opium-Eating in New York." *Harper's Weekly*, May 23, 1857, 321–22.

"The Opium Habit." *Medical and Surgical Reporter* 20 (May 8, 1869): 364.

"Opium in China and the United States." *Missionary Herald*, August 1872, 260–61.

"Opium in the Philippines." *Watchman*, August 25, 1904, 5.

"Opium Joints." *Massachusetts Ploughman*, May 19, 1883, 2.

"Opium 'Joints' in the Black Hills." *Chambers's Journal* 5, no. 250 (October 13, 1888): 654–55.

"The Opium Madness." *Arthur's Illustrated Home Magazine*, February 1879, 80–81.

"Opium Smokers." *Saturday Evening Post*, September 25, 1875, 7.

"Opium-Smoking." *Philadelphia Medical Times* 14, no. 4 (November 17, 1883): 142–44.

"Opium Smoking as a Therapeutic Means." *Journal of the American Medical Association* (July 26, 1884): 100–101.

"Opium Smoking in China." *Boston Medical and Surgical Journal* 26, no. 16 (May 25, 1842): 245–49.

"Opium—The Poor Child's Nurse." *Harper's Weekly*, January 29, 1859, 80.

"The Opium Trade." *Evangelist*, August 28, 1862, 1.

"The Opium Trade." *Gleason's Pictorial*, October 22, 1853, 272.

"The Opium Trade." *Hunt's Merchants' Magazine and Commercial Review*, July 1850, 28–33.

"The Opium War, and Its Justice." *Christian Examiner*, May 1841, 223–37.

O'Shaughnessy, W. B. "On the Preparations of the Indian Hemp, or Gunjah, (*Cannabis Indica*)." *Provincial Medical Journal And Retrospect of the Medical Sciences* 123 (February 4, 1843): 363–69.

"Other Societies." *Baptist Missionary Magazine*, February 1841, 51–54.

"Our Book Table: The Opium Habit." *Old Guard*, November 1868, 876–77.

Our Special Correspondent. "Happy Days in Hollywood." *Vanity Fair*, May 1922, 73.

A Patient, "Original Communications: Opium and Alcohol." *New York Medical Times* 3, no. 2 (November 1853): 37–46.

Paulson, David. "Management of the Victims of Drug Habits." *Medical Standard* 24, no. 3 (March 1901): 130–32.

Pearson, C. B. "Is Morphine 'Happy Dust' to the Addict?" *Medical Council* 23, no. 12 (December 1918): 919–22.

Pearson, C. B. "The Treatment of Morphinism." *Medical Times*, August 1914, 245–46.

"Periscope: Gangrene following Morphine Injections." *Medical and Surgical Reporter* 62, no. 12 (March 22, 1890): 346–48.

"Persian Opium." *American Journal of Pharmacy* (September 1880): 462–64.

Pettey, George E. "A Rational Basis for the Treatment of Narcotic Drug Addiction." *New York Medical Journal* 92, no. 19 (November 5, 1910): 915–17.

"Philadelphia Hospital." *American Medical Intelligencer* 3, no. 16 (November 15, 1839): 246–52.

[Phillips, Willard]. "Confessions of an English Opium-Eater." *North American Review*, January 1824, 90–98.

Pierson, Mrs. Delavan L. "Indian Peyote Worship." *Southern Workman*, April 1915, 241–46.

Pierson, Rev. Isaac. "Opium in China." *Missionary Herald*, March 1877, 75–78.

"Pinakidia." *Southern Literary Messenger*, August 1836, 573–82.

Prentiss, D. W., and Francis P. Morgan. "Anhalonium Lewinii (Mescal Buttons)." *Therapeutic Gazette* 11, no. 9 (September 16, 1895): 577–85.

Prentiss D. W., and Francis P. Morgan. "Mescal Buttons." *Transactions of the Association of American Physicians* 11 (Philadelphia, 1896): 289–309.

Price, Theodore H., and Richard Spillane. "The Commissioner of Internal Revenue as a Policeman." *Outlook*, November 27, 1918, 498–505.

"Proceedings of the New Orleans Session: Addendum: Report of the Committee on the Narcotic Drug Situation in the United States." *Journal of the American Medical Association* 74, no. 19 (May 8, 1920): 1324–28.

"Proofs that the People of the Southern Climes have a Much Stronger Propensity to Heating and Intoxicating Liquors and Drugs than Those of the Northern." *Literary Magazine, and American Register*, April 1804, 73–79.

"Psychic Effects of Hasheesh." *Medical and Surgical Reporter* 59, no. 19 (November 10, 1888): 604.

"Psychology of Opium and Hasheesh: Opium." *Dial*, September 1860, 556–65.

"Publisher's Desk." *Rural New-Yorker*, June 19, 1909, 618.

"Relations Between the Clerical and Medical Professions: The Christian Examiner and the Hydropathic Delusion." *Boston Medical and Surgical Journal* 38, no. 26 (July 26, 1848): 513–20.

"Remarks on the Opium Habit." *Medical and Surgical Reporter* 37, no. 22 (December 1, 1877): 436–37.

"Reminiscences of Coleridge." *North American Review* 65, no. 137 (October 1847): 401–40.

"Report of the Committee on the Narcotic Drug Situation in the United States." *Journal of the American Medical Association* 74 (May 8, 1920): 1324–28.

"Report of the Special Committee on Public Health of the Greater City of New York." *New York State Journal of Medicine* 20, no. 4 (April 1920): 115–20.

"Review." *Philadelphia Medical and Physical Journal* 1, no. 3 (1805): 175–87.

"Review of New Books." *Graham's Magazine*, November 1847, 274–76.

"Review: Trotter's View of the Nervous Temperament." *New-York Medical and Philosophical Journal and Review* 1, no. 2 (June 1809): 233–62.

Robbins, Mrs. E. V. "Chinese Slave Girls: A Bit of History." *Overland Monthly*, January 1908, 100–102.

Roberts, J. D. "Opium Habit in the Negro." *North Carolina Medical Journal* 16, no. 4 (October 1885): 206–7.

Rousseau, J. C. "Sketches on Venereal Complaints." *American Medical Recorder* 3, no. 2 (April 1820): 171–84.

[Ruschenberger, William S. W.]. "Notes and Commentaries, on a Voyage to China." *Southern Literary Messenger*, November 1853, 676–95.

S. "Reid on Nervous Affections." *Portico*, July/August 1817, 15–22.

"Sanitary Legislation. Court Decisions," *Public Health Reports* 31, no. 19 (May 12, 1916): 1203–7.

*Saturday Evening Post*, September 11, 1830, 2.

Seeger, C. L. "Opium Eating." *Boston Medical and Surgical Journal* 9, no. 8 (October 2, 1833): 117–20.

Semple, R. H. "Lecture on Vegetable Poisons." *Pharmaceutical Journal* 2, no. 7 (January 1, 1843): 429–42.

Seymour, Gertrude. "Peyote Worship—An Indian Cult and a Powerful Drug." *Red Man*, June 1916, 341–51.

Shew, Joel. "Dangers of Drugs—Opium." *Water-Cure Journal*, September 1855, 50–52.

Shipman, A. B. "Accidents from Taking Strychnine." *Boston Medical and Surgical Journal* 41, no. 6 (September 12, 1849): 113–14.

Shipman, A. B. "Case of Poisoning with Opium." *American Journal of the Medical Sciences* (August 1840): 508–9.

Shipman, E. W. "The Promiscuous Use of Opium in Vermont." *Transactions of the Vermont State Medical Society, for the Year 1890* (Burlington, Vt.: The Society, 1890): 72–77.

Sigmond, G. G. "Influence of Opium Eating on Health and Longevity." *American Journal of the Medical Sciences* (February 1838): 523.

"The Silver Lining to an Opium Cloud." *Puck*, August 12, 1885, 370.

Simonton, Thomas G. "The Increase of the Use of Cocaine among the Laity of Pittsburg." *Philadelphia Medical Journal* 11, no. 13 (March 28, 1903): 556–60.

Slack, David B. "Opium in Cholera, Dysentery and Diarrhœa." *Boston Medical and Surgical Journal* 3, no. 33 (September 28, 1830): 530–32.

Smith, James McCune. "On the Influence of Opium upon the Catamenial Functions." *New York Journal of Medicine* 2 (January 1844): 56–58.

"Society Proceedings." *Medical Gazette*, January 21, 1882, 27–29.

"Solving the Narcotic Problem." *Druggists Circular* 67, no. 4 (April 1923): 141–42, 150.

"Something Besides Tobacco." *Beadle's Monthly*, August 1866, 135–40.

Squibb, Edward R. "Materia Medica and Pharmacy." *American Medical Times* 1, no. 13 (September 29, 1860): 230–31.

Staats, Dr. Barent P. "A Case of Poisoning by Opium Successfully Treated by Cold Affusions." *New-York Medical and Physical Journal* 3, no. 4 (October–December 1824): 473.

"State of Medicine in Turkey." *Eclectic Journal of Medicine* 2, no. 5 (March 1838): 169–84.

"State of Medicine in Turkey, from Madden's Travels." *New York Medical and Physical Journal* 2 (January 1830): 399–414.

Stoughton, E. W. "The Opium Trade—England and China." *Hunt's Merchants' Magazine*, May 1840, 394–413.

"Summary of Events." *Friend*, October 1, 1904, 96.

"Taking Laudanum." *Journal of Health* 1, no. 11 (February 10, 1830): 161–63.

"Taking Physic." *Hall's Journal of Health* 8, no. 10 (October 1861): 241–42.

[Taylor, Bayard]. "The Vision of Hasheesh." *Putnam's Monthly*, April 1854, 402–8.

Terry, Dr. C. E. "Drug Addictions, A Public Health Problem." *American Journal of Public Health* 4, no. 1 (January 1914): 28–37.

Terry, C. E. "Six Months of the Harrison Act." *American Journal of Public Health* 6, no. 10 (October 1916): 1087–92.

Terry, Charles E. "Narcotic Drug Addiction and Rational Administration." *American Medicine* 26, no. 1 (January 1920): 29–35.

"Thomas De Quincey." *Harper's New Monthly Magazine*, July 1850, 145–50.

"Thomas De Quincey." *Saturday Evening Post*, July 28, 1877, 4.

"Thomas De Quincey." *Yale Literary Magazine*, April 1851, 225–30.

"Thomas De Quincey and His Works." *Eclectic Magazine of Foreign Literature, Science, and Art*, July 1854, 289–99.

"Thomas de Quincey and His Works." *Graham's Magazine*, September 1854, 272–84.

Thwing, Edward P. "American Life as Related to Inebriety." *Quarterly Journal of Inebriety* 10, no. 1 (January 1888): 43–50.

"Travels." *Analytical Review*, January 1793, 26–35.

Tuckerman, H. T. "Something about Wine." *Knickerbocker*, August 1858, 148–58.

"Turkish Opium Takers." *American Phrenological Journal* (1848): 197–98.

Tyndall, D. W. "Opium." *Prairie Farmer*, September 21, 1867, 179.

Uhle, Dr. Charles P. "Health Department." *Godey's Lady's Book and Magazine*, June 1870, 573–74.

"Use of Opium in the United States." *American Journal of Pharmacy* 37 (September 1865): 393.

"Use of Opium in this Country." *Medical and Surgical Reporter* 12, no. 27 (April 15, 1865): 438.

G.H.V., "Opium and the Opium Trade." *American Quarterly Register and Magazine*, May 1848, 158–68.

Van Buren, W. H. "Amputation of the Thigh, and Subsequent Amputation at the Hip-Joint, Followed by Perfect Recovery." *New-York Journal of Medicine* 7 (July 1851): 50–65.

[Vivian, Thomas J.]. "John Chinaman in San Francisco." *Scribner's Monthly*, October 1876, 862–72.

"Von Hammer's *History of the Assassins*." *Foreign Quarterly Review* 1 (November 1827): 449–72.

"Von Hammer's *History of the Assassins*." *Museum of Foreign Literature and Science*, May 1828, 1–11.

"Von Hammer's History of the Assassins." *Port Folio*, 2 (1827): 361–71.

W. "The Destruction of Opium in Canton." *Monthly Miscellany*, January 1840, 36–39.

Ward, Julius H. "The North American Review." *North American Review*, January 1915, 123–34.

Watson, I. A. "Caution in the Use of Chloral Hydrate." *Medical and Surgical Reporter* 26, no. 4 (January 27, 1872): 77–79.

Waugh, W. F. "Opium Inebriety." *Quarterly Journal of Inebriety* 16, no. 4 (October 1894): 310–24.

Weiss, Louis. "A Drug Store in the Far West." *American Journal of Pharmacy* (November 1877): 561–64.

Wharton, Francis. "China and the Chinese Peace." *Hunt's Merchants' Magazine*, March 1843, 205–26.

Wharton, Francis. "East India, and the Opium Trade." *Hunt's Merchants' Magazine*, January 1841, 9–22.

"What Is, and What Might Be." *American Socialist*, March 13, 1879, 81–82.

"What Shall They Do to Be Saved?" *Harper's New Monthly Magazine*, August 1867, 377–87.

Wilbert, M. I. "Some Early Botanical and Herb Gardens." *American Journal of Pharmacy* 80 (September 1908): 412–27.

Wilhite, W. D. "The Opium Habit: A Narrative of Personal Experience." *Southern Medical Record* 13, no. 7 (July 20, 1883): 246–48.

Williams, Edward Huntington. "The Drug-Habit Menace in the South." *Medical Record* (February 7, 1914): 247–49.

Wilson, Jno. Stainback. "Health Department." *Godey's Lady's Book and Magazine*, November 1858, 466–68.

Wilson, Jno. Stainback. "Health Department." *Godey's Lady's Book and Magazine*, March 1861, 272–73.

Winterburn, Geo. W. "A Seductive Drug." *American Medical Journal* 12, no. 3 (March 1884): 116–17.

Wong Chin Foo. "The Chinese in New York." *Cosmopolitan*, June 1888, 297–311.

Woodman, Walter. "Cocaine for Sleeplessness." *Boston Medical and Surgical Journal* 112, no. 12 (March 19, 1885): 287.

"The World-Wide Kingdom." *Baptist Missionary Magazine*, May 1909, 155–59.

Wright, Hamilton. "The International Opium Commission." *American Journal of International Law* 3, no. 3 (July 1909): 648–73.

Young, J. "Medical and Obstetrical Cases." *American Journal of the Medical Sciences* (April 1852): 426–32.

"Youngs v. Youngs." *Northeastern Reporter* 22 (August 9, 1889–January 24, 1890): 806–09.

## Television Episode

Moser, James E., writer. *Dragnet*. Season 2, episode 4, "The Big Seventeen." Directed by Jack Webb, featuring Jack Webb, Herbert Ellis, and Willis Bouchey. Aired November 6, 1952. NBC.

## Government Sources

*Annual Report of the Commissioner of Indian Affairs to the Secretary of the Interior for the Year 1886*. Washington: Government Printing Office, 1886.

California State Senate. Special Committee on Chinese Immigration. *Chinese Immigration: The Social, Moral, and Political Effect of Chinese Immigration*. Sacramento: State Printing Office, 1876.

*Fifty-Seventh Annual Report of the Commissioner of Indian Affairs to the Secretary of the Interior*. Washington: Government Printing Office, 1888.

Harrison Narcotic Act, 38 Stat. 785 (1914).

*Importation and Use of Opium: Hearings Before the Committee on Ways and Means of the House of Representatives*, 61st Congress, 3d Session, on H. R. 25240, H. R. 25241, H. R. 25242, and H. R. 28971 (December 14, 1910, and January 11, 1911) (statement of Dr. Christopher Koch, Vice President, State Pharmaceutical Examining Board of Pennsylvania; Chairman, Legislative Committee, Philadelphia Association of Retail Druggists). Washington: Government Printing Office, 1911.

Palmer, Aaron H. *Memoir, Geographical, Political, and Commercial, on the Present state, productive resources, and capabilities for commerce, of Siberia, Manchuria, and the Asiatic islands of the Northern Pacific ocean; and on the importance of opening commercial intercourse with those countries, &c*. Senate, 30th Congress, 1st Session, Miscellaneous No. 80. [Washington, D. C.], 1848.

*Prohibition of Use of Peyote*. House of Representatives, 65th Congress, 2d Session, Report No. 560 (May 13, 1918).

U.S. Congress. Senate. *Illicit Narcotics Traffic, New York, N. Y. Hearings Before the Subcommittee on Improvements in the Federal Criminal Code of the Committee on the Judiciary, United States Senate, 84th Congress, 1st session, on the Causes, Treatment, and Rehabilitation of Drug Addicts, Pursuant to S. Res. 67. September 19, 20, and 21, 1955, Part 5*. Washington: Government Printing Office, 1956.

U.S. Department of Commerce. Bureau of the Census. *We the Americans: Blacks*. Washington, D. C.: U.S. Government Printing Office, 1993.

United States Internal Revenue, Treasury Department. *Traffic in Narcotic Drugs: Report of Special Committee of Investigation Appointed March 25, 1918, by the Secretary of the Treasury.* Washington: Government Printing Office, 1919.

Wright, Hamilton. *Report on the International Opium Commission and on the Opium Problem as Seen within the United States and Its Possessions.* S. Doc. No. 377, 61st Congress, 2d session, 1909–1910. Washington: Government Printing Office, 1910.

## Court Decisions

*Ex parte Yung Jon*, 28 F. 308 (D. Ore. 1886).
*United States v. Doremus*, 249 U.S. 86 (1919).
*United States v. Jin Fuey Moy*, 241 U.S. 394 (1916).
*Webb et al. v. United States*, 249 U.S. 96 (1919).

## Primary Newspaper Articles

*Adams Sentinel* [Gettysburg, Pa.]. "Opium Eaters." October 10, 1842.
*Arizona Republican.* "The Cocaine Habit Remains Unchecked." June 30, 1909.
*Atlanta Constitution.* "Stripes for Cocaine Sellers." November 15, 1907.
*Baltimore Sun.* "The State vs. James Wilson." February 14, 1840.
*Baltimore Sun.* "Eating Opium." February 1, 1841.
*Baltimore Sun.* "City Court—February Term." February 13, 1841.
*Baltimore Sun.* "Slavery Convention." December 6, 1841.
*Baltimore Sun.* "Hasheesh Candy." December 12, 1863.
*Baltimore Sun.* "Mr. Binns's Curious Experiences." March 6, 1884.
*Baltimore Sun.* "Wild Negro Runs Amuck." April 20, 1909.
*Banner-Democrat* [Lake Providence, La.]. December 22, 1900.
Barn[e]s, L. "The Late Rev. G. W. Brush." *Delaware* [Ohio] *Gazette.* January 31, 1868.
*Boston Daily Globe.* "Opium-Eating Did It." May 4, 1887.
*Boston Post.* "Intemperance in Maine." February 10, 1879.
*Boston Recorder.* "England and China." July 10, 1840.
*Bridgeport* [Conn.] *Times and Evening Farmer.* "Specter Among Negroes of South Now Cocaine." July 20, 1909.
*Bristol* [Tenn.] *Herald Courier.* "Yankee Medico to Attend Opium Meet." October 29, 1908.
*Brooklyn Daily Eagle.* "Inquest." February 5, 1855.
*Brooklyn Daily Eagle.* "Opium Joints: How Life Is Dreamed Away in One of Them." July 8, 1882.
Bryan, Bill. "14 Are Facing Charges Tied to Trafficking of Heroin Here." *St. Louis Post-Dispatch*, September 27, 2001.
*Burlington* [Vt.] *Daily News.* "The Cocaine Habit." July 6, 1909.
*Butte* [Mont.] *Miner.* "The Opium Fiend." October 9, 1877.
*Californian* [Salinas, Calif.]. "Effects of Mexican Loco Weeds." March 2, 1905.
*Chicago Daily Tribune.* "A Victim of Morphia." August 20, 1877.
*Chicago Daily Tribune.* "The Boy's Mother." February 8, 1900.
*Chicago Tribune.* "A Law That Is Cruel only to Be Kind." March 11, 1915.
*Cincinnati Enquirer.* "The Thing 'Ladies' Get Tight On." July 27, 1869.
*Citrograph* [Redlands, Calif.]. "Two Republics." January 13, 1900.
*Colored American* [New York, N. Y.]. "Our Brethren in the Free States." April 22, 1837.
*Colored American* [New York, N. Y.]. "Can't Take Care of Themselves." March 15, 1838.
Crane, Stephen. "Dope Smokers." *Atlanta Constitution*, May 17, 1896.
[Crane, Stephen]. "Opium's Varied Dreams." *Sun* [New York, N. Y.]. May 17, 1896.
*Daily City News* [New Castle, Pa.]. "Rendered Insane by Cocaine." June 27, 1888.
*Daily Inter Ocean* [Chicago, Ill.]. "His Own Story." December 31, 1887.
*Daily Inter Ocean* [Chicago, Ill.]. "Mrs. Meyers Fined for Theft." August 24, 1899.

*Daily Missoulian* [Mont.]. "Tocsin of Battle Is Sounded." November 7, 1909.

*Daily Morning Post* [Pittsburgh, Pa.]. "Local Matters." May 20, 1850.

*Daily Republican* [Monongahela City, Pa.]. "The Victims of Morphine." September 13, 1883.

*El Paso Herald.* "Crazed by a Weed, Man Murders." January 2, 1913.

*El Paso Herald.* "Policeman Lassoes a Drug Crazed Mexican." January 28, 1914.

*El Paso Herald.* "Poisonous Weeds Of Mexico Cause Death." May 9, 1914.

*Evening Star* [Washington, D. C.]. "Washington News and Gossip." September 10, 1880.

*Evening Sun* [Baltimore, Md.]. "Expect Good from Drug Law Decision." March 4, 1919.

*Evening Times* [Grand Forks, N. D.]. March 25, 1909.

*Evening Times* [Grand Forks, N. D.]. "Cocaine Habit American Curse." July 19, 1909.

Foster, Abby K. "A Female Impostor." *Liberator* [Boston, Mass.], August 5, 1853.

Fraser, C. Gerald. "Harlem Response Mixed." *New York Times,* January 5, 1973.

*Frederick Douglass' Paper* [Rochester, N. Y.]. "Speech of Mr. Miller, of N. Jersey, on the Expediency of Recognizing the Independence of Liberia." March 25, 1853.

Gifford, Rev. O. T. "China-Town, San Francisco." *Lebanon* [Pa.] *Daily News.* February 21, 1883.

*Great Falls* [Mont.] *Tribune.* "Carnival of Negro Crime." February 4, 1909.

*Herald* [Los Angeles, Calif.]. "Oriental Vice." June 19, 1897.

*Holton* [Kan.] *Recorder and Express.* "The City of the Golden Gate." July 8, 1875.

*The Independent.* "Abuse of Sedatives and Narcotics." March 6, 1890.

*The Independent.* "Book Table: The Opium Habit." May 13, 1869.

Cook, Clarence. "More About the Permanent Free Picture Gallery." *The Independent,* August 23, 1855.

*The Independent* [Santa Barbara, Calif.]. "Mexico Makes War on Brain-Destroying Weed." June 3, 1907.

*Indianapolis Journal.* "One of Cleveland's Vetoes." August 13, 1888.

*Inter Ocean* [Chicago, Ill.]. "Opium." August 17, 1874.

*Iola* [Kan.] *Daily Register.* "Cocaine Habit Race Menace." July 20, 1909.

*Jackson* [Miss.] *Daily News.* "Cocaine a Menace to Southern Negroes." July 20, 1909.

*Knoxville* [Tenn.] *Daily Chronicle.* June 22, 1881, p. 2.

*Lancaster* [Pa.] *Examiner.* "The Poisons We Indulge In." March 21, 1855.

*Lancaster* [S. C.] *Ledger.* "Dangers of Using Ether and Chloroform—Extraordinary Revelations of Dentists—Sympathy for Dr. Beale." January 17, 1855.

*Lancaster* [S. C.] *News.* "Cocaine Gets in Its Deadly Work." September 30, 1913.

*Liberator* [Boston, Mass.]. June 18, 1852.

*Long Branch* [N. J.] *Record.* "Southern View of Race Riot." October 19, 1906.

*Long-Island Star.* "The Turks." May 7, 1829.

*Los Angeles Express.* "Hindu Blames Cigaret for Prison Sentence." February 21, 1913.

*Los Angeles Herald.* May 20, 1875.

*Los Angeles Times.* "Senate Votes Stiffer Dope Penalties." June 8, 1953.

*Marion* [Ohio] *Daily Star.* "Admits He Led Mob." September 30, 1913.

*Memphis Avalanche.* "The Opium Habit." August 23, 1885.

*Memphis Daily Appeal.* "Local Paragraphs." May 24, 1879.

*Memphis Daily Appeal.* "Local Paragraphs." June 17, 1879.

*Memphis Daily Appeal.* "Opium Smoking." June 28, 1879.

*Nashville Tennessean.* "To the Manhood of Tennessee." June 17, 1908.

*Nashville Tennessean.* "Who Killed Margaret Lear?" June 17, 1908.

*Nashville Tennessean.* "The Negro Vote an Annoying Factor." July 28, 1911.

*National Era* [Washington, D. C.]. "Literary Notices." April 7, 1853.

*National Era* [Washington, D. C.]. "Appetite for Stimulants—Policy of Prohibition." April 19, 1855.

*New-Haven Gazette and the Connecticut Magazine.* "New-Haven, June 21." June 21, 1787.

*New-Haven Gazette, and the Connecticut Magazine.* "To the Publisher of the Weekly Magazine." June 12, 1788.

*New-Haven Gazette, and the Connecticut Magazine.* "From the Memoirs of Baron de Tott, on the Turks and Tartars." October 2, 1788.

*New York Daily Herald.* "Miscellaneous: Hasheesh Candy." September 5, 1862.

*New-York Daily Times.* "New-York City." April 14, 1852.

*New-York Daily Times.* "Literary: Samuel Taylor Coleridge." June 4, 1853.

*New York Herald.* "The Opium Eaters of New York." July 14, 1869.

*New-York Mirror.* "Cure of an Opium-Eater." December 6, 1834, pp. 177–78.

*New-York Mirror.* "Reports of Societies: Eating Opium." March 28, 1840, p. 317.

*New-York Observer.* "Slavery and the Opium Trade." March 24, 1853, p. 93.

*New-York Observer.* "Opium Eating." April 12, 1855, p. 117.

*New-York Times.* February 10, 1860.

*New-York Times.* "Disorderly Men and Women—A Hasheesh Eater." October 28, 1866.

*New-York Times.* "Law Reports: A Depraved Appetite." October 31, 1866.

*New-York Times.* "Chinese in New-York: How They Live, and Where." December 26, 1873.

*New-York Times.* "Opium Smoking in Nevada." July 29, 1877.

*New-York Times.* "The Opium Habit's Power." December 30, 1877.

*New-York Times.* "Topics in the Sagebrush." February 21, 1881.

*New-York Times.* "A Day's Death Record." January 8, 1882.

*New-York Times.* "Philadelphia's Opium Parlor." August 29, 1882.

*New-York Times.* "A New Charge." May 13, 1883.

*New-York Times.* "Mr. Binns Tries Hasheesh." March 7, 1884.

*New-York Times.* "The 'Big Flat' Raided." December 8, 1884.

*New-York Times.* "An Unhappy Household." June 18, 1887.

*New York Times.* "Boy Cocaine Snuffers Hunted by the Police." January 8, 1907.

*New York Times.* "Cocaine User Shoots 7." December 6, 1907.

*New York Times.* "Ex-Inspector Byrnes Ill." February 1, 1910.

*New York Times.* "Caught Using Heroin." June 3, 1913.

*New York Times.* "Say Drug Habit Grips the Nation." December 5, 1913.

*New York Times.* "Poorer Drug Users in Pitiful Plight." April 15, 1915.

*New York Times.* "Wants New Laws for Drug Traffic." November 28, 1917.

*New York Tribune.* "Opium and Its Consumers." July 10, 1877.

*News-Advocate* [Price, Utah]. "Senate Passes Narcotic Bill." January 25, 1917.

*North-Carolina Free Press* [Halifax, N. C.]. "Opium Eater." June 25, 1824.

*Oregon Journal.* "Legality of Sale of Cannabis Question." March 14, 1915.

*Pennsylvania Gazette.* "From the *New England Weekly Journal*, May 12." June 25, 1741.

*Pennsylvania Gazette.* "To the Printers of the Pennsylvania Gazette." August 31, 1769.

*Pennsylvania Packet.* "Memoirs of the Baron de Tott . . ." December 4, 1788.

*Pittsburgh Weekly Gazette.* "The Thing 'Ladies' Get Tight On." July 24, 1869.

*Record-Journal* [Meriden, Conn.]. "Negro Was Crazed by Cocaine." April 20, 1909.

*Record-Union* [Sacramento, Calif.]. "Victim of a Chinese Opium Den." June 10, 1886.

*Record-Union* [Sacramento, Calif.]. "Voice of the Press: A Spurious Article." December 31, 1897.

*River Press* [Fort Benton, Mont.]. "Demoniacal Dens." January 19, 1881.

*Roanoke* [N. C.] *Advocate.* "Intoxicating effects of Wild Hemp." August 23, 1832.

Rosebault, Charles J. "The Opium Habit." *Fort Worth Daily Gazette.* July 11, 1887.

*Sacramento Bee.* "Pipes and Drugs to Burn." January 23, 1913.

*San Francisco Call.* "Foes of Opium Evil Return from Holland." February 21, 1912.

*San Francisco Chronicle.* "The Opium Dens." November 16, 1875.

*San Francisco Chronicle.* "A Growing Evil." July 25, 1881.

*San Francisco Chronicle.* "The Chinese Curse." February 9, 1894.

*San Francisco Examiner.* "Order No. 1254—Prohibiting Opium smoking dens." November 24, 1875.

*San Francisco Examiner.* "Opium Delegate Named." March 21, 1911.

*Santa Barbara Daily News and the Independent.* "Mrs. Finger Is Taken Today by Death." December 4, 1913.

Scofield, J. S. "Opium Eating." *New-York Daily Times,* November 4, 1852.

Seelye, Katharine Q. "In Heroin Crisis, White Families Seek Gentler War on Drugs." *New York Times,* October 30, 2015.

*South-Carolina Gazette.* "Charlestown." July 8, 1732.

*South-Carolina Gazette.* "Advertisements." August 22, 1743.

*St. Louis Post-Dispatch.* "Opium Eating in Chicago." September 17, 1880.

*St. Louis Post-Dispatch.* "Delightful Drug." December 25, 1892.

*Staunton* [Va.] *Daily Leader.* "Negro Given Five Years in Jail." August 11, 1908.

*Stockton Daily Independent.* "Opium. A 'Fiend' Talks to a Reporter About It." August 28, 1883.

Sullivan, Caryn. "Parents—Lock Up Your Prescription Drugs." *TwinCitiesPioneerPress.com,* May 26, 2011. https://www.twincities.com/2011/05/26/caryn-sullivan-parents-lock-up-your-prescriptions-drugs/.

*Sun* [New York, N. Y.]. "Mott Street Picketed." May 11, 1883.

*Sun* [New York, N. Y.]. "Negro Cocaine Fiends." November 2, 1902.

*Susquehanna Democrat* [Wilkes-Barre, Pa.]. "Foreign News: Constantinople." May 14, 1824.

*Tampa Tribune.* "Abolish the Dives; Jail the Vagrants." September 25, 1906.

*Times-Picayune* [New Orleans, La.]. "Opium." April 4, 1840.

*Tioga Eagle* [Wellsboro, Pa.]. "Late and Important from China." March 25, 1840.

*Vermont Watchman & State Journal.* "The Hashish: Singular Effects of an Oriental Drug." May 31, 1849.

*Virginia City* [Nev.] *Territorial Enterprise.* "Chinese Vices." April 7, 1877.

*Weekly Gleaner* [Winston-Salem, N. C.]. "Miscellany: Opium Eaters." September 29, 1829.

Weigle, Gilbert G. "Cupid Guides Addicts' Way to New Life." *San Francisco Examiner.* October 19, 1920.

*Wilmington* [N. C.] *Journal.* "Whiskey Root." October 16, 1857.

## Dissertations

Ahmad, Diana Lynn. "'Caves of Oblivion': Opium Dens and Exclusion Laws, 1850–1882." PhD diss., University of Missouri-Columbia, 1997.

Aikens, Kristina. "A Pharmacy of Her Own: Victorian Women and the Figure of the Opiate." PhD diss., Tufts University, 2008.

Armstrong, Katherine McVane. "Thy Will Lord, Not Mine: Parents, Grief, and Child Death in the Antebellum South." PhD diss., Emory University, 2011.

Charles, Catherine A. "Doctors and Addicts: A Case Study of Demedicalization." PhD diss., Columbia University, 1979.

Flowe, Douglas J. "'Tell the Whole White World': Crime, Violence, and Black Men in Early Migration New York City, 1890–1917." PhD diss., University of Rochester, 2014.

Gabriel, Joseph Michael. "Gods and Monsters: Drugs, Addiction, and the Origins of Narcotic Control in the Nineteenth-Century Urban North." PhD diss., Rutgers University, 2006.

Guba, David Alan Jr. "Empire of Illusion: The Rise and Fall of Hashish in Nineteenth-century France." PhD diss., Temple University, 2018.

Humphries, Lance Lee. "Robert Gilmor Jr. (1774–1848): Baltimore Collector and American Art Patron." PhD diss., University of Virginia, 1998.

Hur, Hyungju. "Staging Modern Statehood: World Exhibitions and the Rhetoric of Publishing in Late Qing China, 1851–1910." PhD diss., University of Illinois, 2012.

Lowe, Sharon. "Behind the Soothing Mist: Women and Opiate Use in the Mining West, 1860–1900." PhD diss., Union Institute and University, 2006.

Mark, Gregory Yee. "Political, Economic and Racial Influences on America's First Drug Laws." PhD diss., University of California, Berkeley, 1978.

Norwood, Dael A. "Trading in Liberty: The Politics of the American China Trade, ca. 1784–1862." PhD diss., Princeton University, 2012.

Seiler, Lars-Winfried. "The Development of an Anti-Opium Ideology in Late Nineteenth Century America." PhD diss., University of South Carolina, 2004.

Zou, Zhen. "'Smoke Gets in Your Eyes': American Writers on the Opium Issue in China, 1840–1860." PhD diss., Purdue University, 2006.

## Archives

Dr. James Carmichael Papers, 1816–1832 and n.d. Letter dated July 2, 1824. Accession #11373. Special Collections Department, University of Virginia Library.

Sylvanus Cobb, Letters, 1827–1867. Sylvanus Cobb Jr. to Robert, October 30, 1867. Clifton Waller Barrett Library, Accession #7507, 7507-a. Special Collections Department, University of Virginia Library.

Richard Dorsey Papers. MS 1764. H. Furlong Baldwin Library, Maryland Center for History and Culture.

Charles Edward French diaries, 1851–1904. P-787, 6 reels (microfilm). Massachusetts Historical Society.

John Harrison Records. Amb.4258. Day Book, 1800–1801. Historical Society of Pennsylvania.

Homans Family Correspondence, 1850–1938, bulk (1862–1864). MssCol 1427. Manuscripts and Archives Division, New York Public Library, Astor, Lenox and Tilden Foundations.

Rufus King Papers, 1766–1899 (Bulk 1783–1826). MS 1660. Southgate to King, July 19, 1800. Vol. 33 Letterbook, American Letters of Introduction to Rufus King, 1796–1802. New-York Historical Society.

Thomas Handasyd Perkins Papers. Perkins & Co. letter, Canton, August 7, 1819. P-334, 17 reels. Massachusetts Historical Society.

Powel Family Papers, 1681–1938, Collection 1582. Elizabeth Powel letter to Bushrod Washington, June 22, 1785. Series 3b, Box 4, Folder 3. Historical Society of Pennsylvania.

Rush Family Papers. Collection LCP.in.HSP134. J. Swaine to Richard Dorsey, July 6, 1809. Volume 16, page 114, Library Company of Philadelphia on deposit at Historical Society of Pennsylvania.

Sarah Waln Recipe Book. Am.1743, Historical Society of Pennsylvania.

George Edward Woodberry papers concerning Edgar Allan Poe, 1829–1928. MS Am 790.5 (46). Houghton Library, Harvard University.

# INDEX

*For the benefit of digital users, indexed terms that span two pages (e.g., 52–53) may, on occasion, appear on only one of those pages.*